Baillière's
CLINICAL
NEUROLOGY
INTERNATIONAL PRACTICE AND RESEARCH

Baillière's

CLINICAL NEUROLOGY

INTERNATIONAL PRACTICE AND RESEARCH

Volume 1/Number 3
November 1992

Unusual Dementias

M. N. ROSSOR
Guest Editor

Baillière Tindall
London Philadelphia Sydney Tokyo Toronto

This book is printed on acid-free paper.

Baillière Tindall   24–28 Oval Road,
W.B. Saunders   London NW1 7DX

The Curtis Center, Independence Square West,
Philadelphia, PA 19106–3399, USA

55 Horner Avenue
Toronto, Ontario M8Z 4X6, Canada

Harcourt Brace Jovanovich Group (Australia) Pty Ltd,
30–52 Smidmore Street, Marrickville, NSW 2204, Australia

Harcourt Brace Jovanovich Japan, Inc
Ichibancho Central Building, 22–1 Ichibancho
Chiyoda-ku, Tokyo 102, Japan

C V WM 220

ISSN 0961–0421

ISBN 0–7020–1631–4 (single copy)

Baillière's Clinical Neurology is published three times each year by Baillière Tindall.
Prices for Volume 1 (1992) are:

TERRITORY	ANNUAL SUBSCRIPTION	SINGLE ISSUE
Europe including UK	£65.00 post free	£27.50 post free
All other countries	Consult your local Harcourt Brace Jovanovich office	

The editor of this publication is Catriona Byres, Baillière Tindall,
24–28 Oval Road, London NW1 7DX.

Typeset by Phoenix Photosetting, Chatham.
Printed and bound in Great Britain by Mackays of Chatham PLC, Chatham, Kent.

Contributors to this issue

JEREMY BROWN MA, MRCP, Department of Neurology, St Mary's Hospital, Praed Street, London, W2 1NY, UK.

ARNE BRUN MD, PhD, Professor, Department of Pathology, Division of Neuropathology, University Hospital, S-22185 Lund, Sweden.

JOHN COLLINGE BSc, MB, Ch.B, MRCP, Senior Clinical Research Fellow, Department of Biochemistry and Molecular Genetics, St Mary's Hospital Medical School and Honorary Senior Registrar in Neurology, St Mary's Hospital, London, UK.

LARS GUSTAFSON MD, PhD, Professor, Department of Psychogeriatrics, University of Lund, P. O. Box 638, S-22009 Lund, Sweden.

JOHN KEW MRCP(UK), Department of Neurology, Institute of Psychiatry, De Crespigny Park, Denmark Hill, London, SE5 8AF, UK.

PETER L. LANTOS MD, PhD, DSc, FRCPath, Professor of Neuropathology, Institute of Psychiatry and Honorary Consultant, Bethlem Royal and Maudsley Hospital Special Health Authority, Honorary Consultant, King's College School of Medicine & Dentistry, and St Thomas' Hospital.

NIGEL LEIGH PhD, FRCP, Department of Neurology, Institute of Psychiatry and King's College of Medicine and Dentistry, De Crespigny Park, Denmark Hill, London, SE5 8AF, UK.

GRAHAM LENNOX BA, MRCP, Lecturer in Clinical Neurology, University of Nottingham Medical School, Nottingham, NG7 2UH, UK.

C. D. MARSDEN DSc, FRCP, FRS, Professor of Neurology, Institute of Neurology, The National Hospital for Neurology & Neurosurgery, Queen Square, London, WC1N 3BG, UK.

M-MARSEL MESULAM MD, Division of Neuroscience and Behavioral Neurology, Harvard Neurology Department and the Dana Research Institute of the Beth Israel Hospital, Boston, MA, USA.

MARK S. PALMER MA, DPhil, Research Fellow, Department of Biochemistry and Molecular Genetics, St Mary's Hospital Medical School, Norfolk Place, London, W2 1PG, UK.

ULLA PASSANT MD, Department of Psychiatry, rCBF-lab, University Hospital, S-22185 Lund, Sweden.

MARTIN N. ROSSOR MA, MD, FRCP, Consultant Neurologist, St Mary's Hospital, Praed Street, London, W2 1NY, Honorary Consultant Neurologist, The National Hospital for Neurology and Neurosurgery, Senior Lecturer, The Institute of Neurology, Queen Square, London, WC1N 3BG, UK.

P. D. THOMPSON MB, PhD, FRACP, Honorary Senior Lecturer, Institute of Neurology, The National Hospital for Neurology & Neurosurgery, Queen Square, London, WC1N 3BG, UK.

SANDRA WEINTRAUB PhD, Division of Neuroscience and Behavioral Neurology, Harvard Neurology Department and the Dana Research Institute of the Beth Israel Hospital, Boston, MA, USA.

Table of contents

Foreword

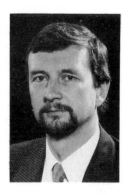

The diseases covered in this book are confined to the degenerative dementias; some of which have only been clearly delineated over the last 5 to 10 years. Degenerative dementias associated with other neurological diseases, such as Huntington's disease, progressive supranuclear palsy, Parkinson's disease, etc. have not been covered as these are commonly considered under other titles. Since this volume does not pretend to be comprehensive, there are many degenerative dementias not covered and some of these are represented by only the odd case report. An explanation of the title *Unusual Dementias* is also necessary, as one might have expected inclusion of a host of unusual dementias due to infections, as in AIDS dementia, auto-immune vasculitides and the diverse metabolic disturbances seen particularly in paediatric neurology, but some of which, for example, metachromatic leucodystrophy, may present in adulthood as dementia. Space does not permit such a comprehensive review and the intention of the series editors was to cover the growing points in the degenerative dementias, rather than attempt to be comprehensive. The suggested title, vulnerable to the charge of inaccuracy, is brief and reflects this growing point of neurology.

Alzheimer's disease is the commonest of the degenerative dementias and a significant proportion of these are autosomal dominant familial diseases. Some of these pedigrees have been associated with mutations in the amyloid precursor protein (APP) gene, although to date these appear to be extremely rare. This particular group of familial Alzheimer's disease is discussed in Chapter 3. Similar molecular genetic advances have revolutionized our understanding of the spongiform encephalopathies, now referred to as the prion dementias, covered in Chapter 8. Some of the topics covered are defined primarily by the clinical syndrome, such as primary progressive dysphasia (Chapter 6), whereas others are largely defined by the neuropathology, such as corticobasal degeneration and Lewy body dementia (Chapters 9 and 10). For other examples the clinical and neuropathological entities are less clear. Frontal lobe dementia refers to groups of patients with predominant frontal symptomatology and in whom the neuropathological changes are predominantly anterior. However, within the clinical rubric of frontal lobe dementia or dementia of frontal lobe type, there may be many neuropathological substrates which include frontal lobe degeneration, Pick's disease with Pick bodies, or spongiform encephalopathy. The term 'frontal lobe dementia' is used quite widely with reference both to a clinical and a neuropathological entity. In this volume the term 'frontal lobe dementia' is used, but not abbreviated. The clinical syndrome referred to as 'dementia of the frontal lobe type' (DFLT) is often used interchangeably with the clinical syndrome of frontal lobe dementia. The term 'frontal lobe degeneration', abbreviated in this text to FLD, has been used to describe more specifically the pathological entity described by Brun and Gustafson (see Chapter 5) and which is associated with a frontal lobe syndrome. The variety of terms and abbreviations that are now used in the literature attests to the difficulties in according distinct nosological status to these different diseases. Hopefully, with the advances in molecular neuropathology and molecular genetics, many of these difficulties will be resolved.

M. N. ROSSOR

Acknowledgements

I would like to thank Carolyn Croft for preparation of typescripts and editorial assistance.

1

Introduction

M. N. ROSSOR

Dementia is predominantly a syndrome of later life, with prevalence estimates of 5% in those above the age of 65 years and 20% in those above the age of 80 years. However, it is also encountered in many neurological diseases in early and middle life. Dementia, defined as multiple domains of cognitive impairment with intact arousal, is a syndrome with a large variety of causes encompassing infections, trauma, and genetic, metabolic and neoplastic disease. To the clinical neurologist many of these causes are obvious and dementia may be only one distinct feature amongst many, albeit an important diagnostic aid. Alternatively, dementia may occur as a fixed deficit after encephalitis or hypoxia and trauma. It is, however, in the group of diseases which are referred to as the primary degenerative dementias that it is the salient feature, and it is also this group which is the most commonly encountered in clinical neurology. Alzheimer's disease (see Chapter 3) is by far and away the commonest disease in this group. The epidemiological importance became apparent from studies in the 1960s and early 1970s; the term Alzheimer's disease had been reserved for the rarer cases of early onset dementia associated with senile plaques and neurofibrillary tangles, whereas senile dementia was considered separately, often as a rather vague entity. It was, however, demonstrated that the histopathological abnormalities of senile plaques and neurofibrillary tangles were common to such patients irrespective of their ages (Blessed et al, 1968). The distinction between Alzheimer's disease and senile dementia of the Alzheimer type remained dependent upon an arbitrary age of 65 years. More recently the term Alzheimer's disease has been used regardless of age, although still recognizing that clinical and neuropathological differences may be apparent between the early and late onset groups.

The early epidemiological studies, which were largely based on retrospective autopsy series in elderly psychogeriatric populations, established that Alzheimer's disease was the major cause of dementia, accounting for approximately 50% of cases, with mixed vascular and Alzheimer's disease accounting for 20% and vascular dementia a further 15%, and the final 15% comprising a miscellaneous group which included tumours, normal pressure hydrocephalus and other degenerative dementias such as Pick's disease (Blessed et al, 1968; Tomlinson et al, 1970). The last 20 years has seen a considerable refinement in the differential diagnosis of vascular and degenerative dementia. Vascular dementia in early studies referred largely

Baillière's Clinical Neurology—
Vol. 1, No. 3, November 1992
ISBN 0–7020–1631–4

to those patients with multiple cortical infarcts, and a broad association was observed between the total volume of infarcted cerebral tissue and the development of the clinical syndrome of dementia. Increasingly, however, the role of small vessel disease has been recognized and the importance of small lacunar subcortical infarcts or diffuse white matter ischaemia has been established. It is, however, within the group of degenerative dementias that most advances have been seen in the last 10 years, and it is with this latter group that this book is concerned.

Twenty years ago the vast majority of cases of clinically diagnosed degenerative dementia would have been labelled as Alzheimer's disease. Even now the use of the National Institute of Neurological and Communicative Disorders and Stroke-Alzheimer's Disease and Related Disorders Association (NINCDS-ADRDA) criteria (McKhann et al, 1984) permits most cases to fall within the category of probable Alzheimer's disease. The relatively few cases that come to autopsy may be found to have sufficient plaques and tangles to support the diagnosis of Alzheimer's disease, although since these histopathological features are found to a minor extent in normal old age the diagnosis is not always secure. In response to this uncertainty, further criteria have been developed based on the neuropathological findings (Khachaturian, 1985), and even the gold standard of neuropathology is now seen to be variable (Tierney et al, 1988).

The remaining non-Alzheimer cases may have had recognized neuronal inclusions permitting a more specific diagnosis, such as Pick's disease, or they may have been part of a readily recognized neurodegenerative disorder in which dementia plays a prominent part, such as Huntington's disease or progressive supranuclear palsy. Many would have had non-specific features of neuronal loss and the diagnosis could not be refined further (Kim et al, 1981).

It has, however, always seemed unlikely that the differential diagnosis of degenerative dementia could be reduced to that of Alzheimer's disease, Pick's disease and a few other miscellaneous non-specific entities. Dementia as a clinical syndrome of general impairment of cognitive function is likely to occur in a wide variety of conditions in which the neural network is disrupted, either at a functional level with metabolic failure of synaptic transmission, or in conditions which result in structural disintegration, as with many of the degenerative dementias. Moreover, a substantial proportion of human genes are expressed in the brain and so the majority of physiological molecules, many of which are implicated in disease, are also found in the brain. It can be argued, therefore, that the number of diseases causing dementia should be far greater than the number of diagnoses currently available to the clinician. If this is accepted, why is there a paucity of recognized non-Alzheimer dementias? First, Alzheimer's disease may not be a single nosological entity, but rather neurofibrillary tangles and senile plaques may represent a common tissue response to a variety of stresses and insults. Thus senile plaques, neurofibrillary tangles, disordered tau metabolism and amyloid deposition would all be seen as a final common pathway of many different diseases. Secondly, within the group of non-specific dementias there may be a multitude of distinct diseases and, in addition, many of the elderly Alzheimer disease patients may in fact represent a variety of diseases which coincidentally develop senile plaques and neurofibrillary tangles. There is some evidence for both of these explanations and there is no doubt that a rapidly increasing number of degenerative dementias are now recognized and that these are not the rarities previously thought.

What has brought about this revolution in the differential diagnosis of dementia? There is no doubt that the realization of the clinical and sociological importance of dementia and the subsequent focused research funding are now reaping their rewards. This has allowed the application of new biological techniques to the refinement of classification and diagnosis. A number of syndromes have been delineated by detailed neuropsychological assessment, such as the focal atrophies and frontal lobe dementias (Chapters 6 and 5). Although by definition dementia involves a multifocal impairment of cognitive dysfunction, the topology of this dysfunction may vary considerably. The earlier definitions of global impairment of cognitive function invited the criticism that if the impairment were indeed global, then individual dementia syndromes could not be recognized. Although patients' cortical function may indeed become global with increasing severity, in many instances the initial pattern, with focal emphasis and islands of preservation, may remain until very late in the disease.

The improved neuroimaging facilities provided by magnetic resonance imaging (MRI) and positron emission tomography (PET) have underpinned the different patterns of cerebral cortical involvement. Selective atrophy of the hippocampus may be seen with MRI scanning in Alzheimer's disease (Kesslak et al, 1991). PET scanning with either oxygen-15 or 2-fluorodeoxyglucose to determine regional metabolic rate may show a characteristic pattern of posterior biparietal-bitemporal hypometabolism in Alzheimer's disease (Frackowiak et al, 1981) and frontal hypometabolism in Pick's disease.

Advances in neuropathology have also made major contributions to the differential diagnosis of degenerative dementia. One of the most important has been the introduction of immunohistochemistry, which has allowed specific immunostaining for β A4 amyloid, prion protein, ubiquitin and tau, all of which are important in delineating the various dementias described in this volume. Comprehensive neuropathological examination has allowed revision of prevalence estimates for some of the degenerative dementias; in particular, frontal lobe degeneration and cortical Lewy body disease may be far more common than previously believed. It is likely that there are some geographical differences. For example, frontal lobe degeneration (Chapter 5) is seen to be the second commonest dementia in Sweden and is common in the Manchester series (Neary et al, 1986). By contrast, in the Nottingham series cortical Lewy body disease is seen to be the second commonest (Chapter 9). In addition to possible regional variations, differences in sampling, particularly with respect to age, are important. The neuropathological criteria themselves may also differ and inevitably there is a subjective element, as shown by a recent study of the reproducibility of the neuropathological diagnosis of Alzheimer's disease (Braak and Braak, 1991).

Finally, however, it is now seen that the neuropathological features that may occur with a given disease can vary considerably, as exemplified by the hereditary spongiform encephalopathy, or prion disease, associated with the 144 base pair insert in the prion protein gene (Chapter 8). The histological features in this family show considerable variability and, most importantly, in one member none of the classical histopathological features of spongiform change was found; this case would previously have been classified as a non-specific dementia (Collinge et al, 1990). This particular family was diagnosed on the basis of the genetic abnormality and highlights the third important advance which has had a major impact on the degenerative dementias, namely molecular genetics.

The techniques of molecular genetics have allowed, by linkage analysis and more successfully by analysis of candidate genes, detailed study of a substantial number of neurological diseases. Striking examples are Duchenne's muscular dystrophy, dystrophia myotonica, Friedreich's ataxia and Huntington's disease, although in the latter two conditions only polymorphic markers which lie close to the disease locus have been found. Many of the degenerative dementias may be familial, and molecular genetic analysis has been particularly successful in the prion dementias (Chapter 8) and in familial Alzheimer's disease (Chapter 3). This approach is also ideally suited to the familial cases of frontal lobe degeneration (Chapter 5) and Pick's disease (Chapter 4). The molecular genetic approach also circumvents the objection that the variable clinical expression and features on neuroimaging need not necessarily reflect distinct diseases, but merely the chance anatomical distribution of the disease process.

In Chapter 2 a neuropathology overview is provided and attention drawn to the generality of neuronal loss and the presence of neuronal inclusion bodies in these diseases. Both of these features might be viewed as inevitable consequences of diseases affecting post-mitotic cells. Although there is an opportunity for neuronal remodelling, there is no opportunity for regeneration. Thus neuronal loss would be an expected feature, and if inclusion bodies represent accumulated proteins which are not disposed of by the cell then this can also be seen as a natural consequence of the longevity of neurones and their inability to regenerate. The diseases discussed here are essentially those of middle age and beyond, with only rare exceptions occurring in the third decade. Subtle changes in gene expression and protein production or failure of catabolism may give rise to accumulation of unwanted metabolic products over the time course of the human life span.

At present the combination of clinical features and neuropathology are the primary means of diagnosis. It is generally assumed that the distribution of the histopathology determines the clinical features. Thus the frontal lobe features of frontal lobe dementia, the language disturbance of primary progressive dysphasia and Pick's disease with temporal atrophy, and the memory impairment, visuospatial disturbance and fluent dysphasia of Alzheimer's disease all reflect the characteristic distributions of pathology in these diseases. It is probable that, within these area of selective vulnerability, the particular neurones damaged, for example the pyramidal cells in

Alzheimer's disease, and the precise nature of the cellular failure will also determine the clinical features, but this remains to be demonstrated. Since the neuropathological features, both in terms of the distribution and the type of inclusion bodies, are central to the diagnosis, it is not surprising that diseases with associated inclusion bodies have been those which were the earliest to be delineated, such as Alzheimer's disease and Pick's disease, and which are most commonly diagnosed. However, the recent impact of molecular genetics has called into question the reliability of diagnoses based upon neuropathology alone. For example, the 144 base pair insert family (Chapter 8) exhibits both classical spongiform change and non-specific features within the same family. Similarly a variety of inclusion bodies can be found with defined genetic defects; cortical Lewy bodies have been observed together with senile plaques and neurofibrillary tangles in one autopsied case of familial Alzheimer's disease with the amyloid precursor protein (APP) 717 valine to isoleucine mutation (Lantos et al, 1992), and neurofibrillary tangles have been observed in a family with the codon 198 mutation in the prion protein gene (Ghetti et al, 1989), suggesting that inclusions may not be specific and may represent a relatively limited response of neurones to a variety of insults. Further support for the possible non-specific nature of some inclusions is provided by the observation of patients who may have a combination of histological features, such as an overlap of cortical Lewy bodies and Alzheimer histopathology (see Chapter 9) or the overlap of Pick's disease and Alzheimer's disease (Smith and Lantos, 1983). It is also an intriguing feature of the degenerative dementias that many occur both on a familial and sporadic basis; for example, reports of Alzheimer's disease, frontal lobe degeneration, prion disease and Pick's disease and increasingly other degenerative dementias such as Lewy body dementia occurring on a familial basis are being published. In general, the familial cases behave as an autosomal dominant disease. This common combination of sporadic and familial examples of these unusual dementias would also argue for a multifactorial aetiology, with the disease expression and the neuropathological features representing a final common pathway of tissue response.

Molecular genetics clearly has the opportunity to provide a gold standard for diagnosis; if the disease is associated with a particular mutation and this mutation is found in an affected patient, then an unequivocal diagnosis can be made regardless of the clinical or neuropathological features. Nevertheless, such a diagnostic formulation is inadequate for clinical management. First, the presence of a disease mutation does not necessarily equate with the disease and one cannot assume full penetrance. For example, the Prion Protein (PrP) 200 lysine mutation has been described in elderly family members without overt disease (Goldfarb et al, 1990). Secondly, the phenotypic variability that is commonly observed is important in disease management. Thus the neuropathological substrate may be associated with particular clinical features or lead to defined therapeutic strategies; the clinical features unique to that individual patient need to be formulated clearly in order to understand the everyday disability experienced.

How then should the clinician approach a patient with dementia? A

careful history and clinical examination will need to include neuropsychological assessment in addition to the more commonly used rating scales, as
only in this way will the precise pattern of cognitive impairment be established. Routine investigations to exclude systemic disease such as vitamin
B_{12} or thyroid deficiency and neurosyphilis are necessary, together with
neuroimaging using either computerized tomography (CT) or MRI to
exclude neoplasia and normal pressure hydrocephalus. The more difficult
question is how far to investigate the remaining cases of degenerative
dementia in whom at the present time there is no prospect of treatment. The
electroencephalogram may be valuable in the differential diagnosis, being
relatively normal in Pick's disease and frontal lobe degeneration, but
abnormal early in Alzheimer's disease. Examination of the cerebrospinal
fluid (CSF) may be helpful to exclude the rare inflammatory causes such as
vasculitides or cases of multiple sclerosis presenting purely with cognitive
impairment, although the CSF is unlikely to be abnormal in these instances
if the MRI is normal. Screening for PrP and APP gene mutations in familial
cases is now a valuable diagnostic adjunct, and it is always worth seeking a
family history carefully as this is not always immediately obvious. Cerebral
biopsy has undoubtedly contributed to our understanding of the histological
substrates of degenerative dementia with cerebral atrophy (Neary et al,
1986) and a specific diagnosis can be anticipated from biopsy, but these
rarely lead to treatment (Hulette et al, 1992). It is likely for the present time
that cerebral biopsy will be reserved for those atypical cases which are
thought unlikely to be due to one of the degenerative dementias and in
which a suspected infective or inflammatory component might lead to
specific treatment.

FUTURE PROSPECTS

Research into dementia in the last decade has been dramatic in parallel with
the pace of research in the neurosciences. Indeed, research in this area has
provided important insights into basic neuroscience; for example, the search
for the derivation of the βA4 amyloid in Alzheimer's disease led to the
cloning of the APP gene and the discovery of APP as a ubiquitous
transmembrane molecule, the physiological functions of which are still
being elucidated. Cases of degenerative dementia also provide models of
selective neuronal damage in which the consequent neuropsychological
deficits can be dissected. An example is the demonstration of a category-
specific and modality-specific dysphasia in a patient with left focal temporal
atrophy, supporting the view for parallel modality-specific meaning systems
in the brain (McCarthy and Warrington, 1988). Research effort will not only
see a refined nosology in this area, but hopefully also the development of
rational treatment. To date the emphasis has been on the development of
neurotransmitter replacement therapies, which have been successful in
Parkinson's disease, but the future is likely to see the development of
treatments specifically designed to prevent the molecular pathology. The
amyloid deposition in cases of Alzheimer's disease and the conversion of

prion protein from the cellular to the scrapie form are the best candidates at the present. The degenerative dementias represented here as the unusual dementias have become a growing point in neurology, and it is to be hoped that their management will also become more optimistic as we move into the next century.

REFERENCES

Blessed G, Tomlinson BE & Roth M (1968) The association between quantitative measures of dementia and of senile change in the cerebral grey matter of elderly subjects. *British Journal of Psychiatry* **114:** 797–811.

Braak H & Braak E (1991) Neuropathological staging of Alzheimer-related changes. *Acta Neuropathologica* **82:** 239–259.

Collinge J, Owen F, Poulter M et al (1990) Prion dementia without characteristic pathology. *Lancet* **336:** 7–9.

Frackowiak RSJ, Pozzilli C, Legg NJ et al (1981) Regional cerebral oxygen supply and utilization in dementia. A clinical and physiological study with oxygen-15 and positron tomography. *Brain* **104:** 753–778.

Ghetti B, Tagliavini F, Masters CL et al (1989) Gerstmann–Straussler–Scheinker disease. II. Neurofibrillary tangles and plaques with PrP-amyloid coexist in an affected family. *Neurology* **39:** 1453–1461.

Goldfarb LG, Mitrova E, Brown P, Toh BK & Gajdusek DC (1990) Mutation in codon 200 of scrapie amyloid protein gene in two clusters of Creutzfeldt–Jakob disease in Slovakia. *Lancet* **336:** 514–515.

Hulette CM, Earl NL & Craine BJ (1992) Evaluation of cerebral biopsies for the diagnosis of dementia. *Archives of Neurology* **49:** 28–31.

Kesslak JP, Nalcioglu O & Cotman CW (1991) Quantification of magnetic resonance scans for hippocampal and parahippocampal atrophy in Alzheimer's disease. *Neurology* **41:** 51–54.

Khachaturian ZS (1985) Diagnosis of Alzheimer's disease. *Archives of Neurology* **42:** 1097–1105.

Kim RC, Collins GH, Parisi JE, Wright AW & Chu YB (1981) Familial dementia of adult onset with pathological findings of a 'non specific' nature. *Brain* **104:** 61–78.

Lantos PL, Luthert PJ, Hanger D et al (1992) Familial Alzheimer's disease with the amyloid precursor protein 717 mutation and sporadic Alzheimer's disease have the same cytoskeletal pathology. *Neuroscience Letters* **137:** 221–224.

McCarthy RA & Warrington EK (1988) Evidence of modality-specific meaning systems in the brain. *Nature* **334:** 428–430.

McKhann G, Drachman D, Folstein M et al (1984) Clinical diagnosis of Alzheimer's disease: Report of the NINCDS/ADRDA workgroup under the auspices of the Department of Health and Human Services Task Force on Alzheimer's disease. *Neurology* **34:** 939–944.

Neary D, Snowden JS, Bowen DM et al (1986) Cerebral biopsy in the investigation of presenile dementia due to cerebral atrophy. *Journal of Neurology, Neurosurgery and Psychiatry* **49:** 157–162.

Smith DA & Lantos PL (1983) A case of combined Pick's disease and Alzheimer's disease. *Journal of Neurology, Neurosurgery and Psychiatry* **46:** 675–677.

Tierney MC, Fisher RH, Lewis AJ et al (1988) The NINCDS-ADRDA Work Group criteria for the clinical diagnosis of probable Alzheimer's disease: A clinicopathologic study of 57 cases. *Neurology* **38:** 359–364.

Tomlinson BE, Blessed G & Roth M (1970) Observations on the brains of demented old people. *Journal of the Neurological Sciences* **11:** 205–242.

2

Neuropathology of unusual dementias: an overview

P. L. LANTOS

The importance of dementias in the ageing populations of industrialized countries is difficult to overstate. It is therefore not surprising that neuro-degenerative diseases, which are the cerebral substrates of most dementias, represent one of the fastest developing areas of biomedical research. Indeed, progress has been spectacular in this field. For the practising neuro-pathologist, two developments have been particularly relevant. First is the increased understanding of the cellular and molecular mechanisms which underlie neuronal degeneration and death, the cellular phenomena forming the final common pathway of all neurodegenerative disorders. As the thrust of scientific enquiry combined modern investigative techniques of immuno-cytochemistry, quantitative morphometry, electron microscopy, molecular biology, molecular genetics and protein chemistry with traditional neuro-histology, our knowledge of pathogenesis has expanded from tissues through cells to molecules. The second development flows from the first and is the realization that neurodegenerative diseases are complex, and hetero-geneity is the rule, rather than the exception, even within a single disease entity. This complexity and heterogeneity presents the neuropathologist with considerable diagnostic problems. Confronted with an unusual case, the challenge lies in the choice: to attempt to define a new entity, a subtype, an atypical form, or merely to describe the case as neurodegenerative disease 'not otherwise specified'.

DIAGNOSTIC PROBLEMS OF NEURODEGENERATIVE DISEASE

In general, the histological features of neurodegenerative diseases can be classified in three groups. The first is the formation of abnormal structures, either intracellular or extracellular. The intracellular structures are usually intraneuronal and intracytoplasmic (e.g. neurofibrillary tangles, Pick bodies, Lewy bodies), although oligodendroglial inclusions have also been described in multiple system atrophy (Papp et al, 1989). Extracellular lesions, like senile plaques, may reach considerable size and interfere with the proper organization and function of tissue, rather than cell. Intracellular inclusions may become extracellular, as neurofibrillary tangles do, after the death of the

Baillière's Clinical Neurology—
Vol. 1, No. 3, November 1992
ISBN 0–7020–1631–4

host neurone, with change in their morphology and antigenicity (Tabaton et al, 1991). Neuronal and synaptic loss forms the second group; these negative features are equally important in the diagnosis of neurodegenerative diseases, although they are more difficult to assess than the 'positive' abnormalities of the first group. The third group of histological abnormalities covers glial and vascular changes. It would be an oversimplification to state that these are secondary alterations consequent upon neuronal damage. Whilst astrocytic and microglial response is normally associated with neuronal loss and tissue destruction, the role of these cells, for example, in the formation of amyloid has not been established. Thus the histological spectrum of neurodegenerative diseases is complex and variable. The diagnosis of these disorders is further complicated by the fact that these abnormalities in most cases are not specific to a particular disease entity: many of them occur in ageing and in other neurological disorders. One of the hallmark lesions of Alzheimer's disease, the neurofibrillary tangle, develops in ageing, dementia pugilistica, Down's syndrome, the amyotrophic lateral sclerosis–parkinsonism and dementia complex of Guam, some sporadic cases of motor neurone disease, post encephalitic parkinsonism, progressive supranuclear palsy and subacute sclerosing panencephalitis (for review, see Lantos, 1990). More recently, they have also been described in myotonic dystrophy, as a sign of progeria (Kiuchi et al, 1991).

The occurrence of neuronal inclusions in the brain of intellectually intact elderly people raises the necessity of quantitation. Although neurodegeneration most often follows a pattern of selective neuronal vulnerability, for example, the pigmented nuclei of the brainstem in Parkinson's disease, or the hippocampus in Alzheimer's disease, a more diffuse involvement of the brain is likely to occur. This has been known in Alzheimer's disease and Creutzfeldt–Jakob disease, but a more diffuse pathology in Parkinson's, Huntington's and motor neurone diseases has been only more recently realized. The severity of the neurodegenerative process may show considerable variation from one area to another and for this reason, comprehensive and standardized sampling is a prerequisite of diagnostic accuracy. This is particularly true in cases of unusual dementias.

ALZHEIMER'S DISEASE

Diagnostic criteria

Before considering the problems of atypical and familial cases, it is important to emphasize that even the typical, sporadic cases may present diagnostic problems. Since none of the histological features of Alzheimer's disease is specific and all occur in ageing, it is not surprising that diagnostic problems still exist. Several attempts have been made to establish diagnostic criteria and, although many problems have been identified, not all the controversial issues have been solved. The proposed set of criteria hinges on the presence and number of neurofibrillary tangles and senile plaques, the two hallmark lesions of Alzheimer's disease, whilst much less consideration is given to neuronal and synaptic loss. Interestingly, it was the realization that dementias may occur in the absence of Alzheimer-type pathology or other pathognomonic lesions which directed the attention to less obvious changes and resulted in the definition of the neuropathology of unusual cases.

A workshop convened by the Medical Research Council suggested only minimum data for research, although recommended the quantitation of plaques and tangles in standardized preparations, without specifying any numerical criteria (Wilcock et al, 1989). North American neuropathologists have proposed age-related diagnostic criteria which are biased in favour of plaques. In patients under the age of 50 years, there should be at least 2–5 tangles and plaques anywhere in the neocortex per square millimetre. In the age groups 50–65, 66–75 and over 75 years, the number of plaques per field should exceed 8, 10 and 15, respectively. The requirement for tangles is more vague: in the two youngest groups some neurofibrillary tangles may be present, whilst in the over 75 group tangles may be absent (Khachaturian, 1985). These recommendations are weakened by the suggestion that the figures can be revised downward, according to one opinion by 50%, if there is a positive clinical history of Alzheimer's disease. Defining Alzheimer's disease as a predominantly hippocampal affliction, Ball et al (1985) suggested that more than 20 tangle-bearing neurones/mm^3 or fewer than 5600 neurones in the same volume of tissue should be diagnostic. However, in the experience of Anderson and Hubbard (1985) this threshold for tangle content at around 0.36% of neurone is too low and would include about 30% of mentally normal elderly people. A recent set of recommendations by the Consortium to Establish a Register for Alzheimer's Disease has introduced the concept of probability, similar to clinical diagnosis, into the neuro-pathological diagnosis of Alzheimer's disease. Thus, according to the severity of plaque formation, the presence of clinical evidence of dementia and the presence or absence of other neuropathological lesions likely to cause dementia, definite, probable and possible cases are distinguished (Mirra et al, 1991).

The proposal ignores neurofibrillary tangles, and the degree of plaque formation remains vague in terms of mild, moderate and severe. It is becoming increasingly clear that quantitation is meaningful only if neuro-pathologists adhere to a standardized methodology, including sampling, fixation, section thickness, staining technique, etc. A multicentre study reviewing the practices of 11 different laboratories found that subjective assessment is currently a more reliable index of comparing cases from various centres than quantitative values which depend greatly on the tech-nique used (Duyckaerts et al, 1990). A similar survey of more than 100, mainly North American neuropathologists has revealed wide variations in the method of examination and in the use of quantitative diagnostic criteria (Wisniewski et al, 1989). Moreover, the agreement between clinical and pathological diagnoses varies considerably, from 64 to 86%, depending upon the neuropathological criteria applied (Tierney et al, 1988).

In order to understand variations in the severity and distribution of Alzheimer-type changes, the study of the sequential development of Alzheimer's disease is of paramount importance. The investigations of the early stages of the disease present considerable problems, since the overwhelming majority of patients die at an advanced stage and the precise onset of dementia, which of course is not simultaneous with the beginning of neurodegeneration, is difficult, if not impossible to establish. Our knowledge of the early stages of Alzheimer's disease is derived from three sources: cases of dementia, non-demented ageing brains and Down's syndrome. These neuropathological assessments, which will not be considered here, have been instrumental in elucidating several morphological and molecular aspects of pathogenesis. On a practical level, a neuropathological staging of Alzheimer's changes has been proposed. This may not explain the vagaries of distribution but helps to chart the relentless progress of the disease. In a large series of brains from non-demented and demented individuals, the distributions of amyloid deposits and neurofibrillary tangles were analysed. The distribution pattern and packing density of amyloid deposits proved to be of limited significance in defining disease stages. The distribution of neuritic plaques showed considerable variation, not only within a particular cytoarchitectural unit but also from individual to individual. Neurofibrillary tangles and neuropil threads, however, indicated the progress of pathology and allowed six stages to be distinguished (Braak and Braak, 1991). In the earliest two, so-called transentorhinal stages, neurofibrillary changes affected the transentorhinal layer Pre-α neurones, whilst in the limbic stages (stages III and IV), the degenerative process spread to the proper entorhinal cortex. In stages V and VI, the so-called isocortical stages, neurofibrillary changes destroyed practically all isocortical association areas. Neuropathological studies of so-called preclinical, incipient and mild cases of Alzheimer's disease (Crystal et al, 1988; Katzman et al, 1988; Hubbard et al, 1990; Morris et al, 1991) are not only useful in diagnostic practice, but also in the theoretical consideration of pathogenesis.

Considering the diagnostic problems of Alzheimer's disease in general, it is hardly surprising that the unusual cases pose considerable difficulties for the neuropathologists. With increasing knowledge of the genetic background of Alzheimer's disease, sporadic and familial forms can be distinguished, the latter representing between 10 and 50% of all cases (see Chapter 3). Atypical and combined cases exist both in the sporadic and familial variety, although much less is known about the latter.

Atypical and combined cases

The clinical heterogeneity of Alzheimer's disease has long been recognized and originally clear distinction was made between the early onset, presenile Alzheimer's disease and the senile dementia of the Alzheimer type. Although these two forms are now regarded as part of the same disease spectrum and a cut-off point at 65 years of age is both arbitrary and misleading, there are obvious neuropathological and neurochemical differences between early and late onset cases (Rossor et al, 1984; Tomlinson and Corsellis, 1984). Reviewing 121 consecutive patients with Alzheimer-type dementia, Mayeux et al (1985) distinguished four subgroups: benign cases, showing little or no progression; the myoclonic subgroup with early onset, severe intellectual impairment and frequent mutism; the extrapyramidal patients in whom the severe intellectual decline is complicated by neurological signs and psychotic symptoms; and finally the classical subgroup which is characterized by gradual progression of mental and functional decline. The clinical heterogeneity of Alzheimer's disease has been recently reviewed (Rossor, 1991).

The neuropathological subtypes corresponding to the clinical subgroups are being gradually defined. Patients with extrapyramidal signs may have some parkinsonian pathology, ranging from classical Parkinson's disease through cortical Lewy body disease to non-specific loss of neurones in the substantia nigra. Out of 20 neuropathologically verified cases of Alzheimer's disease, 11 showed Lewy body formation, neuronal loss and gliosis in the pigmented nuclei of the brainstem, whilst eight brains also had Lewy bodies in the nucleus basalis of Meynert and three in the cortex (Ditter and Mirra, 1987). The neuropathological correlates of parkinsonism may be hetero-geneous: coexistent Parkinson's disease, non-specific degenerative changes in the substantia nigra and no obvious nigral abnormalities have all been observed in a study of the natural history and pathogenesis of parkinsonism in Alzheimer's disease (Morris et al, 1989). Cases without nigral pathology have indicated that extranigral lesions possibly affecting mesocortical dopaminergic pathways may contribute to the development of parkinson-ism. Patients who develop spastic paresis and ataxia at post-mortem examination show degeneration of the corticospinal tracts and severe involvement of the cerebellum by plaque formation, in addition to classical Alzheimer pathology elsewhere in the brain (Aikawa et al, 1985). Myo-clonus is associated with severe course, early onset and mutism, and often these cases are familial. In a juvenile case of Alzheimer's disease starting at the age of 34 years and lasting 6 years, myoclonic jerks, generalized convulsions, dysarthria and ataxia developed. The presence of kuru-like plaques in the cerebellum, amyloid angiopathy and grumose degeneration in the dentate nucleus were additional features, and the grumose change was thought to be responsible for the myoclonus (Ishino et al, 1984).

It is not unusual to find a predominance of one or the other hallmark lesion of Alzheimer's disease and refer to these cases as plaque–or tangle-predominant forms. In extreme cases no neurofibrillary tangles may be present: Terry et al (1987), examining 60 cases over the age of 74 years, reported an absence of tangles in 30%. They compared various clinical and pathological parameters of this group (Group B) with the majority of cases which had both tangles and plaques (Group A): these included degree of dementia, rate of progression, age at death, brain weight, cerebral hemi-spheric weight, cell counts from the frontal, temporal and parietal cortices, the number of neocortical plaques, the number of plaques and tangles in the hippocampus, and the levels of neocortical choline acetyltransferase and somatostatin. No significant differences were found in any of these indices, apart from increased numbers of plaques in the mid-frontal and superior temporal cortex in Group A. Similarly, the pathological abnormalities were, in general, more severe in Group A, but they did not attain statistical significance. Thus, the authors concluded that the disease is the same with or without neurofibrillary tangles, although their presence, not surprisingly, is associated with greater severity.

A further example of heterogeneity of Alzheimer's disease is the focal manifestations of clinical signs or symptoms which are often matched by localized accentuation of neuropathology. The disease process usually spares the primary sensory and motor cortex and consequently lacks the related symptomatology. In a case of early onset dementia with slowly progressive hemiparesis, neuropathology showed severe involvement of the somatosensory cortex by plaque and tangle formation. A further unusual feature was the normal somatostatin-like immunoreactivity, whilst choline acetyltransferase activity was reduced in all regions (Jagust et al, 1990). Progressive visual impairment leading to cortical blindness has also been reported in association with Alzheimer's disease. The occipital lobe was severely affected by Alzheimer-type pathology, although the lesions in the primary visual cortex were not specifically described (Faden and Townsend, 1976). In seven cases of senile dementia, laminar neuronal loss and gliosis exclusively occurred in the CA1 area of the hippocampus, entorhinal cortex and medial occipitotemporal cortex. The subcortical white matter showed extensive fibrillary gliosis. The number of both neurofibrillary tangles and senile plaques exceeded that of controls. The clinical picture was dominated by personality changes in addition to cognitive impairment. The authors regarded these cases as a variant of Alzheimer-type senile dementia, despite the unusual clinical and pathological features (Mizutani et al, 1990).

These cases illustrate the clinical and neuropathological heterogeneity of Alzheimer's disease. Whilst with improving clinicopathological correlation it has been possible to find the pathological bases of unusual clinical symptomatology, the mechanism whereby certain areas are affected by degenerative changes in some cases, but not in others, remains to be elucidated.

Alzheimer's disease may present in combination with cerebral vascular disease; the incidence of these combined cases is so high (Tomlinson et al, 1970) that they hardly qualify as unusual. However, the coexistence of Alzheimer's disease with other neurodegenerative disorders could present clinical and pathological diagnostic problems and should be considered. Combined cases of Alzheimer's and Pick's disease have been reported (for review, see Smith and Lantos, 1983). However, Pick body-like inclusions have been described in the granular neurones of the dentate fascia in over half of Alzheimer cases (Dickson et al, 1986a). Although their distribution, histology, ultrastructure and immunocytochemistry were similar to those of Pick's disease, the authors ruled out that these cases represented combined Alzheimer's and Pick's disease. More likely, their finding could support the hypothesis that the pathological changes characteristic of Alzheimer's disease and Pick's disease may represent a spectrum of related neuro-degenerative disorders (Morris et al, 1984). Alzheimer's disease may occur with extensive Lewy body formation and localized spongiform change of the neuropil (Hansen et al, 1989). Although this latter abnormality may not represent a form of transmissible spongiform encephalopathy, concomitant occurrence of Creutzfeldt–Jakob and Alzheimer's diseases has also been reported (Powers et al, 1991). The combination of Alzheimer-type neuropathology with Lewy bodies and motor neurone disease will be discussed later.

Familial cases

Recently, interest has focused on familial cases, since genetic linkage studies have revealed point mutations in the gene coding for the amyloid precursor protein (see Chapter 3). Although there are several reports on the neuropathology of familial Alzheimer's disease, a systematic and quantitative comparative analysis with sporadic cases is still missing.

Neuropathological examination of four brains out of 51 affected members in a Canadian family did not reveal any unusual histological features (Nee et al, 1983). Earlier, however, cerebellar amyloid plaques had been described (Pro et al, 1979) which shared morphological features with those in kuru and in some cases of Creutzfeldt–Jakob disease (Azzarelli et al, 1985). The presence of these cerebellar plaques in familial Alzheimer's disease is variable: out of 17 autopsies carried out in two large Belgian families, 11 cases in the first family showed only typical Alzheimer-type pathology with occasional cerebellar plaques, whilst all six cases of the second family had developed amyloid plaques in the cerebellum. These stained positively with antibodies to βA4 protein, but were negative for prion protein (Martin et al, 1991). The plaques of familial cases have greater propensity to fuse together than those of sporadic cases, particularly in the cingulate cortex, presubiculum and striatum. Familial cases also had many compact plaques which appeared to be associated with severe amyloid angiopathy in the globus pallidus (Iseki et al, 1990). Neurofibrillary tangles and plaques have been quantified in hippocampal areas CA1–CA4, subiculum, presubiculum and dentate gyrus in three pedigrees. The highest density of plaques and tangles occurred in CA1 and CA2 areas (Figure 1), whilst virtually no lesions were present in the presubiculum. The three pedigrees did not show any overall differences in total densities, but statistical analyses revealed that an uncommon type of plaque develops more frequently in two pedigrees. This plaque type with a marked amyloid core, but no argyrophilic dendrites, was restricted to CA4 area. The importance of these findings is that they highlight the heterogeneity of distribution and morphology of Alzheimer lesions between different families and even between members of the same family (Struble et al, 1991).

The presence of vacuolar or 'spongy' change in some cases is a more controversial phenomenon and may raise diagnostic problems in distinguishing Alzheimer's disease from Creutzfeldt–Jakob disease. In four cases of autosomal dominant Alzheimer's disease, the patients developed not only severe dementia, but also myoclonus and mutism before death. The temporal and frontal cortex had undergone vacuolar change, but lack of astrocytosis and different distribution of lesions as well as the abundance of plaques and tangles excluded the diagnosis of Creutzfeldt–Jakob disease (Duffy et al, 1988).

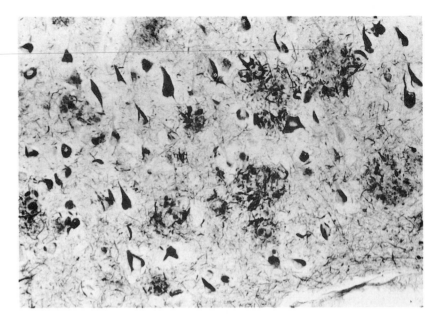

Figure 1. Senile plaques, neurofibrillary tangles and abnormal neurites in the hippocampus of a case of familial Alzheimer's disease. (Modified Bielschowsky silver impregnation; × 500, reduced to 69% on reproduction.)

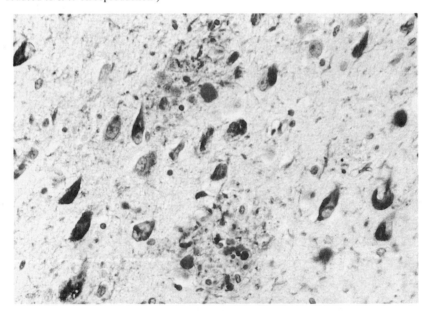

Figure 2. Plaques and tangles in the hippocampus of a patient with valine to isoleucine mutation at codon 717 of the amyloid precursor protein. (Immunostaining with tau antibody (by courtesy of Professor B. H. Anderton, Institute of Psychiatry, London), using the avidin–biotin complex method; × 500, reduced to 69% on reproduction.)

The neuropathology of a familial case with a valine to isoleucine mutation at codon 717 of the amyloid precursor protein has shown abundant neurofibrillary abnormalities in the forms of tangles, plaque neurites and neuropil threads, in addition to moderately severe deposition of βA4 protein both in the substance of the brain and the vessels walls. Interestingly, many Lewy bodies were also seen in the cortex and subcortical grey matter. Detailed immunocytochemical study, using antibodies to βA4 protein, tau (Figure 2), phosphorylated neurofilament epitopes and ubiquitin, as well as biochemical fractionation and Western blot analysis for the abnormally phosphorylated form of tau (A68), did not show substantial differences between familial and sporadic cases (Lantos et al, 1992). These findings imply that an abnormality of the amyloid precursor protein metabolism is responsible not only for the deposition of βA4 protein but also for cytoskeletal pathology.

PICK'S DISEASE

Typical Pick's disease is not difficult to recognize and even the macroscopic appearances may be diagnostic (Chapter 4). Severe lobar atrophy affecting the frontal or temporal lobes or both, and the relatively well-preserved posterior part of the superior temporal gyrus contrasting with its severely damaged neighbours are highly suggestive of Pick's disease. Histology expels any lingering doubts: characteristic Pick bodies in neurones (Figure 3), large,

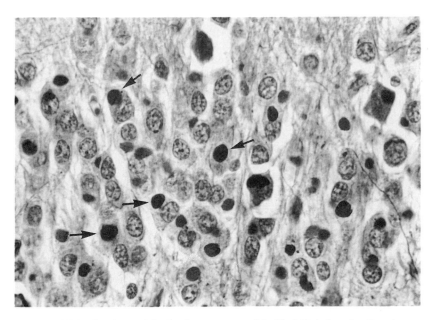

Figure 3. Pick bodies (arrows) in the dentate gyrus. (Modified Bielschowsky silver impregnation; × 800, reduced to 69% on reproduction.)

swollen Pick cells, neuronal loss and astrocytosis secure the diagnosis (for review, see Lantos, 1990). Despite the lobar nature of atrophy, Pick bodies are extensively distributed throughout the brain and they have been observed in areas as remote from the frontotemporal cortex as the olfactory bulb (Yoshimura, 1988) and locus coeruleus (Forno et al, 1989). Of the histological hallmarks of Pick's disease, Pick bodies are usually associated with this condition, although similar structures have been observed in Down's syndrome (Pogacar and Rubio, 1982), tuberous sclerosis (Hirano et al, 1968) and experimental kuru (Lampert et al, 1969). By contrast, swollen, chromatolytic neurones have been described in other neurodegenerative diseases (Clark et al, 1986) and are consequently less pathognomonic of the disease. Ultrastructurally, Pick bodies are composed of two types of filaments: straight tubular filaments with a diameter of 15 nm, and fibrils with constrictions at every 160 nm. These structures resemble the straight and paired helical filaments of neurofibrillary tangles, respectively (Yoshimura, 1989). Immunocytochemistry has confirmed this similarity: neurofibrillary tangles and Pick bodies are both associated with identical phosphorylated neurofilament epitopes (Ulrich et al, 1987). Moreover, both subtypes of filamentous structures in Pick bodies and the occasional transitional form are all immunoreactive with antibodies to tau (Kato and Nakamura, 1990) and to ubiquitin (Lowe et al, 1988).

Based on the involvement of subcortical structures and the distribution and composition of neuronal inclusions, classical and generalized variants of Pick's disease can be distinguished. In this second group, subcortical structures also become atrophied and contain neuronal inclusions (Munoz-Garcia and Ludwin, 1984). However, variations exist in the distribution and severity of pathology, and these atypical cases may present considerable diagnostic problems. Constantinidis et al (1974) have distinguished three groups based on neuropathological features. One-third of the cases showed the classical histological features, whilst the second group had swollen cells in the gliosed and atrophic cortex. In the third group, which comprised slightly more than one-third of the cases, the atrophied cortex displayed astrocytosis, but contained neither swollen Pick cells, nor Pick bodies (Figure 4). This third group, lacking both histological hallmarks of Pick's disease, causes most diagnostic problems and has similarities with so-called progressive subcortical gliosis (Neumann and Cohn, 1967).

In four cases with clinical features of Pick's disease, the brains showed severe atrophy of the caudate nucleus in addition to atrophy of the fronto-temporal regions. Histologically, however, there were neither Pick cells nor Pick inclusions, although severe neuronal loss and astrocytosis of the affected areas, and myelin pallor in the deep white matter and subcortical gliosis were all seen. Moreover, sometimes spongiform change in cortical layer 2 had developed. Despite a confusing profusion of synonyms to describe these changes, the authors consider these cases, on the basis of clinical, macroscopic and histological features, to fall within the spectrum of Pick's disease and suggest the descriptive term of 'lobar atrophy without Pick bodies and Pick cells' (Hulette and Crain, 1990).

The heterogeneity of Pick's disease is further demonstrated by the

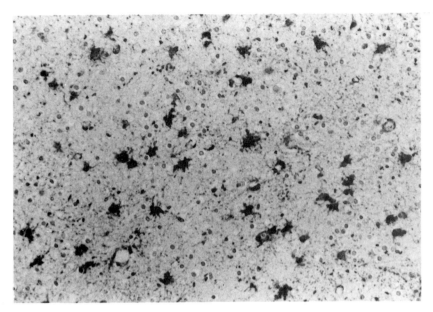

Figure 4. Subcortical gliosis: immunocytochemistry for GFAP shows astrocytosis in the sub-cortical white matter of frontal lobe. (Avidin–biotin complex; × 300, reduced to 69% on reproduction.)

presence or absence of striatopallidonigral degeneration. That there is a selective and substantial neuronal loss in the substantia nigra has been established by a morphometric study (Uchihara et al, 1990). The frequency and degree of striatopallidonigral degeneration have been assessed in a clinicopathological study of 41 cases of Pick's disease (Kosaka et al, 1991). About 41% of the cases had definite evidence of striatopallidonigral degeneration: the striatum, particularly the caudate nucleus, was most frequently and most severely affected, whilst the external segment of the globus pallidus suffered least often and least severely. The medial to central portion of the substantia nigra appeared to be more vulnerable than the rest. In comparing the severely and moderately affected group with that of the mildly degenerate and normal striatopallidonigral system group, several differences had emerged. The former had more female cases, longer duration of the disease and more advanced cases. The brains in this group were more atrophied with a frontal emphasis and atypical cases, including those without Pick bodies, were more common. Moreover, striatonigral degeneration and olivopontocerebellar atrophy in association with Pick's disease has also been described (Horoupian and Dickson, 1991); the oligodendroglial intracytoplasmic inclusions found in this case had been reported in multiple system atrophy (Papp et al, 1989). A case clinically resembling amyotrophic lateral sclerosis had Pick's disease with unusual features: in addition to degeneration of the substantia nigra, some of the neurones in the endplate of the hippocampus contained 'compound' Pick bodies characterized by an eosinophilic core (Sam et al, 1991). Cases of dementia have been reported in which swollen chromatolytic neurones extensively occurred in the setting of cortical degeneration. The brains had moderate to marked atrophy of the frontal regions, and the histological abnormalities affected the anterior parts of the brain. The authors considered these cases to represent an early stage in the pathogenetic process and suggested that an attempt should be made to distinguish pathogenetically distinct subgroups which have been classified together under the diagnosis of Pick's disease (Clark et al, 1986).

Familial cases are known to occur and the best documented case is a large Dutch family with 25 clinically diagnosed cases. Of these, 14 had been confirmed by autopsy. The disease is most likely to be transmitted by a dominant gene (Groen and Endtz, 1982). More recently, familial forms of progressive subcortical gliosis have been reported, segregated as an autosomal dominant trait, and the diagnosis was confirmed by neuropathology in six cases from two kindreds (Lanska et al, 1991).

FRONTAL LOBE DEMENTIA

Two independent research groups from Lund (Gustafson et al, 1985) and Manchester (Neary et al, 1986) have defined frontal lobe dementia as an entity distinct from Alzheimer's disease. Frontal lobe dementia has an earlier onset, affects both sexes equally and nearly half of the patients have a family history. The importance of this new entity has been recognized, since it is more common than previously considered. The ratio of frontal lobe dementia or dementia of frontal lobe type (DFLT) to Alzheimer's disease is approximately 1:4 in the British series (Neary, 1990). Parallel with the clinical investigations, the neuropathology of these cases has been established. In a large series of 158 cases of organic dementia, 16 cases (10%) appeared to form a separate group, termed frontal lobe degeneration of non-Alzheimer's type FLD (Chapter 5). The neuropathology was defined in these cases by the lack of any specific lesions typical of other neurodegenerative disorders. The degeneration of the grey matter, affecting the frontal lobes most severely, was characterized by neuronal loss, mild astrocytosis and superficial spongiosis. Senile plaques, neurofibrillary tangles and amyloid angiopathy were absent or occurred very mildly in senile patients. Similarly, typical Pick inclusions were not found, although large, swollen chromatolytic cells were occasionally seen. In addition to the frontal lobe, the anterior half of the temporal lobe showed milder changes and the parieto-occipital region was less affected. The hippocampus, amygdala and nucleus basalis of Meynert were only slightly damaged, and there was no preferential involvement of any hippocampal area. The striatum also showed mild abnormalities in most cases, but the caudate nucleus, thalamus and most of the brainstem had been spared. Mild neuronal loss in the substantia nigra was noted (Brun, 1987). Deposition of βA4 protein was reported in the brain of two elderly patients, but this phenomenon was regarded as a consequence of ageing rather than an expression of specific pathology (Mann and Jones, 1990). In addition, the white matter was also affected as a result of cortical degeneration (Englund and Brun, 1987). These white matter abnormalities consisted of myelin loss and astrocytosis, and were similar to those seen in Pick's disease, but differed from the changes of Alzheimer's, Binswanger's and Creutzfeldt–Jakob diseases. Moreover, these studies have revealed the lack not only of neuropathological features, but also of neurochemical abnormalities associated with Alzheimer's disease (Neary et al, 1986).

Thus the type and distribution of abnormalities clearly distinguishes frontal lobe degeneration from Alzheimer's disease. However, its relationship to Pick's disease is more controversial. If we accept the view that Pick's disease is a well-defined lobar atrophy characterized not only by neuronal loss and astrocytosis, but Pick inclusions and Pick cells, then the differential diagnosis should not present serious problems. However, if Pick's disease is regarded, as now is increasingly the case, as a histological spectrum of abnormalities ranging from the typical picture to cases in which neither neuronal inclusions nor Pick cells may be found, then the neuropathologist faces considerable difficulties. For this reason it has been suggested that whilst frontal lobe dementia has to be clearly distinguished from Alzheimer's disease, both on clinical and pathological grounds, the same demarcation from Pick's disease is not possible, and indeed frontal lobe dementia may represent forms of Pick's disease (Neary et al, 1988).

In a review of 460 demented patients, 14 had neuronal loss and astrocytosis in multiple sites including the frontoparietal cortex, but no neuronal inclusions and virtually no senile plaques. These cases, which were termed 'dementia lacking distinctive pathology', presented with memory loss and personality changes, developed dysarthria and dysphagia later and died within 2–7 years. The psychometric findings in some patients were consistent with frontal lobe dementia and there was a family history of dementia and neurological disease in eight patients (Knopman et al, 1990).

Reviewing the neuropathology of patients with frontal lobe dementia, Brun and Gustafson (1991) have distinguished four groups: group 1 had severe Alzheimer's disease; group 2 had selective bilateral incomplete infarctions of the white matter; group 3 had Binswanger's disease; and group 4, the largest cohort, suffered from frontal lobe degeneration of non-Alzheimer type as previously described (Brun, 1987).

Although not frontal in distribution, it is worthwhile to consider here those cases which are characterized by the widespread occurrence of argyrophilic grains in the neuropil of the cerebral cortex in the absence of any Alzheimer-type pathology (Braak and Braak, 1987, 1989). Since these argyrophilic grains were the sole abnormalities in ten out of 80 brains of demented patients, the authors assumed that these lesions could be the morphological substrate of an unknown, dementing disease. These structures also occur in the subcortical grey matter, are filamentous and stain positively with the monoclonal antibody Alz-50 (Itagaki et al, 1989). In some cases these argyrophilic grains, together with neuropil threads and neurofibrillary tangles, occur in the hippocampus, entorhinal cortex, locus coeruleus, substantia nigra, subthalamic nucleus and inferior olives and are composed of straight tubulofilamentous structures of 25 nm in diameter, similar to those seen in progressive supranuclear palsy. These findings suggest that late onset dementia with argyrophilic grains associated with subcortical tangles and neuropil threads may represent an atypical form of progressive supranuclear palsy (Masliah et al, 1991).

LOBAR ATROPHY

Pick's disease and frontal lobe degeneration of non-Alzheimer type are lobar atrophies. In addition, other forms of focal atrophy exist and cases with slowly progressive aphasia have been described (Wechsler, 1977; Mesulam, 1982) (see Chapter 6).

Primary progressive aphasia is a clinical term introduced by Mesulam (1982), who reviewed six patients with this language disturbance. Some of the patients also had focal atrophy of the perisylvian region on imaging. Since then there have been several reports but in only 13 cases were post-mortem examinations carried out (Lippa et al, 1991). The first case reported by Wechsler (1977) showed loss of large cortical neurones, astrocytosis and spongiform change asymmetrically affecting the dominant hemisphere.

Whilst the clinical entity appears to have been established, the underlying neuropathology remains debatable. However, it is reasonable to assume that the pathological process associated with primary progressive aphasia is not a single, well-defined entity, but a heterogeneous mixture of lesions. These may include focal accentuation of Alzheimer's disease (Poeck and Luzzati, 1988; Green et al, 1990) or Pick's disease (Wechsler et al, 1982; Graff-Radford et al, 1990). Spongiform change may occur (Wechsler, 1977), and two cases were reported with focal change in cortical layer 2 and astrocytosis in the deeper layers (Kirshner et al, 1987). This appearance may present problems in differential diagnosis from Creutzfeldt–Jakob disease, although these patients did not suffer from dementia. Primary progressive aphasia may also be associated with focal neuronal achromasia (Lippa et al, 1991). The presence of these cells in this case raised the possibility of Pick's disease and corticobasal degeneration, although the overall appearance fell between the two. This case further underlines the neuropathological heterogeneity of primary progressive aphasia.

MOTOR NEURONE DISEASE AND DEMENTIA

The association between motor neurone disease and dementia was originally recognized as part of the dementia-parkinsonism complex of Guam (Hirano et al, 1961a, 1961b) and since then cases have been reported both from Western countries and from Japan (see Chapter 7). The occurrence of dementia with motor neurone disease raises two important questions. First, what is the neuropathological substrate of the patient's mental impairment? Second, how do the cerebral changes found in these cases correlate with other neurodegenerative disorders in general and with the frontal lobe dementia of non-Alzheimer type in particular? In other words, do these cases represent a new nosological entity or merely form a subgroup of motor neurone disease?

With increasing interest in these cases, the brain has been subjected to more thorough neuropathological examination involving not only special neurohistological techniques, but also immunocytochemistry, electron microscopy and quantitative assessments in order to establish the cerebral pathology which may exist outside the motor system and may be responsible for dementia. An early review of 26 cases revealed non-specific, mild changes throughout the central nervous system without evidence of vascular disease or primary degenerative dementia, but with the pathology of motor neurone disease (Mitsuyama, 1984). These findings have been confirmed in a larger series of 34 Japanese cases which have revealed a mild to moderate degree of glial proliferation, subcortical gliosis and a moderate degree of status spongiosus of the superficial cortex, mainly in the frontotemporal area. Severe loss of pigmented neurones in the substantia nigra occurred in half of the patients and mild neuronal loss was seen in the frontotemporal cortex. No Pick cells, Pick inclusions, neurofibrillary changes or senile plaques were seen. Brain weight was reduced, but this tissue loss was not as severe as in Alzheimer's, Pick's or Creutzfeldt–Jakob disease. The hypoglossal nucleus and the anterior horns of the spinal cord showed degenerative changes, but demyelination of the lateral tracts of the cord was not obvious. The muscles suffered neurogenic atrophy (Morita et al, 1987). The abnormalities in the brain were similar to those seen in progressive subcortical gliosis and several research workers concentrated on glial changes. Glial fibrillary acidic protein (GFAP) immunocytochemistry revealed abnormal clusters of positively stained reactive astrocytes in the precentral cortex (Kamo et al, 1987) and widespread astrocytosis in the subcortical white matter (Kushner et al, 1991).

However, these changes are unlikely to explain fully the dementia associated with motor neurone disease and cortical involvement in these cases may be more extensive than previously thought. A morphometric study revealed substantial reduction in the number of cortical neurones, particularly those larger than $90 \, \mu m^2$. The pattern of neuronal loss differed from Alzheimer's disease in that the substantia innominata was spared and neither choline acetyltransferase nor somatostatin was reduced (Horoupian et al, 1984). There was also attrition of the dendritic tree of pyramidal cells. A recent study has also shown neuronal loss, gliosis and spongiosis in the upper layers of the frontal and temporal lobes and dendritic abnormalities of the surviving neurones, including reduced dendritic trees, proximal dendritic varicosities, amputation of dendrites and depletion of spines. The authors thought that these dendritic changes could contribute to the pathogenesis of dementia (Ferrer et al, 1991). A further important development in the elucidation of cortical pathology in motor neurone disease has been the demonstration of ubiquitin-positive structures in the cortex.

Although ubiquitin-positive inclusions in the motor cortex had already been demonstrated (Lowe et al, 1989, Leigh et al, 1991), they were only recently described in both the hippocampus and entorhinal cortex (Okamoto et al, 1991). The hippocampal and neocortical inclusions are not argyrophilic and do not react with antibodies which label neurofibrillary tangles and Pick bodies. Moreover, the inclusions in dentate granule cells were present only in patients with dementia, but not in typical cases of amyotrophic lateral sclerosis (Wightman et al, 1992). Despite cortical involvement, the neuro-pathology of these cases is still considerably different from the abnormalities of Alzheimer's disease. However, the amyotrophic lateral sclerosis and parkinsonism–dementia complex of Guam may represent a link between the different pathologies of motor neurone disease and Alzheimer's disease. Recent investigations have revealed that this complex and geographically well-demarcated disorder has virtually all the histological abnormalities of Alzheimer's disease, including neurofibrillary tangles, granulovacuolar degeneration, Hirano bodies, cell loss in the basal forebrain and cortical atrophy, although senile plaques are absent or rare (Perl et al, 1991).

Whilst the neuropathological basis of dementia with motor neurone disease is being elucidated, the nosological status of these cases remains controversial. Several authors have considered that these cases represent a new entity (Mitsuyama, 1984; Morita et al, 1987), whilst the majority view holds that they are a variant of an already defined neurodegenerative disease. The superficial histological resemblance to Creutzfeldt–Jakob disease has raised the possible association with spongiform encepha-lopathies (see Chapter 8). Although there are no Pick cells and Pick inclusions, the overall neuropathology has similarities with progressive subcortical gliosis, which itself was considered to be an atypical mani-festation of Pick's disease. The clinical and pathological findings of a recent study have pointed to a relationship between dementia with motor neurone disease and dementia of the frontal lobe type (Neary et al, 1990). However, there is solid clinical and pathological evidence for the involvement of the motor system, and the similarities with non-demented cases of motor neurone disease clearly outweigh the differences. These cases with dementia are thus likely to represent a variant of motor neurone disease and further immunocytochemical and morphometric studies are likely to confirm this view.

PRION DISEASES

Increasing knowledge of a group of transmissible dementias has been reflected in the frequent changes of names designated to these disorders. Slow virus diseases, indicating the putative causative agent, was replaced by the descriptive name of spongiform encephalopathies. Now with the eluci-dation of their molecular pathology, the term prion disease is increasingly gaining ground. Seven diseases belong to this group: three occur in man (Creutzfeldt–Jakob disease, Gerstmann–Sträussler–Scheinker disease and kuru) and four in animals (scrapie, mink encephalopathy, chronic wasting disease of deer and elk, and bovine spongiform encephalopathy). There are at least three reasons for the increased interest, both scientific and public, in spongiform encephalopathies. First, there has been a spectacular progress in the understanding of the cellular and molecular pathology as well as the genetic background of these diseases. Secondly, they are transmissible and cases of iatrogenic transmission by stereotactic surgery, corneal transplant, dural graft and pituitary hormone treatment have been reported. Thirdly, the identification of bovine spongiform encephalopathy, transmitted to cattle from sheep by infected foodstuffs, has raised wider issues of public health. Various aspects of spongiform encephalopathies, including their molecular biology, genetics and neuropathology have been recently reviewed (Brown et al, 1991; Prusiner, 1991; Will, 1991; Lantos, 1992; see also Chapter 8).

The neuropathology of Creutzfeldt–Jakob disease appears straightforward and is characterized by the classical triad of spongiform change, neuronal loss and astrocytosis of the cerebral cortex and deep grey matter. The distribution and severity of these changes may vary substantially. Cortical, corticospinal, corticostriatal, corticostriatospinal and cerebellar forms can be distinguished according to the pattern of lesions. More importantly, the severity of abnormalities may vary even within the same brain, and a severely affected stretch of the cortical ribbon may alternate with relatively well-preserved areas. The white matter may also be affected by spongiosis, loss of myelin and astrocytic proliferation.

The second human spongiform encephalopathy, Gerstmann–Sträussler–Scheinker disease, has somewhat different neuropathology: there is extensive amyloid plaque formation and spongiform change. The cerebellum is usually most severely affected and the plaques may have single or multiple cores, but the neuritic components are sparse or absent. The amyloid is clearly different from that of Alzheimer's disease: it does not give positive reaction with antibodies to $\beta A4$ protein, but is immunoreactive with antisera against prion protein 27–30. Spongiform change is not as extensive and severe as in Creutzfeldt–Jakob disease.

The third human disease is kuru, which had been propagated by cannibalism in the Highlands of Papua New Guinea. The cerebral hemispheres show changes similar to those in Creutzfeldt–Jakob disease, whilst in the atrophied cerebellum there is loss of Purkinje and granule cells, astrocytosis and fibrillary gliosis, and amyloid plaque formation.

Whilst the typical cases of spongiform encephalopathies do not present any diagnostic problems for the neuropathologist, unusual cases also exist. The so-called amyotrophic form shows clinical and pathological differences from the classical cases of Creutzfeldt–Jakob disease: the duration of the illness is longer and the typical spongiform change in the brain is absent (Salazar et al, 1983). However, the transmission of one case (Connolly et al, 1988) has confirmed that this is a variant of Creutzfeldt–Jakob disease. None the less, it was only recently realized, with the introduction of molecular genetics, that the genetic abnormality typical of inherited human spongiform encephalopathies may be associated with atypical pathology (Figure 5). A man of 36 years of age had a 144 base pair insertion in the open reading

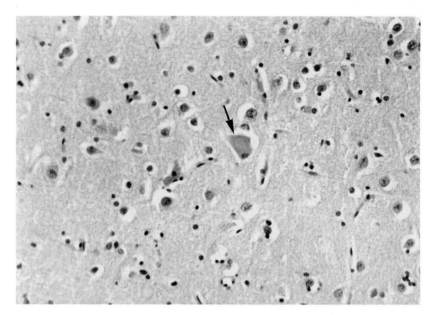

Figure 5. Swollen, achromatic neurone (arrow) in the cortex of a man of 36 years of age who had a 144 bp insertion in the open reading frame of the prion protein gene. No typical histological abnormalities of spongiform encephalopathy are seen. (Haematoxylin and eosin; × 300, reduced to 69% on reproduction.)

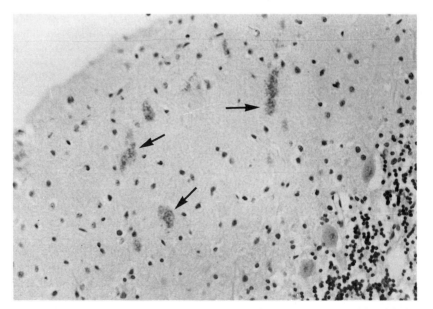

Figure 6. Positive immunostaining (arrows) with an antibody to prion protein (by courtesy of Dr J. Hope, Institute for Animal Health, Edinburgh) in the molecular layer of the cerebellum. (Avidin–biotin complex; × 300, reduced to 69% on reproduction.)

frame of the prion protein gene, identical to that previously described in a family with neuropathologically confirmed familial Creutzfeldt–Jakob disease, but neuropathological examination did not show any of the typical changes of spongiform encephalopathies (Collinge et al, 1990). This case raises important issues. First, the true incidence of transmissible dementias is likely to have been underestimated, since cases without the histological hallmarks of the disease might have gone undiagnosed. From this it follows that genetic screening and immunohistochemical demonstration of the abnormal isoform of prion protein should complement traditional neuro-histology to establish the true incidence of these diseases (Figure 6). Secondly, the genetic basis of transmissible spongiform encephalopathies is likely to be more extensive than previously realized. Thirdly, the convenient descriptive term of spongiform encephalopathy may have to be abandoned in favour of prior disease.

LEWY BODY DEMENTIA

The association of dementia with Parkinson's disease has long been estab-lished and only its frequency has been disputed. According to a conservative estimate one in five Parkinson's patients becomes demented, but only thorough investigation could ascertain the true incidence of dementia (Brown and Marsden, 1984). The concept of neuropathological changes responsible for this dementia has undergone dramatic revision during the last decade. For a long time it has been accepted that Alzheimer-type pathology in the cortex forms the neurohistological basis of the patient's cognitive impairment; indeed, the degree of dementia correlates well with the severity of Alzheimer-type pathology in the cortex in cases without features of diffuse Lewy body disease (Paulus and Jellinger, 1991).

It was the observation of cortical Lewy bodies which transformed the view of the pathogenesis of dementia in Parkinson's disease (see Chapter 9). In a study of 55 cases of Parkinson's disease, three groups could be distinguished according to the frequency and distribution of Lewy bodies and Alzheimer-type changes. In Group A, four patients had progressive dementia and developed not only Alzheimer-type pathology, but also many Lewy bodies in the cortex. These occurred predominantly in the small and medium-sized pyramidal neurones of the fifth and sixth layers of the temporal, frontal, insular and cingulate cortex (Figure 7). The distribution of Lewy bodies in the brainstem was usual and the term diffuse Lewy body disease was introduced to describe those cases. In Group B (15 cases), patients had classical parkinsonism and Lewy bodies in the diencephalon and brainstem, whilst cortical Lewy bodies and Alzheimer lesions were less frequent in the cortex than in the previous group. However, demented patients (seven out of 15) had more cortical Lewy bodies and Alzheimer changes than non-demented patients. Group C (36 cases) did not develop dementia, the cerebral cortex was spared of Lewy bodies, and Alzheimer pathology was in accordance with the patients' ages. Lewy bodies occurred in the di-encephalon and brainstem (Yoshimura, 1983). Consequently, Groups A, B

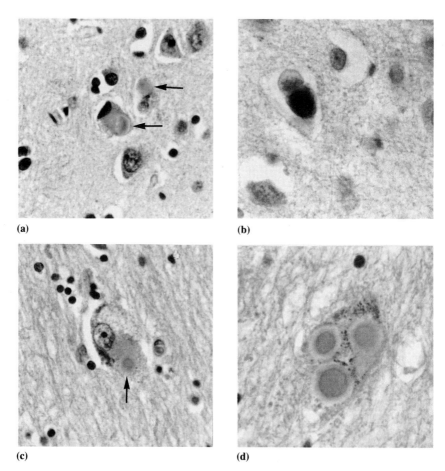

Figure 7. (a) Cortical Lewy bodies (arrows) in the frontal lobe. (Haematoxylin and eosin; ×800.) (b) Cortical Lewy body immunostained with ubiquitin antibody. (Avidin–biotin complex; ×1250.) (c) Lewy body (arrow) in a neurone of the nucleus basalis of Meynert. (Haematoxylin and eosin; ×800.) (d) Lewy bodies in a neurone of the substantia nigra. (Haematoxylin and eosin; ×1250.) (All reduced to 60% on reproduction.)

and C were termed diffuse, transitional and brainstem-type of Lewy body disease, respectively, and only this last was equated with classical idiopathic Parkinson's disease (Kosaka et al, 1984). The precise neuropathological basis of dementia has, however, remained controversial in relation to cortical versus subcortical pathology and Lewy bodies versus Alzheimer lesions. A large clinicopathological study revealed that in diffuse Lewy body disease, cortical lesions, Lewy bodies and Alzheimer changes were responsible for the dementia. In one-quarter of cases with brainstem-type Lewy body disease Alzheimer type pathology was responsible for the dementia, whilst, in the majority, degeneration of the subcortical nuclei, particularly the nucleus basalis of Meynert contributed to intellectual impairment

(Kosaka et al, 1988). Thus the importance of subcortical pathology was emphasized in the cause of dementia in Parkinson's disease (de la Monte et al, 1989). However, using antibodies to ubiquitin, which identify cortical Lewy bodies with greater accuracy than traditional histological stains, a quantitative neuropathological study revealed that the severity of dementia is related to cortical Lewy body density, whilst subcortical pathology plays a less important role. Senile plaques were common, but neurofibrillary tangles rare (Lennox et al, 1989). As distinct from diffuse Lewy body disease, a clinically and neuropathologically defined form of Lewy body dementia was recently described in the elderly (Perry et al, 1990). Clinically, these cases did not fulfil the diagnostic criteria of either Alzheimer's or Parkinson's disease. Many cases were diagnosed as multi-infarct dementia, but autopsy did not confirm the diagnosis. Neuropathological examination, however, revealed Lewy body formation and selective neuronal loss in the brainstem and other subcortical nuclei, and Lewy bodies in the neocortex and limbic cortex, but at a frequency well below that reported in diffuse Lewy body disease. Many senile plaques and few neurofibrillary tangles were seen. Thus the authors contend that the clinical and neuropathological features are different, both from those in Parkinson's and Alzheimer's disease, and that these cases may represent a distinct neurodegenerative disorder in which mental symptoms dominate over signs of movement disability. They form the second most common single cause of dementia after Alzheimer's disease in the elderly (Perry et al, 1989). Hansen et al (1990) reported cortical and subcortical Lewy bodies in 13 cases out of 36 verified cases of Alzheimer's disease and considered them to form clinically and pathologically a distinct subset of Alzheimer's disease, the so-called Lewy body variant. Neuropathologically these cases showed gross pallor of the substantia nigra, greater neuronal loss in the locus coeruleus, substantia nigra and substantia innominata and fewer midfrontal tangles than pure Alzheimer's disease. They also had a higher incidence of spongiform vacuolization in the medial temporal lobe and lower neocortical choline acetyltransferase activities. The number of neurofibrillary tangles in the entorhinal cortex was higher than in controls, but lower than in Alzheimer's disease (Hansen et al, 1991). The dementia in these cases is likely to result from the combined factors of neuronal loss of subcortical projection nuclei (substantia nigra, locus coeruleus and nucleus basalis of Meynert), cortical Lewy bodies, spongiform vacuolization of the medial temporal lobe and Alzheimer-type pathology.

It is of great theoretical importance to distinguish diffuse Lewy body disease from mixed Parkinson's disease and Alzheimer's disease. The senile plaques of diffuse Lewy body disease are characterized by amyloid deposits and few or no neuritic components. Moreover, there is no significant neuritic change in the neuropil (Dickson et al, 1989). Interestingly, it is hippocampal degeneration which differentiates diffuse Lewy body disease from Alzheimer's disease. Immunocytochemistry with antibodies to ubiquitin has demonstrated immunoreactive neurites in the CA2 and CA3 region of the hippocampus in diffuse Lewy body disease and these ubiquitin-positive structures were absent in Alzheimer's disease, normal elderly individuals and in Parkinson's disease. Further immunocytochemical characterization by double-labelling showed that only a small fraction stained with antibodies to neurofilaments or Alz-50, but no staining was seen with an antibody to Alzheimer neurofibrillary tangles. This staining pattern is different from that of Alzheimer's disease, in which neurites are immunoreactive with all these antibodies, and thus the neuritic degeneration in the CA2–3 region of the hippocampus is a specific histopathological feature of diffuse Lewy body disease (Dickson et al, 1991). Immunocytochemistry has also shown differences between Lewy bodies of diffuse Lewy body disease and of idiopathic Parkinson's disease, in that only the former gave positive reaction with antibodies to tau protein (Galloway et al, 1989).

Recent investigations have revealed that Lewy bodies may occur well beyond the traditional topographical territory of Parkinson's disease and represent the histological hallmark of Lewy body diseases. Within these, idiopathic Parkinson's disease and diffuse Lewy body disease may represent opposite ends of the spectrum, whilst senile dementia of the Lewy type may occupy the intermediate stage. Whilst the neuropathological substrate of dementia in these conditions has been, to some extent, clarified, further studies are needed to establish the full range of cortical pathology and its relation to subcortical changes. Lewy bodies, which have attracted so much attention recently, are likely to be one of the several histological abnormalities which contribute to the pathogenesis of dementia.

CORTICOBASAL DEGENERATION

Recently interest has focused on corticobasal degeneration, also referred to as corticonigral and corticodentatonigral degeneration (see Chapter 10). Originally the clinical and pathological features of this disorder were reported in three patients by Rebeiz et al (1968), who termed the disease 'corticodentatonigral degeneration with neuronal achromasia'. Clinically the cases resembled progressive supranuclear palsy, whilst some of the pathological features were similar to those of Pick's disease. Cortical atrophy developed in the posterior frontal, paraolfactory and parietal regions, whilst the rest of the brain remained relatively well preserved. Neurones of the substantia nigra were depleted in all three cases and the dentate nuclei showed degeneration in two. In the atrophied areas there was severe neuronal loss, with the presence of abnormal, swollen, chromatolytic cells (Figure 8). In the fourth case, reported by Scully (1985), post-mortem findings showed frontal atrophy with large, swollen, pale cells. In a report of three further cases, the entity of corticobasal degeneration has been more clearly defined (Gibb et al, 1989). Neuropathological examination revealed frontoparietal atrophy characterized by cortical cell loss, gliosis and Pick cells, but neither hippocampal pathology nor Pick bodies were observed. In addition, neuronal loss and gliosis occurred in the thalamus, lentiform nucleus, red nucleus, subthalamic nucleus, midbrain tegmentum, substantia nigra and locus coeruleus. Neuronal inclusions in the substantia nigra (Figure 9), termed corticobasal inclusions, were similar to the neuro-

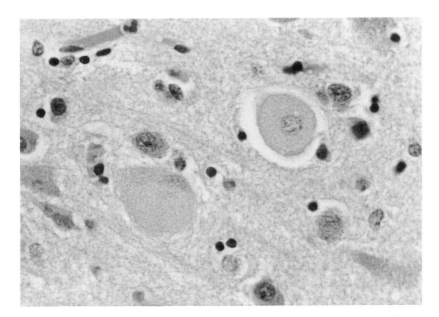

Figure 8. Swollen, achromatic neurones in the frontal lobe of a case of corticobasal degeneration. (Haematoxylin and eosin; × 800, reduced to 69% on reproduction.)

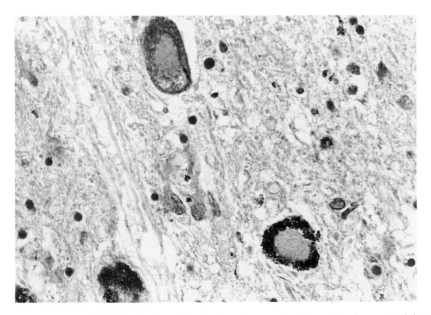

Figure 9. Neuronal inclusions in the substantia nigra show moderately positive immunostaining with an antibody to tau protein (by courtesy of Professor B. H. Anderton, Institute of Psychiatry, London). (× 800, reduced to 69% on reproduction.)

fibrillary tangles of progressive supranuclear palsy, whilst other, pale inclusions, shared features with the pale body of Parkinson's disease, but Lewy bodies and neurofibrillary tangles were usually absent. Some nigral inclusions were similar to those found in Pick's disease. The authors concluded that, despite some histological similarities to Pick's disease, the distribution of neuronal loss and the corticobasal inclusions are unique to corticobasal degeneration and justify this disorder as a nosological entity. Immunocytochemistry with monoclonal antibodies to neurofilaments reveal that various inclusions in corticobasal degeneration share antigenic determinants with both neurofilaments and neurofibrillary tangles (Gibb et al, 1989). One of these antibodies, RT97, is specific for phosphorylated epitopes. Interestingly, Dickson et al (1986b) have earlier reported positive staining of ballooned neurones in neurodegenerative disorders, including Pick's disease and in a single case of corticobasal degeneration. More recently 15 cases have been reported with corticobasal ganglionic degeneration, but post-mortem examination was carried out only in two cases. These revealed swollen, achromatic neurones and degeneration in the cerebral cortex and substantia nigra. Moreover, biochemical analysis of one case showed severe, diffuse loss of dopamine in the striatum. The authors suggest that this condition occurs more frequently than hitherto thought, but the definitive diagnosis depends upon neuropathological examination (Riley et al, 1991).

Two further cases reported by Lippa et al (1990) showed the usual histological features and immunocytochemistry revealed the presence of phosphorylated epitopes in the swollen cortical neurones. In addition tau-positive neurones were described in the superficial cortical layers; these inclusions were ubiquitin negative, did not contain phosphorylated neurofilament epitopes and were not argyrophilic in Bodian's silver impregnation. In their distribution and staining properties they did differ from both Pick and Lewy bodies and may be unique to corticonigral degeneration (Paulus and Selim, 1990). Recently a previously unreported type of neuritic degeneration has been described in four cases: concentric clusters of short stubby neurites, containing straight filaments of 15–18 nm in diameter and resembling senile plaques but without amyloid deposition, are present in the cortex (Mattiace et al, 1991).

Views concerning the nosological entity of corticobasal degeneration are divided. Whilst Alzheimer's disease and Parkinson's disease do not represent, neuropathologically, serious differential diagnostic problems, the separation from progressive supranuclear palsy and Pick's disease may be more difficult. The similarities and differences with these other two neurodegenerative disorders have been reviewed (Gibb et al, 1989). Neurofibrillary tangles are not, unlike in progressive supranuclear palsy, a prominent feature of corticobasal degeneration. However, they may occur, and light microscopic differences may not be obvious. Moreover, they are immunohistochemically more similar to tangles in progressive supranuclear palsy than to those in Alzheimer's disease: they are tau positive, but ubiquitin negative (Paulus and Selim, 1990). Whilst the substantia nigra is affected in both conditions, the corticobasal inclusions are absent in progressive supranuclear palsy and the involvement of the dentate is also different in the two conditions. The pathological similarities with Pick's disease are striking, although in corticobasal degeneration no typical Pick bodies occur. However, small tau-positive inclusions have been demonstrated in the upper layers of the cortex. Conversely, Pick's disease has been described without typical inclusions, and the substantia nigra may also be involved in Pick's disease, creating considerable differential diagnostic problems. Thus, corticobasal degeneration, may share both clinical and pathological features with other neurodegenerative diseases. It is therefore essential to examine fully these cases and to characterize both the clinical symptomatology and neuropathological spectrum of lesions. Positron emission tomography promisingly shows a unique pattern of regional cortical oxygen hypometabolism and striatal fluorodopa uptake (Sawle et al, 1991). Further immunocytochemical and molecular biological investigation may help to clarify further corticobasal degeneration and its relationship to other neurodegenerative diseases.

CONCLUSIONS

Recent developments in clinical investigations, neuropathology and molecular biology have been instrumental in advancing our knowledge of neurodegenerative disorders which underlie dementias. From this progress, several trends have clearly emerged.

First, increasingly sophisticated methods, both at clinical and neuropathological levels, have enabled new nosological entities to be defined. At the same time, it was realized that most neurodegenerative diseases are heterogeneous both clinically and neuropathologically. Comprehensive neurohistological studies, using quantitative morphometry and immunocytochemistry, have revealed that a spectrum of cellular abnormalities may exist within the same nosological entity: at one end of the spectrum all the histological hallmarks may be present, whilst at the other only non-specific changes may occur. An example for the latter is the so-called Pick's disease without Pick bodies and Pick cells, and the question may arise whether these form frustes qualify to be diagnosed as Pick's disease or whether they merge imperceptibly with the frontal lobe dementia of non-Alzheimer type. Thus there are clearly two conflicting trends between attempts to define new nosological entities and the recent realization of the heterogeneity of neurodegenerative disorders. The introduction of molecular genetics into research has also increased this heterogeneity. Our insight into familial forms of several of these diseases has increased and new mutations have been found. Mutation in the prion protein gene, for example, may be associated with highly atypical or, more precisely, non-specific minimal neuropathology.

A cardinal, common feature of most neurodegenerative disorders is the presence of intracellular inclusions, usually associated with abnormalities of the cytoskeleton. Our knowledge of the existence and distribution of these structures has expanded in recent years. Neurofibrillary abnormalities have long been known to occur in Alzheimer's disease, not only in the form of tangles, but also in the neurites of senile plaques. However, their existence in neuropil threads has only recently gained attention. Similarly, the presence of Lewy bodies in the pigmented neurones of the brainstem has been long considered to be the 'core' pathology of Parkinson's disease, yet their widespread occurrence in the cortex has been noted only 10 years ago. New types of inclusions have been also described, their presence highlighted by immunocytochemistry. Ubiquitin-positive structures in the hippocampus and neocortex in motor neurone disease and neuronal inclusions in cortico-basal degeneration are the examples. Moreover, abnormal cytoskeletal inclusions have been described, for the first time not only in nerve cells but also in glia: oligodendroglial inclusions, noted in Gallyas' silver impregnation, were subsequently characterized by both immunocytochemistry and electron microscopy in multiple system atrophy (Papp et al, 1989). The importance of these developments is twofold. They help to define nosological entities and to focus the attention of molecular biologists and protein chemists on future research priorities. Indeed, in each case our knowledge of the morphology, antigenicity and biochemical composition of these inclusions has considerably increased.

Of the diseases considered here, βA4 protein deposition with consequent cerebral amyloidosis is a pathognomonic event only in Alzheimer's disease. There is now increasing evidence, from genetic studies (Goate et al, 1991), from neuropathological investigations (Lantos et al, 1992) and from experiments with transgenic mice (Quon et al, 1991), to suggest that mutation in the amyloid precursor protein gene and the subsequent βA4 deposition is the primary pathogenetic event which initiates all the other cellular pathologies. Of course, βA4 deposition may occur in ageing and its presence in elderly patients with non-Alzheimer pathologies reflects this phenomenon.

It has also been realized that cellular inclusions are not static, either structurally or antigenically. That neuronal inclusions may have a life cycle has best been demonstrated for neurofibrillary tangles. Although the earliest changes and the precise sequence of their formation are not known, the structural and antigenic differences which exist between intracellular and extracellular forms have been established (Tabaton et al, 1991).

A further important development in studies on neurodegenerative diseases has been the discovery that degenerative processes, hitherto considered to affect only or predominantly subcortical systems, involve the cortex. Lewy bodies may occur extensively in the cortex and there are cortical abnormalities in motor neurone disease. Progressive supranuclear palsy, although not considered in this volume, also affects the cortex; neuronal loss and the formation of neuropil threads have now been well recognized. The involvement of the cortex in these diseases has an important clinical implication: the concept of subcortical dementia has to be reassessed. The pathological basis of subcortical dementias has been controversial. Severe and extensive involvement of subcortical structures is unlikely to spare the cortex completely, since these structures are connected, directly or indirectly, with the cortex. However, if the cortex is directly affected, the dementia associated with these diseases is not purely subcortical. Thus neuropathological development may stimulate neuropsychiatrists and neuropsychologists to clarify the concept of subcortical dementia.

The above developments convincingly show that neurodegenerative diseases in general, but particularly those which underlie unusual dementias, remain a fascinating and controversial field of neuroscience. For the neuropathologists it is occasionally easier to exclude diseases than to give a positive diagnosis. This apparent uncertainty may be disappointing for the clinicians, who expect an unequivocal neuropathological diagnosis and a precise neuroanatomical correlation for each and every one of the clinical signs and symptoms. At present many problems remain unresolved and prevent this achievement. However, the collaboration between clinicians, neuropathologists and basic neuroscientists holds the promise of elucidating further the causes and developments of neurodegenerative diseases.

Acknowledgements

The author wishes to thank Dr N. J. Cairns and Mr A. Chadwick, members of the MRC Alzheimer's Disease Brain Bank, for their help, and Mrs Elizabeth Kemp for secretarial assistance.

REFERENCES

Aikawa H, Suzuki K, Iwasaki Y & Iizuka R (1985) Atypical Alzheimer's disease with spastic paresis and ataxia. *Annals of Neurology* **17:** 297–300.

Anderson JM & Hubbard BM (1985) Definition of Alzheimer's disease. *Lancet* **i:** 408.

Azzarelli B, Muller J, Ghetti B & Dyken M (1985) Cerebellar plaques in familial Alzheimer's disease (Gerstmann–Sträussler–Scheinker variant?). *Acta Neuropathologica* **65:** 235–246.

Ball MJ, Fisman M, Hachinski V et al (1985) A new definition of Alzheimer's disease: a hippocampal dementia. *Lancet* **i:** 14–16.

Braak H & Braak E (1987) Argyrophilic grains: characteristic pathology of cerebral cortex in cases of adult onset dementia without Alzheimer changes. *Neuroscience Letters* **76:** 124–127.

Braak H & Braak E (1989) Cortical and subcortical argyrophilic grains characterize a disease associated with adult onset dementia. *Neuropathology and Applied Neurobiology* **15:** 13–26.

Braak H & Braak E (1991) Neuropathological staging of Alzheimer-related changes. *Acta Neuropathologica* **82:** 239–259.

Brown P, Goldfarb LG & Gajdusek DC (1991) The new biology of spongiform encephalopathy: infectious amyloidoses with a genetic twist. *Lancet* **i:** 1019–1022.

Brown RG & Marsden CD (1984) How common is dementia in Parkinson's disease. *Lancet* **ii:** 1262–1265.

Brun A (1987) Frontal lobe degeneration of non-Alzheimer type. I. Neuropathology. *Archives of Gerontology and Geriatrics* **6:** 193–208.

Brun A & Gustafson L (1991) Psychopathology and frontal lobe involvement in organic dementia. In Iqbal K, McLachlan DRC, Winsblad B & Wisniewski HM (eds) *Alzheimer's Disease Basic Mechanisms, Diagnosis and Therapeutic Strategies*, pp 27–33. Chichester: Wiley.

Clark AW, Manz HJ, White CL et al (1986) Cortical degeneration with swollen chromatolytic neurons: its relationship to Pick's disease. *Journal of Neuropathology and Experimental Neurology* **45:** 268–284.

Collinge J, Owen F, Poulter M et al (1990) Prion dementia without characteristic pathology. *Lancet* ii: 7–9.

Connolly JH, Allen IV & Dermott E (1988) Transmissible agent in the amyotrophic form of Creutzfeldt–Jakob disease. *Journal of Neurology, Neurosurgery, and Psychiatry* 51: 1459–1460.

Constantinidis J, Richard J & Tissot R (1974) Pick's Disease. Histological and clinical correlations. *European Neurology* 11: 208–217.

Crystal H, Dickson D, Fuld P et al (1988) Clinico-pathologic studies in dementia: nondemented subjects with pathologically confirmed Alzheimer's disease. *Neurology* 38: 1682–1687.

Dickson DW, Yen S-H, Horoupian DS (1986a) Pick body-like inclusions in the dentate fascia of the hippocampus in Alzheimer's disease. *Acta Neuropathologica* 71: 38–45.

Dickson DW, Yen S-H, Suzuki KI et al (1986b) Ballooned neurones in select neuro-degenerative diseases contain phosphorylated neurofilament epitopes. *Acta Neuropathologica* 71: 216–223.

Dickson DW, Crystal H, Mattiace LA et al (1989) Diffuse Lewy body disease: light and electron microscopic immunocytochemistry of senile plaques. *Acta Neuropathologica* 78: 572–584.

Dickson DW, Ruan D, Crystal H et al (1991) Hippocampal degeneration differentiates diffuse Lewy body disease (DLBD) from Alzheimer's disease: light and electron microscopic immunocytochemistry of CA2–3 neurites specific to DLBD. *Neurology* 41: 1402–1409.

Ditter SM & Mirra SS (1987) Neuropathologic and clinical features of Parkinson's disease in Alzheimer's disease patients. *Neurology* 37: 754–760.

Duffy P, Mayeux R & Kupsky W (1988) Familial Alzheimer's disease with myoclonus and 'spongy change'. *Archives of Neurology* 45: 1097–1100.

Duyckaerts C, Delaère P, Hauw J-J et al (1990) Rating of the lesions in senile dementia of the Alzheimer type: concordance between laboratories. *Journal of the Neurological Sciences* 97: 295–323.

Englund E & Brun A (1987) Frontal lobe degeneration of non-Alzheimer type. IV. White matter changes. *Archives of Gerontology and Geriatrics* 6: 235–243.

Faden AI & Townsend JJ (1976) Myoclonus in Alzheimer's disease. A confusing sign. *Archives of Neurology* 33: 278–280.

Ferrer I, Roig C, Espino A, Peiro G & Guiu MX (1991) Dementia of frontal lobe type and motor neuron disease. A Golgi study of the frontal cortex. *Journal of Neurology, Neuro-surgery and Psychiatry* 54: 932–934.

Forno LS, Eng LF & Selkoe DJ (1989) Pick bodies in the locus ceruleus. *Acta Neuropathologica* 79: 10–17.

Galloway PG, Bergeron C & Perry G (1989) The presence of tau distinguishes Lewy bodies of diffuse Lewy body disease from those of idopathic Parkinson disease. *Neuroscience Letters* 100: 6–10.

Gibb WRG, Luthert PJ & Marsden CD (1989) Corticobasal degeneration. *Brain* 112: 1171–1192.

Goate A, Chartier-Harlin M-C, Mullan M et al (1991) Segregation of a missense mutation in the amyloid precursor protein gene with familial Alzheimer's disease. *Nature* 349: 704–706.

Graff-Radford NR, Damasio AR, Hyman BT et al (1990) Progressive aphasia in a patient with Pick's disease: a neuropsychological, radiologic, and anatomic study. *Neurology* 40: 620–625.

Green J, Morris JC, Sandson J, McKeel DW Jr & Miller JW (1990) Progressive aphasia a precursor of global dementia? *Neurology* 40: 423–429.

Groen JJ & Endtz LJ (1982) Hereditary Pick's disease. Second re-examination of a large family and discussion of other hereditary cases, with particular reference to electroencepha-lography and computerized tomography. *Brain* 105: 443–459.

Gustafson L, Brun A, Holmkvist AF & Risberg J (1985) Regional cerebral blood flow in degenerative frontal lobe dementia of non-Alzheimer type. *Journal of Cerebral Blood Flow and Metabolism* 5 (supplement 1): 141–142.

Hansen LA, Masliah E, Terry RD & Mirra SS (1989) A neuropathological subset of Alzheimer's disease with concomitant Lewy body disease and spongiform change. *Acta Neuropathologica* 78: 194–201.

Hansen L, Salmon D, Galasko D et al (1990) The Lewy body variant of Alzheimer's disease: a clinical and pathologic entity. *Neurology* 40: 1–8.

Hansen LA, Masliah E, Quijada-Fawcett S & Rexin D (1991) Entorhinal neurofibrillary tangles in Alzheimer disease with Lewy bodies. *Neuroscience Letters* **129:** 269–272.

Hirano A, Kurland LT, Krooth RS & Lessell S (1961a) Parkinsonism–dementia complex, an endemic disease on the island of Guam. *Brain* **84:** 642–661.

Hirano A, Malamud N & Kurland LT (1961b) Parkinsonism–dementia complex, an endemic disease on the island of Guam II. Pathological features. *Brain* **84:** 662–679.

Hirano A, Tuazon R & Zimmerman HM (1968) Neurofibrillary changes, granulovacuolar bodies and argentophilic globules observed in tuberous sclerosis. *Acta Neuropathologica* **11:** 257–261.

Horoupian DS & Dickson DW (1991) Striatonigral degeneration, olivopontocerebellar atrophy and 'atypical' Pick disease. *Acta Neuropathologica* **81:** 287–295.

Horoupian DS, Thal L, Katzman R et al (1984) Dementia and motor neuron disease: morphometric, biochemical, and Golgi studies. *Annals of Neurology* **16:** 305–313.

Hubbard BM, Fenton GW & Anderson JM (1990) A quantitative histological study of early clinical and preclinical Alzheimer's disease. *Neuropathology and Applied Neurobiology* **16:** 111–121.

Hullette CM & Crain BJ (1990) Fronto-temporal lobar atrophy without Pick's bodies or Pick's cells: a significant cause of Pick's syndrome. *Journal of Neuropathology and Experimental Neurology* **49:** 275.

Iseki E, Matsushita M, Kosaka K et al (1990) Morphological characteristics of senile plaques in familial Alzheimer's disease. *Acta Neuropathologica* **80:** 227–232.

Ishino H, Higashi S, Chuta M & Ohta H (1984) Juvenile Alzheimer's disease with myoclonus: amyloid plaques and grumose alteration in the cerebellum. *Clinical Neuropathology* **3:** 193–198.

Itagaki S, McGeer PL, Akiyama H et al (1989) A case of adult-onset dementia with argyrophilic grains. *Annals of Neurology* **26:** 685–689.

Jagust WJ, Davies P, Tiller-Borcich JK & Reed BR (1990) Focal Alzheimer's disease. *Neurology* **40:** 14–19.

Kamo H, Haebara H, Akiguchi I et al (1987) A distinctive distribution of reactive astroglia in the precentral cortex in amyotrophic lateral sclerosis. *Acta Neuropathologica* **74:** 33–38.

Kato S & Nakamura H (1990) Presence of two different fibril subtypes in the Pick body: an immunoelectron microscopic study. *Acta Neuropathologica* **81:** 125–129.

Katzman R, Terry R, DeTeresa R et al (1988) Clinical, pathological, and neurochemical changes in dementia: a subgroup with preserved mental status and numerous neocortical plaques. *Annals of Neurology* **23:** 138–144.

Khachaturian ZS (1985) Diagnosis of Alzheimer's disease. *Archives of Neurology* **42:** 1097–1104.

Kirshner HS, Tanridag O, Thurman L & Whetsell WO Jr (1987) Progressive aphasia without dementia: two cases with focal spongiform degeneration. *Annals of Neurology* **22:** 527–532.

Kiuchi A, Otsuka N, Namba Y, Nakano I & Tomonaga M (1991) Presenile appearance of abundant Alzheimer's neurofibrillary tangles without senile plaques in the brain in myotonic dystrophy. *Acta Neuropathologica* **82:** 1–5.

Knopman DS, Mastri AR, Frey WH, Sung JH & Rustan T (1990) Dementia lacking distinctive histologic features: a common non-Alzheimer degenerative dementia. *Neurology* **40:** 251–256.

Kosaka K, Yoshimura M, Ikeda K & Budka H (1984) Diffuse type of Lewy body disease: progressive dementia with abundant cortical Lewy bodies and senile changes of varying degree—a new disease? *Clinical Neuropathology* **3:** 185–192.

Kosaka K, Tsuchiya K & Yoshimura M (1988) Lewy body disease with and without dementia: a clinicopathological study of 35 cases. *Clinical Neuropathology* **7:** 299–305.

Kosaka K, Ikeda K, Kobayashi K & Mehraein P (1991) Striatopallidonigral degeneration in Pick's disease: a clinicopathological study of 41 cases. *Journal of Neurology* **238:** 151–160.

Kushner PD, Stephenson DT & Wright S (1991) Reactive astrogliosis is widespread in the subcortical white matter of amyotrophic lateral sclerosis brain. *Journal of Neuropathology and Experimental Neurology* **50:** 263–277.

Lampert PW, Earle KM, Gibbs CJ Jr & Gajdusek DC (1969) Experimental kuru encephalopathy in chimpanzees and spider monkeys. *Journal of Neuropathology and Experimental Neurology* **28:** 353–370.

Lanska DJ, Currier RD, Cohen M et al (1991) Familial progressive subcortical gliosis. *Journal of Neuropathology and Experimental Neurology* **50:** 305.

Lantos PL (1990) Ageing and dementias. In Weller RO (ed.) *Nervous System, Muscle and Eyes, Systemic Pathology*, 3rd edn, vol. 4, pp 360–396. Edinburgh: Churchill Livingstone.

Lantos PL (1992) From slow virus to prion: a review of transmissible spongiform encephalopathies. *Histopathology* **20:** 1–11.

Lantos PL, Luthert PJ, Hanger D et al (1992) Familial Alzheimer's disease with the amyloid precursor protein position 717 mutation and sporadic Alzheimer's disease have the same cytoskeletal pathology. *Neuroscience Letters* **137:** 221–224.

Leigh PN, Whitwell H, Garofalo O et al (1991) Ubiquitin-immunoreactive intraneuronal inclusions in amyotrophic lateral sclerosis. Morphology, distribution, and specificity. *Brain* **114:** 775–778.

Lennox G, Lowe J, Landon M et al (1989) Diffuse Lewy body disease: correlative neuropathology using anti-ubiquitin immunocytochemistry. *Journal of Neurology, Neurosurgery and Psychiatry* **52:** 1236–1247.

Lippa CF, Smith TW & Fontneau N (1990) Cortical degeneration with neuronal achromasia. A clinicopathologic study of two cases. *Journal of the Neurological Sciences* **98:** 301–310.

Lippa CF, Cohen R, Smith TW & Drachman DA (1991) Primary progressive aphasia with focal neuronal achromasia. *Neurology* **41:** 882–886.

Lowe J, Blanchard A, Morrell K et al (1988) Ubiquitin is a common factor in intermediate filament inclusion bodies of diverse type in man, including those of Parkinson's disease, Pick's disease, and Alzheimer's disease, as well as Rosenthal fibres in cerebellar astrocytomas, cytoplasmic bodies in muscle, and Mallory bodies in alcoholic liver disease. *Journal of Pathology* **155:** 9–15.

Lowe J, Aldridge F, Lennox G et al (1989) Inclusion bodies in motor cortex and brainstem of patients with motor neurone disease are detected by immunocytochemical localisation of ubiquitin. *Neuroscience Letters* **105:** 7–13.

Mann DMA & Jones D (1990) Deposition of amyloid (A4) protein within the brains of persons with dementing disorders other than Alzheimer's disease and Down's syndrome. *Neuroscience Letters* **109:** 68–75.

Martin JJ, Gheuens J, Bruyland M et al (1991) Early-onset Alzheimer's disease in 2 large Belgian families. *Neurology* **41:** 62–68.

Masliah E, Hansen LA, Quijada S et al (1991) Late onset dementia with argyrophilic grains and subcortical tangles or atypical progressive supranuclear palsy? *Annals of Neurology* **29:** 389–396.

Mattiace LA, Wu E, Aronson M & Dickson DW (1991) A new type of neuritic plaque without amyloid in corticonigral degeneration with neuronal achromasia. *Journal of Neuropathology and Experimental Neurology* **50:** 310.

Mayeux R, Stern Y & Spanton S (1985) Heterogeneity in dementia of the Alzheimer type: evidence of subgroups. *Neurology* **35:** 453–461.

Mesulam MM (1982) Slowly progressive aphasia without generalized dementia. *Annals of Neurology* **11:** 592–598.

Mirra SS, Heyman A, McKeel D et al (1991) The Consortium to Establish a Registry for Alzheimer's Disease (CERAD). Part II. Standardization of the neuropathologic assessment of Alzheimer's disease. *Neurology* **41:** 479–486.

Mitsuyama Y (1984) Presenile dementia with motor neuron disease in Japan: clinicopathological review of 26 cases. *Journal of Neurology, Neurosurgery and Psychiatry* **47:** 953–959.

Mizutani T, Amano N, Sasaki H et al (1990) Senile dementia of Alzheimer type characterized by laminar neuronal loss exclusively in the hippocampus, parahippocampus and medial occipitotemporal cortex. *Acta Neuropathologica* **80:** 575–580.

de la Monte SM, Wells SE, Hedley-Whyte T & Growdon JH (1989) Neuropathological distinction between Parkinson's dementia and Parkinson's plus Alzheimer's disease. *Annals of Neurology* **26:** 309–320.

Morita K, Kaiya H, Ikeda T & Namba M (1987) Presenile dementia combined with amyotrophy: a review of 34 Japanese cases. *Archives of Gerontology and Geriatrics* **6:** 263–277.

Morris JC, Cole M, Barber BO & Wright D (1984) Hereditary dysphasic dementia and the Pick–Alzheimer spectrum. *Annals of Neurology* **16:** 455–466.

Morris JC, Drazner M, Fulling K, Grant EA & Goldring J (1989) Clinical and pathological aspects of Parkinsonism in Alzheimer's disease. *Archives of Neurology* **46:** 651–657.

Morris JC, McKeel DW, Storandt M et al (1991) Very mild Alzheimer's disease: informant-based clinical, psychometric, and pathologic distinction from normal aging. *Neurology* **41:** 469–478.

Munoz-Garcia D & Ludwin SK (1984) Classic and generalized variants of Pick's disease: a clinicopathological, ultrastructural, and immunocytochemical comparative study. *Annals of Neurology* **16:** 467–480.

Neary D (1990) Non Alzheimer's disease forms of cerebral atrophy. *Journal of Neurology, Neurosurgery and Psychiatry* **53:** 929–931.

Neary D, Snowden JS, Bowen DM et al (1986) Neuropsychological syndromes in presenile dementia due to cerebral atrophy. *Journal of Neurology, Neurosurgery and Psychiatry* **49:** 163–174.

Neary D, Snowden JS, Northen B & Goulding P (1988) Dementia of frontal lobe type. *Journal of Neurology, Neurosurgery and Psychiatry* **51:** 353–361.

Neary D, Snowden JS, Mann DMA et al (1990) Frontal lobe dementia and motor neuron disease. *Journal of Neurology, Neurosurgery and Psychiatry* **53:** 23–32.

Nee LE, Polinsky RJ, Eldridge R et al (1983) A family with histologically confirmed Alzheimer's disease. *Archives of Neurology* **40:** 203–208.

Neumann MA & Cohn R (1967) Progressive subcortical gliosis, a rare form of presenile dementia. *Brain* **90:** 405–418.

Okamoto K, Hirai S, Yamazaki Y, Sun X & Nakazato Y (1991) New ubiquitin-positive intraneuronal inclusions in the extra-motor cortices in patients with amyotrophic lateral sclerosis. *Neuroscience Letters* **129:** 233–236.

Papp MI, Kahn JE & Lantos PL (1989) Glial cytoplasmic inclusions in the CNS of patients with multiple system atrophy (striatonigral degeneration, olivopontocerebellar atrophy and Shy–Drager syndrome). *Journal of Neurological Sciences* **94:** 79–100.

Paulus W & Jellinger K (1991) The neuropathologic basis of different clinical subgroups of Parkinson's disease. *Journal of Neuropathology and Experimental Neurology* **50:** 743–755.

Paulus W & Selim M (1990) Corticonigral degeneration with neuronal achromasia and basal neurofibrillary tangles. *Acta Neuropathologica* **81:** 89–94.

Perl DP, Steele JC, Loerzel A & Kurland LT (1991) Amyotrophic lateral sclerosis–Parkinsonism dementia complex of Guam as a model of Alzheimer's disease. In Iqbal K, McLachlin DRC, Winblad B & Wisniewski HM (eds) *Alzheimer's Disease: Basic Mechanisms, Diagnosis and Therapeutic Strategies*, pp 375–381. Chichester: Wiley.

Perry RH, Irving D, Blessed G, Perry EK & Fairbairn AF (1989) Clinically and neuropathologically distinct form of dementia in the elderly. *Lancet* **i:** 166.

Perry RH, Irving D, Blessed G et al (1990a) Senile dementia of Lewy body type. A clinically and neuropathologically distinct form of Lewy body dementia in the elderly. *Journal of the Neurological Sciences* **95:** 119–139.

Perry RH, Irving D & Tomlinson BE (1990b) Lewy body prevalence in the aging brain: relationship to neuropsychiatric disorders, Alzheimer-type pathology and catecholaminergic nuclei. *Journal of the Neurological Sciences* **100:** 223–233.

Poeck K & Luzzatti C (1988) Slowly progressive aphasia in three patients. The problem of accompanying neuropsychological deficit. *Brain* **111:** 151–168.

Pogacar S & Rubio A (1982) Morphological features of Pick's and atypical Alzheimer's disease in Down's syndrome. *Acta Neuropathologica* **58:** 249–254.

Powers JM, Liu Y, Hair LS et al (1991) Concomitant Creutzfeldt–Jakob and Alzheimer diseases. *Acta Neuropathologica* **83:** 95–98.

Pro JD, Sumi SM & Smith CH (1979) Amyloid plaques in the cerebellum in presenile familial Alzheimer's disease. *Neurology* **29:** 538–539.

Prusiner SB (1991) Molecular biology of prion diseases. *Science* **252:** 1515–1522.

Quon D, Wang Y, Catalano R, Marian Scardina J, Murakami K & Cordell B (1991) Formation of beta-amyloid protein deposits in brains of transgenic mice. *Nature* **352:** 239–241.

Rebeiz JJ, Kolodny EH & Richardson EP Jr (1968) Corticodentatonigral degeneration with neuronal achromasia. *Archives of Neurology* **18:** 20–33.

Riley DE, Lang AE, Lewis A et al (1990) Cortical-basal ganglionic degeneration. *Neurology* **40:** 1203–1212.

Rossor M (1991) Heterogeneity in Alzheimer's disease. In Ishii T, Allsop D & Selkoe DJ (eds) *Frontiers of Alzheimer Research*, pp 21–32. Amsterdam: Elsevier.

Rossor MN, Iversen LL, Reynolds GP, Mountjoy CQ & Roth M (1984) Neurochemical characteristics of early and late onset types of Alzheimer's disease. *British Medical Journal* **288:** 961–964.

Salazar AM, Masters CL, Gajdusek DC & Gibbs CJ Jr (1983) Syndromes of amyotrophic lateral sclerosis and dementia: relation to transmissible Creutzfeldt–Jakob disease. *Annals of Neurology* **14:** 17–26.

Sam M, Gutmann L, Schochet SS & Doshi H (1991) Pick's disease: a case clinically resembling amyotrophic lateral sclerosis. *Neurology* **41:** 1831–1833.

Sawle GV, Brooks DJ, Marsden CD & Frackowiak RSJ (1991) Corticobasal degeneration—a unique pattern of regional cortical oxygen hypometabolism and striatal fluorodopa uptake demonstrated by positron emission tomography. *Brain* **114:** 541–556.

Scully R (1985) Case records of the Massachusetts General Hospital (Case 38-1985). *New England Journal of Medicine* **313:** 739–748.

Smith DA & Lantos PL (1983) A case of combined Pick's disease and Alzheimer's disease. *Journal of Neurology, Neurosurgery and Psychiatry* **46:** 675–677.

Struble RG, Polinsky RG, Hedreen JC et al (1991) Hippocampal lesions in dominantly inherited Alzheimer's disease. *Journal of Neuropathology and Experimental Neurology* **50:** 82–94.

Tabaton M, Cammarata S, Mancardi G et al (1991) Ultrastructural localization of β-amyloid, τ, and ubiquitin epitopes in extracellular neurofibrillary tangles. *Proceedings of the National Academy of Sciences of the USA* **88:** 2098–2102.

Terry RD, Hansen LA, DeTeresa R et al (1987) Senile dementia of the Alzheimer type without neocortical neurofibrillary tangles. *Journal of Neuropathology and Experimental Neurology* **46:** 262–268.

Tierney MC, Fisher RH, Lewis AJ et al (1988) The NINCDS–ADRDA Work Group criteria for the clinical diagnosis of probable Alzheimer's disease: a clinicopathologic study of 57 cases. *Neurology* **38:** 359–364.

Tomlinson BE & Corsellis JAN (1984) Ageing and dementias. In Hume Adams J, Corsellis JAN & Duchen LW (eds) *Greenfield's Neuropathology*, 4th edn, pp 951–1025. London: Edward Arnold.

Tomlinson BE, Blessed G & Roth M (1970) Observation on the brain of demented old people. *Journal of the Neurological Sciences* **11:** 205–242.

Uchihara T, Tsuchiya K & Kosaka K (1990) Selective loss of nigral neurons in Pick's disease: a morphometric study. *Acta Neuropathologica* **81:** 155–161.

Ulrich J, Haugh M, Anderton BH et al (1987) Alzheimer dementia and Pick's disease: neurofibrillary tangles and Pick bodies are associated with identical phosphorylated neurofilament epitopes. *Acta Neuropathologica* **73:** 240–246.

Wechsler AF (1977) Presenile dementia presenting as aphasia. *Journal of Neurology, Neurosurgery and Psychiatry* **40:** 303–305.

Wechsler AF, Verify MA, Rosenschein S, Fried I & Scheibel AB (1982) Pick's disease. A clinical, computed tomographic, and histologic study with Golgi impregnation observations. *Archives of Neurology* **39:** 287–290.

Wightman G, Anderson VER, Martin J et al (1992) Hippocampal and neocortical ubiquitin immunoreactive inclusions in amyotrophic lateral sclerosis with dementia. *Neuroscience Letters* **139:** 269–274.

Wilcock GK, Hope RA, Brooks DN et al (1989) Recommended minimum data to be collected in research studies on Alzheimer's disease. *Journal of Neurology, Neurosurgery and Psychiatry* **52:** 693–700.

Will RG (1991) The spongiform encephalopathies. *Journal of Neurology, Neurosurgery and Psychiatry* **54:** 761–763.

Wisniewski HM, Rabe A, Zigman W & Silverman W (1989) Neuropathological diagnosis of Alzheimer disease. *Journal of Neuropathology and Experimental Neurology* **48:** 606–609.

Yoshimura N (1983) Cortical changes in the parkinsonian brain: a contribution to the delineation of 'diffuse Lewy body disease'. *Journal of Neurology* **229:** 17–32.

Yoshimura N (1988) Olfactory bulb involvement in Pick's disease. *Acta Neuropathologica* **77:** 202–205.

Yoshimura N (1989) Topography of Pick body distribution in Pick's disease: a contribution to understanding the relationship between Pick's and Alzheimer's diseases. *Clinical Neuropathology* **8:** 1–6.

3

Familial Alzheimer's disease

M. N. ROSSOR

Controversy about the precise nosological status has surrounded Alzheimer's disease since its first description in 1907 (Alzheimer, 1911). Initially there was concern about the relationship between presenile dementia and later onset cases which showed overlap with apparent normal old age. The clinicopathological studies of the 1960s (Blessed et al, 1968), however, established the qualitative identity between Alzheimer's disease and senile dementia of the Alzheimer type, and in the last decade the term 'Alzheimer's disease' has been used regardless of age. However, recent detailed clinical and neuropathological studies of Alzheimer's disease have drawn attention to the many different features that might serve to identify subgroups. Thus the original attempt to distinguish between presenile Alzheimer's disease and a late onset senile dementia has recently redirected attention to differences dependent upon age of onset. These can be observed at the clinical, histopathological and neurochemical level (Chui et al, 1985; Mayeux et al, 1985; Rossor, 1991), although these may only show an association with age without necessarily implying biological subtypes. A group of patients have prominent extrapyramidal features, some of whom may be found to have diffuse Lewy bodies in the cerebral cortex and basal ganglia, the Lewy body variant of Alzheimer's disease (Hansen et al, 1990). Other patients may be identified by a striking focal onset with dysphasia, Balint's syndrome or cortical sensory loss with hemiparesis. One of the earliest subdivisions of Alzheimer's disease, however, was the recognition that it may be an autosomal dominant familial disease. Early reports of probable Alzheimer's disease with a familial component included those of Lua (1920), Meggendorfer (1925), Flugel (1929), Schottky (1932) and Scheele (1933). It was, however, the study of Lowenberg and Waggoner (1934) that reported in detail a clearly autosomal dominant pedigree with histologically proven Alzheimer's disease. They also drew attention to a number of the features that are common to subsequent publications, including the early age of onset and prominent myoclonus and seizures. Since then many extensive pedigrees have been published, all of which show autosomal dominant inheritance (Nee et al, 1983; Martin et al, 1991). Initially, familial Alzheimer's disease (FAD) was thought to be rare, but epidemiological surveys have suggested that it constitutes a major component of Alzheimer's disease and indeed some authors consider that all are familial. Estimates vary (see below) but clearly there is a significant

Baillière's Clinical Neurology—
Vol. 1, No. 3, November 1992
ISBN 0–7020–1631–4

genetic factor in the development of Alzheimer's disease. This applies not only to young onset cases, which have formed the majority of published FAD pedigrees, but also to the late onset cases. It is now clear that FAD is itself heterogeneous, with more than one chromosomal locus. The discovery of mutations in the amyloid precursor protein (APP) gene has paved the way for detailed analysis of FAD. Although APP mutation families are very rare (only ten published pedigrees to date), the screening of specific genetic markers will bring a precision to epidemiological surveys. It also establishes the biological heterogeneity of Alzheimer's disease, which is likely to apply to sporadic as well as familial cases. Indeed the presence of Alzheimer-type histopathological changes in normal old age would argue that the entity referred to as Alzheimer's disease represents a final common pathway of a variety of neuronal insults.

EPIDEMIOLOGY

Many pedigrees with multiple members affected by Alzheimer's disease have now been reported in the literature and a substantial number of publications confirm the familial clustering of Alzheimer's disease (Sjogren, 1952; Larsson et al, 1963; Akesson, 1969; Heston et al, 1981; Whalley et al, 1982; Heyman et al, 1984; reviewed by Li et al, 1991). What, however, is the proportion of cases of Alzheimer's disease which are familial? Epidemiological studies indicate that the majority are of late onset and sporadic (Rocca et al, 1990; Fratiglioni et al, 1991). Moreover there is a major problem with such studies which imply a genetic basis on the prevalence of the family history amongst probands. Sampling bias is important and in one study a similar prevalence of family history was found amongst relatives of patients with Parkinson's disease as with Alzheimer's disease (Mayeux et al, 1991). Estimates of the prevalence of FAD have ranged from 5% to as high as 100% (Breitner et al, 1988a,b), with the majority suggesting a prevalence in the order of 15–25%. A number of approaches have been utilized.

Case control studies

There have been only a few detailed case control studies to investigate a family history as a risk factor. In the study of Heyman et al (1984), which looked at cases with onset below the age of 70 years, 55% had a family history. In the careful case control study of Amaducci et al (1986), in which two control cases were matched, family history was a major risk factor for the younger onset cases. By contrast in the study of Chandra et al (1987) there was no significant family history, but these were of late onset. Clearly, however, selection biases are an ever present danger with a tendency to study extended families and to overdiagnose amongst family members if one has been affected (Chandra and Schoenberg, 1989; Mayeux et al, 1991). The majority of the many published case control studies have confirmed the increased prevalence of a family history (Shalat et al, 1987; Hofman et al, 1989; Broe et al, 1990; Van Duijn et al, 1991).

Lifetime risk studies

In the population surveys the lifetime risk of developing Alzheimer's disease in first-degree relatives of those affected has been studied. If the disease is genetic and behaves as an autosomal dominant then it is anticipated that the lifetime risk would approach 50%. Many authors have found lifetime risks of less than 25% (Larsson et al, 1963; Heston et al, 1981; Sadovnick et al, 1989), although in some studies there was no obvious increased risk (Chandra et al, 1987). However since Alzheimer's disease is predominantly a disease of late life, more recent studies have adjusted for early death amongst family members using Caplan–Meier life table methods and making allowance for those patients who were too young to have developed the disease. Some of the problems in modelling have been discussed by Tzourio et al (1991). A number of studies using these methods have indicated a cumulative risk for Alzheimer's disease of nearly 50% by the age of 90 years, suggesting a strong genetic component (Breitner and Folstein, 1984; Breitner et al, 1986a,b, 1988a; Mohs et al, 1987; Huff et al, 1988). This compares with a cumulative risk of 10% for Alzheimer's disease in first-degree relatives of controls. Indeed from the known incidence rate in the Rochester community study it can be predicted that 16% of any control population would have a family history for dementia (Chandra and Schoenberg, 1989).

Twin studies

The comparison of concordance rates for Alzheimer's disease in mono-zygotic compared with dizygotic twin pairs can provide information on relative genetic and environmental factors. There have been a number of case studies of both concordant and discordant monozygotic and dizygotic twin pairs for Alzheimer's disease (Davidson and Robertson, 1955; Hunter et al, 1972; Cook et al, 1981; Embry and Lippman, 1985). Nee et al (1987) recently reviewed 22 twin pairs, of which 17 were monozygotic. They found similar concordance rates between monozygotic (41%) and dizygotic (40%) twins. This would argue for major environmental factors in the development of the disease. However, this was clearly a biased sample as dizygotic twins are far more prevalent than monozygotic twins in the general population, suggesting an ascertainment bias. Moreover in some instances there is a very long gap between the age of onset in concordant twin pairs, as long as 10 years in some pairs (Nee et al, 1987), which makes interpretation difficult. This can be contrasted with other diseases, such as Huntington's disease in which ages of onset are very similar and monozygotic twins are concordant (Sudarsky et al, 1983). The ideal study here is that of neuropathologically supported studies of twin pairs in a randomly sampled population; an ideal which has yet to be met. The wide difference in age of onset of Alzheimer's disease in monozygotic twins argues for important environmental factors causing either sporadic disease, or as a major epigenetic influence on age of onset. A recent review of twin studies (Breitner et al, 1990) draws attention to the variety of drawbacks of ascertainment bias, difficulties of diagnosis and lack of neuropathological confirmation. The ideal to assess the prevalence and importance of genetic factors would be the identification of linked markers or specific genetic defects and assessment of their prevalence in the general population.

MOLECULAR GENETICS

Chromosome 21 linkage and the APP gene

Trisomy 21 Down's syndrome has provided an important model for Alzheimer's disease. The association of Alzheimer's disease histopathology with Down's syndrome has been recognized for many decades (Ropper and Williams, 1980) and it is now generally accepted that Down's individuals will develop Alzheimer histopathology in their forties and fifties, usually with a superadded loss of cognitive function (Oliver and Holland, 1986). The development of Alzheimer-type histopathology starts early with the deposition of preamyloid diffuse plaques as early as the second decade (Mann et al, 1990). In view of this association between trisomy 21 Down's syndrome and senile plaques and neurofibrillary tangles, it was logical to focus early linkage studies on chromosome 21 markers. In 1987, St George-Hyslop and colleagues reported linkage of anonymous markers on chromosome 21 to Alzheimer's disease in four kindreds (St George-Hyslop et al, 1987). The markers used were D21S1/S11 and D21S16, both markers on the proximal portion of the long arm of chromosome 21 near to the obligate Down's syndrome region. One of the four kindreds studied was the large family reported by Nee et al (1987) and the German pedigree published by Frommelt et al (1991). Shortly after the publication of chromosome 21 linkage a series of papers were published which detailed the cloning of the amyloid precursor protein (APP) gene and which represented the culmination of a line of research into the origin of βA4 amyloid in Alzheimer's disease (Goldgaber et al, 1987; Kang et al, 1987; Tanzi et al, 1987).

βA4 amyloid is a central component of senile plaques where it is seen in a fibrillary form and confers Congo red staining and birefringence on histological sections. There were initial problems with isolation due to the insolubility of the protein, but it was subsequently shown to be a 39–42 amino acid protein consisting predominantly of a β-pleated structure. The amyloid in senile plaques and the amyloid deposited in cerebral vessels were shown to be identical (Glenner and Wong, 1984). Once the amino acid sequence had been established it was possible to clone the gene, which was found to encode for a much larger molecule, the amyloid precursor protein. This molecule is synthesized in three major forms, with 695, 751 or 770 amino acid residues, depending upon whether a Kunitz protease inhibitor domain is included; these forms result from alternative splicing of the mRNA (for review see Yankner and Mesulam, 1991). The APP molecule spans the membrane (Kang et al, 1987) and the extracellular component is identical to the protease inhibitor, protease nexin-II (Oltersdorf et al, 1989). The normal processing of APP releases nexin-II by cleavage adjacent to the cell surface (Sisodia et al, 1990). The β-amyloid sequence lies within the APP molecule and straddles part of the membrane and extracellular component. This processing would cleave within the β-amyloid molecule, implying that alternative processing must occur to generate the βA4 amyloid deposition in Alzheimer's disease. Recently, an alternative lysosomal–endosomal pathway has been described which can generate βA4 amyloid moieties (Haas et al, 1992). The APP molecule is transported down the axon by fast axonal transport to be incorporated within the membrane, with substantial amounts found in relation to synapses. Although the precise physiological function of APP is not known, it is a widely conserved molecule throughout evolution and expressed in many tissues throughout the body; it is not confined to the brain, although the predominant form expressed within the brain lacks the Kunitz protease inhibitor insert.

Considerable interest in the role of APP in Alzheimer's disease was generated when the gene was located to the long arm of chromosome 21 near to the putative FAD locus (Goldgaber et al, 1987; Tanzi et al, 1987). APP thus became a strong candidate gene for FAD and some early evidence was presented to suggest that in some cases of Alzheimer's disease there was an extra copy of the APP gene (Goldgaber et al, 1987). However, in some families of early onset FAD, the APP gene was excluded as the disease locus by obligate crossovers (Van Broeckhoven et al, 1989). Moreover chromosome 21 linkage had not been demonstrated in some, predominantly late onset, families (Schellenberg et al, 1988). A large international collaboration pooled the linkage data from a number of centres and demonstrated that FAD was genetically heterogeneous, with the chromosome 21 linkage confined to the young onset group (St George-Hyslop et al, 1990). The early linkage studies had relied on combining FAD pedigrees and studying linkage as a group. Clearly if the disease is genetically heterogeneous then such linkage studies are severely limited as one might be pooling diseases with quite distinct genetic and chromosomal loci. Linkage studies, however, could still be performed on individual families if the pedigree were large enough and sufficiently informative, since the disease could be assumed to

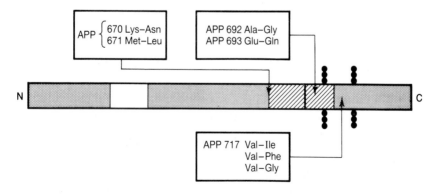

Figure 1. APP mutations in familial dementia.

be genetically homogeneous in that family. One such family, out of some 200 studied by the Alzheimer's Disease Research Group at St Mary's Hospital, London, was sufficiently informative to demonstrate chromosome 21 linkage. More importantly, the APP gene could not be excluded. Direct sequencing was therefore performed of exons 16 and 17 which encode the βA4 amyloid sequence. A cytosine to thymine transition at position 2149 was demonstrated which resulted in a *Bcl*I novel restriction endonuclease site that could be used to show that the mutation segregated with the disease in this family (Goate et al, 1991). Screening DNA from available families revealed an identical mutation in a single US pedigree. The mutation results in a valine to isoleucine substitution at APP 717 (APP 770 transcript) which lies just outside the C-terminus of the βA4 domain within the membrane spanning region. Since then a large number of familial and sporadic cases have been screened and no mutations have been found in sporadic Alzheimer cases, nor in late onset familial cases (Crawford et al, 1991). However, in younger onset cases one further UK family has been discovered; four Japanese families; and recently a large Canadian pedigree described in detail previously by Karlinsky et al (1991) has also been shown to have an identical mutation (Hardy et al, 1991; Karlinsky et al, 1992).

Since the original discovery of the valine to isoleucine mutation, two further mutations have been reported at APP 717. A valine to phenylalanine substitution has been reported in a single kindred from the US (Murrell et al, 1991), and a valine to glycine mutation in a UK family (Chartier-Harlin et al, 1991). At the time of writing only single families with these latter two mutations have been reported. Recently, a double mutation at APP 670/671 (APP 670 lysine ⇒ asparagine/671 methionine ⇒ leucine) has been reported in a clinically diagnosed Swedish FAD pedigree (Mullan et al, 1992). This double mutation lies at the N terminus of the βA4 amyloid domain.

Another mutation in the APP gene had been described in 1990 in patients with hereditary cerebral haemorrhage with amyloidosis of the Dutch type (HCHWA-D). This mutation lies within the βA4 domain at APP 693 and results in a glutamate to glutamine substitution (Levy et al, 1990). In this disease amyloid is deposited in blood vessels, leading to cortical haemorrhages which occur in the fourth and fifth decade. Diffuse amyloid plaques are seen, but not neuritic plaques or neurofibrillary tangles. There is some evidence that these patients develop a superadded dementia (Haan et al, 1990). An adjacent mutation APP 692 alanine ⇒ glycine has been reported in a single family associated with both cerebral haemorrhage and Alzheimer histopathology (Hendriks et al, 1992).

It is not known how these APP mutations lead to Alzheimer's disease. There is no obvious change in the constitutive processing introduced by the mutation of valine to isoleucine (Maruyama et al, 1991), and any changes are likely to be subtle. This is perhaps not surprising since the disease takes some 40 years before it expresses itself. There is also no obvious change in mRNA expression (Harrison et al, 1991). However, these mutations do establish APP mismetabolism as a central mechanism in these families. There are, naturally, many unanswered questions, such as how β-amyloid deposition progresses to the development of neuritic plaques and how the characteristic distribution within the brain occurs. It is not clear why APP 693 glutamate to glutamine should result in cerebral vascular amyloid with diffuse plaques and that APP 717 mutations result in the development of neuritic plaques. It is assumed that the development of neurofibrillary tangles are a secondary phenomenon and there is evidence that these tend to form in the cell bodies of neurones whose processes are involved in senile plaque formation (Hardy and Allsop, 1991). It is also not clear how the β-amyloid deposition leads to cell death, although there is evidence for amyloid neurotoxicity (reviewed by Yankner and Mesulam, 1991). Transgenic mice with the established mutations are being developed, but results are not yet available. Transgenic mice with overexpression of the APP gene do develop amyloid deposition, but as yet without proven neuritic plaques or neurofibrillary tangles (Quon et al, 1991).

Non-chromosome 21-linked FAD

All of the reported APP mutation families have their onset in the forties and early fifties, although it is very unlikely that all young onset FAD pedigrees will have APP mutations. It is also unclear as to whether APP mutations will account for all of the chromosome 21-linked families. Chromosome 21 linkage has been excluded in a number of families, predominantly of late onset (Shellenberg et al, 1988) and those with Volga German ancestry (Bird et al, 1988). Moreover there is some evidence for chromosome 19 linkage in some of the late onset families (Pericak-Vance et al, 1991). A number of candidate genes are being investigated, such as the microtubule-associated protein tau, but as yet there is no other evidence for linkage and no other demonstrated mutations that clearly segregate with the disease. Since it has been established that FAD is genetically heterogeneous, it is not possible to predict how many potential genetic sites, nor indeed how many examples of allelic heterogeneity may be demonstrated. It is probable, but not established, that such heterogeneity underpins the phenotypic heterogeneity that can be observed in FAD.

CLINICAL FEATURES

The clinical details of many pedigrees with FAD have been published (for reviews see St George-Hyslop, 1989; Frommelt et al, 1991; Martin et al, 1991; Rossor et al, 1992). From the available published reports FAD always appears to behave as an autosomal dominant disease, with males and females equally affected and many examples of male to male transmission. In the younger onset families, which constitute the majority of reported pedigrees, there are few indications of non-penetrance, with some possible exceptions (Bird et al, 1988; Fitch et al, 1988), although in the pedigree reported by Patel (1989) no histology was published to confirm the diagnosis. There is also evidence of anticipation of the age of onset in subsequent generations (Nee et al, 1983) which may in part be due to increased awareness amongst the family members.

Various clinical features have been sought which might serve to distinguish the FAD group from sporadic Alzheimer's disease. In general, FAD cases are younger at onset (Heston et al, 1981; Folstein et al, 1983; Huff et al, 1988), however this has not been confirmed in other series (Chui et al, 1985) and may represent censoring of pedigrees by other diseases in the late onset families. Indeed, the age specific incidence in community studies is not bimodal and so clearly there has to be overlap of FAD and sporadic disease with respect to the age at onset (Rocca et al, 1986; Fratiglioni et al, 1991). Aphasia and agraphia have been claimed to identify FAD cases (Folstein and Breitner, 1981), but this has not generally been confirmed (Chui et al, 1985; Cummings et al, 1985). Myoclonus appears to be common amongst familial Alzheimer's disease cases (Risse et al, 1990; Rainero et al, 1992), but this is not specific since it also occurs in sporadic cases. Neuroimaging shows no obvious difference and cases undergoing positron emission tomography (PET) scanning (Polinsky, 1987; Sadovnick et al, 1988; Frommelt et al, 1991) have shown the posterior biparietal-bitemporal hypometabolism that is characteristic of sporadic Alzheimer's disease. A number of epidemiological studies have observed an increased prevalence of thyroid disease (Heyman et al, 1984) and this may be associated with FAD pedigrees, but does not strictly segregate with the disease (Ewins et al, 1991). Zubenko et al (1988) have reported increased platelet membrane fluidity in families with Alzheimer's disease.

Although no features overall serve to distinguish FAD from sporadic cases, it is now clear from the molecular genetic data that this is a heterogeneous disease; the heterogeneity is both genetic, i.e. different loci, and allelic, i.e. different mutations at a single locus. Van Bogaert (1940) first drew attention to the variable clinical pattern that may be observed amongst FAD pedigrees and suggested a classification based on the presence of pyramidal, cerebellopyramidal, cerebellar and extrapyramidal features in addition to the cognitive impairment. Not all of the families reported at that time had neuropathological confirmation, and pyramidal signs, although observed in some families with senile plaques and neurofibrillary tangles (Heston et al, 1966), are atypical. Bird et al (1989) published clinical details on 24 kindreds and presented evidence for clinical and neuropathological variability with groups identified by early or late onset, cultural isolates such as the Volga Germans, those with associated white matter changes, those with tangles and no plaques and a small group with anterior horn cell disease.

A number of extensive pedigrees have been published (Heston et al, 1966; Nee et al, 1983; Foncin et al, 1985; Frommelt et al, 1991; Martin et al, 1991) and some of these have clinical features which set them apart from the common presentation of memory impairment progressing to more generalized cognitive deficits (St George-Hyslop, 1989; Kennedy et al, 1992; Rossor et al, 1992). Some develop myoclonus and early seizures (Lowenberg and Waggoner, 1934; McMenemey et al, 1939; Feldman et al, 1963; Landy and Bain, 1970; Kennedy et al, 1992). In some families myoclonus is very prominent and has been related to spongiform change (Duffy, 1988); it is of interest that myoclonus may also be observed in trisomy 21 Down's syndrome patients (Blumbergs et al, 1981). Some kindreds have displayed prominent extrapyramidal features (Feldman et al, 1963; Frommelt et al, 1991; Goudsmit et al, 1981; Foncin et al, 1985; Fukutani et al, 1989), often late in the course of the disease and in some instances associated with extensive subcortical pathology with neurofibrillary tangles in the basal ganglia (Feldman et al, 1963) or with cortical Lewy body disease (Lantos et al, 1992). Other kindreds have had prominent psychiatric disturbances with aggressiveness, psychosis and depression (Feldman et al, 1963; Foncin et al, 1985; Bird et al, 1989). Pyramidal features are rare, although motor disturbances may occur with dyspraxia. The family reported by Heston et al (1966) and Landry had pyramidal signs, although it is of note that extensor plantar responses are rarely reported. There is one case reported by Fukutani et al (1989) in which choreatic movements were observed. In general, however, pyramidal dysfunction and involuntary movements appear to be rare and there may be overlap with other atypical familial dementias, such as that described by Sumi et al (1992) in which tangles only were observed.

One feature commented on by many authors is the variable age at onset and this was used by Bird et al (1989) to distinguish subgroups of FAD. Many authors have also commented on the similar age of onset within families (Sinex and Myers, 1982; Folstein et al, 1983) and the greater variance of age at onset between, than within, families has been proposed as evidence for allelic heterogeneity (Van Duijn et al, 1991). However, some families demonstrate quite a large range in the age of onset, arguing for important epigenetic influences (Kennedy et al, 1992). It is possible that the genetic heterogeneity will be reflected in the different clinical patterns and there is now an opportunity to explore the range of features seen with the different APP mutations.

APP 717 valine-isoleucine

This is the first APP mutation which was described in one UK and one US family (Goate et al, 1991). Since then it has been reported in three Japanese families (Hardy et al, 1991; Naruse et al, 1991), a further UK family (M. N. Rossor, unpublished data) and in the Canadian family of Irish ancestry originally reported by Karlinsky et al, 1991, 1992). With this mutation the age of onset within families is broadly similar, being 54.9 years for the original UK family F23, 49.4 years for the US family F372, a mean of 51.5 years for the three Japanese families and 47.6 years for the Canadian family. The rate of progression is somewhat more variable. Difficulties in interpretation of familial and sporadic disease is exemplified by the US family, in which there was a phenocopy with onset of cognitive impairment at the age of 60 years but with no mutation present (Mullan et al, personal communication). Dyscalculia is an early feature, noted in the UK family and in the Canadian family (Karlinsky et al, 1991). Another point of interest is the early non-cognitive symptoms such as vertigo, apathy and change of personality reported before cognitive decline in a number of the families. Late features include gait disturbance, rigidity and seizures and the motor features in one case were associated with coexistent Lewy bodies in the cerebral cortex (Lantos et al, 1992).

APP 717 valine-phenylalanine

To date there has only been a single Indiana family described with this mutation (Murrell et al, 1991). The mean age of onset is 43 years, with a duration of approximately 7 years and mean age at death of 50 years. The common mode of presentation is with memory disturbance (Ghetti et al, 1992; Farlow et al, 1992).

APP 717 valine-glycine

As with APP 717 valine-phenylalanine, there is only a single family described, in this instance from England (Chartier-Harlin et al, 1991). The mean age of onset is 52 years, with a wider range from 40 years to the late fifties (Kennedy et al, 1992). As with the other families with APP 717 mutations, the early presentation is with memory impairment and in this family myoclonus, seizures and depression are common accompanying features. One patient underwent neuroimaging which included PET and this showed the characteristic pattern of posterior biparietal bitemporal hypometabolism.

APP 693 glutamate-glutamine

Although this mutation does not result in Alzheimer histopathology, but rather is associated with HCHWA-D, it does represent an example of allelic heterogeneity at the APP locus. The mutation lies outside the membrane but within the βA4-amyloid domain (Levy et al, 1990). Patients with HCHWA-D develop a severe cerebral amyloid angiopathy (see below) which leads to cortical haemorrhages, usually in their forties. Approximately half die from their first bleed and the remainder suffer from recurrent haemorrhage (Wattendorf et al, 1982). In addition to evidence of cortical haemorrhage, magnetic resonance imaging (MRI) may reveal subcortical white matter changes which probably reflect the angiopathy. Moreover patients may develop cognitive impairment over and above the neuropsychological deficits which might arise directly from the cortical haemorrhages (Haan et al, 1990a).

NEUROPATHOLOGY

Some of the reported cases of familial Alzheimer's disease have not included neuropathology, but in the majority that have, all show neocortical senile plaques and neurofibrillary tangles. In those reports in which amyloid angiopathy has been commented upon, its severity and distribution is variable, although many of the earlier studies, which were less extensive, lacked immunohistochemistry and relied on Congo red staining. Some marked variations in neuropathology have been reported within families, for example, in the publications of Grünthal and Wenger (1939, 1940), in which a brother and sister are reported; the brother had abundant senile plaques and neurofibrillary tangles, but the sister, who developed identical clinical features, had none of these. However, without specific genetic markers one cannot exclude clinical phenocopies arising independently.

As with clinical features there have been many attempts to identify histological features in the FAD group which would distinguish them from the sporadic cases. Cerebellar deposits of amyloid in FAD have been commented on by a number of authors (Pro et al, 1979), and Mackenzie et al (1991) found that all of their cases of FAD had cerebellar deposits, but only 50% of sporadic cases. However, this is not specific since in the family described by Frommelt et al (1991) cerebellar deposits were found in a number of individuals, but by no means all. Struble et al (1991) analysed the hippocampal histological features in three of the FAD families of the original chromosome 21 study (St George-Hyslop et al, 1987), namely FAD 1, 2 and 4. All demonstrated amyloid angiopathy, but there were some differences between families; thus in FAD 1 there were very few plaques with neuritic cores compared with the others. However, as with the clinical heterogeneity, differences are difficult to assess in the absence of specific genetic markers. A brief description of the published neuropathology associated with the known mutations is given below.

APP 717 valine-isoleucine

Numerous senile plaques and neurofibrillary tangles with modest amyloid angiopathy were found in both the US and Japanese families. In the Canadian family plaques and tangles and mild angiopathy were reported (Karlinsky et al, 1991). The single autopsied case of the F23 UK family had cortical Lewy bodies (Lantos et al, 1992), which raises interesting questions of whether this represents a concomitant environmental factor, or whether amyloid mismetabolism can lead directly to Lewy body formation. In the single UK case phosphorylated tau was identical to that found in sporadic cases (Lantos et al, 1992).

APP 717 valine-phenylalanine

Senile plaques, neurofibrillary tangles and mild angiopathy were reported in this case and plaques with large amyloid cores were prominent in the hippocampus (Ghetti et al, 1992). This plaque formation is similar to the report of Struble et al (1991).

APP 717 valine-glycine

There is one neuropathological report from this single UK pedigree (Mann et al, 1992). The report concerns a 61-year-old woman; typical changes of senile plaques and neurofibrillary tangles were found, with additional widespread diffuse βA4-amyloid deposits. Immunostaining with anti-PHF (paired helical filament), anti-tau and anti-ubiquitin demonstrated wide-spread tangles and neuritic plaque formation. Anti-βA4 immunostaining revealed severe congophilic angiopathy within meningeal vessels overlying cerebellar and occipital cortices, although this was less severe than in other brain regions. There were no neuronal inclusions other than neurofibrillary tangles.

APP 693 glutamate-glutamine

The neuropathological features of HCHWA-D are characterized by a severe amyloid angiopathy affecting the small and medium-sized vessels of both the cerebral cortex and the leptomeninges. By contrast to Alzheimer's disease there is an absence of cytoskeletal pathology, with no neurofibrillary tangles and no Alz 50 staining of dystrophic neurites. Specific immuno-staining reveals parenchymal preamyloid deposits and, less frequently, amyloid deposits which are fibrillary in nature. Staining with anti-alpha1-antichymotrypsin also stains the senile plaques as it does with Alzheimer's disease (Timmers et al, 1990).

CONCLUSION

At the present time it appears that APP mutations in familial Alzheimer's disease are rare, but FAD in general may be relatively common and the prevalence studies indicate a major genetic factor. It is of interest that Alzheimer's disease shares, with the majority of diseases discussed in this volume (frontal lobe degeneration, Pick's disease, Lewy body dementia and prion disease), a combination of familial and sporadic cases. This may reflect a relatively limited repertoire of neuronal response to injury, with each nosological entity reflecting a final common pathway of response to a variety of pathological processes. The discovery of APP mutations offers a powerful approach to understanding these neurodegenerative diseases. Although very rare, with only ten families reported to date with APP 717 mutations, it has given a major impetus to the search for animal models of Alzheimer's disease. The results from transgenic mice with APP 717 mutations are not yet known, but mice with overexpression of the APP gene (Quon et al, 1991) do show amyloid deposits, although as yet no cases of confirmed senile plaques or neurofibrillary tangles have been published.

It is tempting to speculate that other mutations causing FAD will be found in genes which encode for components of APP metabolic pathways, for example, the putative APP secretase enzyme. Alternatively there might be mutations in genes involved in alternative pathology, such as the phos-phorylation of tau with secondary amyloidogenesis. As the range of genetic markers becomes established, this will serve to underpin the epidemiology and will be particularly powerful in the analysis of the difficult group of late onset disease. This review has concentrated on the younger onset families which have provided the majority of data, but as the study by Farrer et al

(1990) indicates, there is a significant genetic component to the risk of late onset disease.

Within the area of inherited neurological disease, it is frequent to find considerable variability in the clinical expression of identical mutations within a family. Clearly, however, the precise mutation can have a profound influence, as evidenced by HCHWA-D, where a small shift in the site of mutation leads to deposition of amyloid in vessels in such a way as to lead to cortical haemorrhage, a feature not generally seen with Alzheimer's disease despite the angiopathy. Moreover the parenchymal deposits do not have a neuritic component, and the phenotypic expression of mutations other than APP 717 are awaited with interest. If the precise site of mutation can determine the neuropathology and clinical features in this way, then careful longitudinal studies of FAD patients, including those at risk, provide an opportunity to determine the epigenetic factors which will influence disease expression.

It is clear from the example of HCHWA-D that simple amyloid deposition is insufficient to produce the full pattern of Alzheimer's disease, and yet APP mismetabolism triggered by APP 717 mutations is sufficient to trigger the full cascade of cytoskeletal pathology, and in one instance (Lantos et al, 1992) this was accompanied by cortical Lewy body formation. This has major implications for treatment strategies regardless of the primacy of amyloid deposition. Drugs which may interact with amyloid and prevent fibril formation and subsequent cytoskeletal pathology, or which might interact with the enzymes involved in APP metabolism, such as the putative APP secretase, offer obvious strategies. Thus although APP mutation FAD is rare, and as such justifies inclusion in a volume on Unusual Dementias, it may have major implications for understanding Alzheimer's disease in general.

Acknowledgement

The author thanks Dr A Kennedy for preparation of the figure.

REFERENCES

Akesson HO (1969) A population study of senile and arteriosclerotic psychoses. *Human Heredity* **19**: 546–566.

Alzheimer A (1911) Uber eine eigenartige Krankheitsfalle des spateren Alters. *Zeitschrift für die Gesamte Neurologie und Psychiatrie* **4**: 356.

Amaducci LA, Fratiglioni L, Rocca WA et al (1986) Risk factors for clinically diagnosed Alzheimer's disease: a case-control study of an Italian population. *Neurology* **36**: 922–931.

Bird T, Lampe T, Nemens E et al (1988) Familial Alzheimer's Disease in American descendants of the Volga Germans: probable genetic founder effect. *Annals of Neurology* **23**: 25–31.

Bird TD, Sumi SD & Nemens EJ (1989) Phenotypic heterogeneity in familial Alzheimer's disease: a study of 24 kindreds. *Annals of Neurology* **25**: 12–21.

Blessed G, Tomlinson BE & Roth M (1968) The association between quantitative measures of dementia and of senile change in the cerebral grey matter of elderly subjects. *British Journal of Psychiatry* **114**: 797–811.

Blumbergs P, Beran R & Hicks P (1981) Myoclonus in Down's syndrome. Association with Alzheimer's disease. *Archives of Neurology* **38**: 453–545.

Breitner JCS & Folstein MF (1984) Familial Alzheimer's dementia: a prevalent disorder with specific clinical features. *Psychological Medicine* **14**: 63–80.

Breitner JCS, Folstein MF & Murphy EA (1986a) Familial aggregation in Alzheimer dementia. I. A model for the age-dependent expression of an autosomal dominant gene. *Journal of Psychiatric Research* **20**: 31–43.

Breitner JCS, Folstein MF & Murphy EA (1986b) Familial aggregation in Alzheimer dementia. II. Clinical genetic implications of age-dependent onset. *Journal of Psychiatric Research* **20**: 45–55.

Breitner JCS, Murphy EA, Silverman JM, Mohs RC & Davies JL (1988a) Age-dependent expression of familial risk in Alzheimer's disease. *American Journal of Epidemiology* **128**: 536–548.

Breitner JCS, Silverman JS, Mohs RC & David KL (1988b) Familial aggregation in Alzheimer's disease: comparison of risk among relatives of early- and late-onset cases and among male and female relatives in successive generations. *Neurology* **38**: 207–212.

Breitner JCS, Murphy EA, Folstein MF & Magruder-Habib K (1990) Twin studies of Alzheimer's disease: an approach to etiology and prevention. *Neurobiology of Aging* **11**: 641–648.

Broe GA, Henderson AS, Creasy H et al (1990) A case-control study of Alzheimer's disease in Australia. *Neurology* **40**: 1698–1707.

Chandra V & Schoenberg BS (1989) Inheritance of Alzheimer's disease: epidemiologic evidence. *Neuroepidemiology* **8**: 164–174.

Chandra V, Bharucha NE & Schoenberg BS (1986) Pattern of mortality from types of dementia in the United States 1971 and 1973–1978. *Neurology* **36**: 204–208.

Chandra V, Philipose V, Bell PA et al (1987) Case-control study of late onset 'probable Alzheimer's disease'. *Neurology* **37**: 1295–1300.

Chartier-Harlin MC, Crawford F, Houlden H et al (1991) Early-onset Alzheimer's disease caused by mutations at codon 717 of the beta-amyloid precursor protein gene. *Nature* **353**: 844–846.

Chui HC, Teng EL, Henderson VW et al (1985) Clinical subtypes of dementia of the Alzheimer type. *Neurology* **35**: 1544–1550.

Cook RH, Schneck SA & Clark DB (1981) Twins with Alzheimer's disease. *Archives of Neurology* **38**: 300–301.

Crawford F, Hardy J, Mullan M et al (1991) Sequencing of exons 16 and 17 of the beta-amyloid precursor protein gene in 14 families with early onset Alzheimer's disease fails to reveal mutations in the beta-amyloid sequence. *Neuroscience Letters* **133**: 1–2.

Cummings JL, Benson F, Hill MA et al (1985) Aphasia in dementia of the Alzheimer type. *Neurology* **35**: 394–397.

Davidson EA & Robertson EE (1955) Alzheimer's disease with acne rosacea in one of identical twins. *Journal of Neurology, Neurosurgery and Psychiatry* **18**: 72–77.

Duffy P, Mayeaux R & Kupsky W (1988) Familial Alzheimer's disease with myoclonus and 'spongy change'. *Archives of Neurology* **45**: 1097–1100.

Embry C & Lippman S (1985) Presumed Alzheimer's disease beginning at different ages in two twins. *Journal of the American Geriatric Society* **33**: 61–62.

Ewins DL, Rossor MN, Butler J et al (1991) Association between autoimmune thyroid disease and Familial Alzheimer's disease. *Clinical Endocrinology* **35**: 93–96.

Farlow MR, Murrell J, Zeldenrust S, Ghetti B & Benson M (1992) Clinical, neuropathological and molecular genetic characteristics of a family with early-onset Alzheimer's disease. *Neurology* **42** (supplement 3): 720.

Farrer LA, O'Sullivan DM & Cupples LA (1989) Assessment of genetic risk for Alzheimer's disease among first-degree relatives. *Annals of Neurology* **25**: 485–493.

Farrer LA, Myers RH, Cupples LA et al (1990) Transmission and age at onset patterns in familial Alzheimer's disease: evidence for heterogeneity. *Neurology* **40**: 395–403.

Feldman EG, Chandler KA, Levy L & Glasser GH (1963) Familial Alzheimer's disease. *Neurology* **13**: 811–824.

Fitch N, Becker R & Heller A (1988) The inheritance of Alzheimer's disease: a new interpretation. *Annals of Neurology* **23**: 14–19.

Flugel FL (1929) Zur Diagnostik der Alzheimerschen Krankheit. *Zeitschrift für die Gesamte Neurologie und Psychiatrie* **120**: 183.

Folstein MF & Breitner JCS (1981) Language disorder predicts familial Alzheimer's disease. *John Hopkins Medical Journal* **149**: 145–147.

Folstein M, Powell D & Breitner J (1983) The cognitive pattern of familial Alzheimer's disease. Banbury Report 15. Biological Aspects of Alzheimer's disease.

Foncin JE, Salmon D, Supino-Viterbo V et al (1985) Presenile Alzheimer's disease in a large kindred. *Revue Neurologique* **141**: 194–202.

Fratiglioni L, Grut M, Forsell Y et al (1991) Prevalence of Alzheimer's disease and other dementias in an elderly urban population: relationship with age, sex and education. *Neurology* **41**: 1886–1892.

Frommelt P, Schnabel R, Kühne W, Nee LE & Polinsky RJ (1991) Familial Alzheimer's disease: a large, multigeneration German kindred. *Alzheimer Disease and Associated Disorders* **5**: 36–43.

Fukutani Y, Nakamura I, Kobayashi K, Yamaguchi N & Matsubara R (1989) An autopsy case of familial juvenile Alzheimer's disease with extensive involvement of the subcortical gray and white matters. *Acta Neuropathologica* **77**: 329–332.

Ghetti B, Murrell J, Benson MD & Farlow MR (1992) Spectrum of amyloid β-protein immunoreactivity in hereditary Alzheimer disease with a guanine to thymine missense change at position 1924 of the APP gene. *Brain Research* **571**: 133–139.

Glenner GG & Wong CW (1984) Alzheimer's disease: initial report of the purification and characterization of a novel cerebrovascular amyloid protein. *Biochemical and Biophysical Research Communications* **120**: 885–890.

Goate A, Chartier-Harlin MC, Mullan M et al (1991) Segregation of a missense mutation in the amyloid precursor protein gene with familial Alzheimer's disease. *Nature* **349**: 704–706.

Goldgaber D, Lerman ML, McBride OW, Saffiotti V & Gajdusek DC (1987) Characterization and chromosomal localization of a cDNA encoding brain amyloid of Alzheimer's disease. *Science* **235**: 877–880.

Goudsmit J, White BJ, Weitkamp R et al (1981) Familial Alzheimer's disease in two kindreds of the same geographic and ethnic origin. *Journal of the Neurological Sciences* **49**: 79–89.

Grünthal E & Wenger O (1939) Nachweis von Erblichkeit bei der Alzheimerschen Krankheit nebst Bemerkungen über den Alterungsvorgang im Gehirn. *Monatsschrift für Psychiatrie und Neurologie* **101**: 8–25.

Grünthal E & Wenger O (1940) Ergänzende Untersuchungen und Bemerkungen zu der Arbeit: Nachweis von Erblichkeit bei der Alzheimerschen Krankheit. *Monatsschrift für Psychiatrie und Neurologie* **102**: 303–311.

Haan J, Lanser JBK, Zijderveld I, van der Does IGF & Roos RAC (1990) Dementia in Hereditary Cerebral Haemorrhage with Amyloidosis—Dutch type. *Archives of Neurology* **47**: 965–967.

Hansen L, Salmon D, Galasko D et al (1990) The Lewy Body variant of Alzheimer's disease: a clinical and pathologic entity. *Neurology* **40**: 1–8.

Hardy J & Allsop D (1991) Amyloid deposition as the central event in the aetiology of Alzheimer's disease. *Trends in Pharmacological Science* **12**: 383–388.

Hardy J, Mullan M, Chartier-Harlin MC et al (1991) Alzheimer's disease: a new nosology. *Lancet* **327**: 1342–1343.

Harrison PJ, Barton AJL & Pearson RCA (1991) Expression of amyloid β-protein precursor mRNAs in familial Alzheimer's disease. *Neurorep.* **2**: 152–154.

Heston LL, Lowther DLW & Leventhal CM (1966) Alzheimer's disease: a family study. *Archives of Neurology* **15**: 225–233.

Heston LL, Mastri AR, Anderson E & White J (1981) Dementia of the Alzheimer type: clinical genetics, natural history, and associated conditions. *Archives of General Psychiatry* **38**: 1085–1090.

Heyman A, Wilkinson WE, Stafford JA et al (1984) Alzheimer's disease: a study of epidemiological aspects. *Annals of Neurology* **15**: 335–341.

Hofman A, Schulte W, Vanja BA et al (1989) History of dementia and Parkinson's disease in 1st-degree relatives of patients with Alzheimer's disease. *Neurology* **39**: 1589–1592.

Huff FJ, Auerbach J, Chakravarti A & Boller F (1988) Risk of dementia in relatives of patients with Alzheimer's disease. *Neurology* **38**: 786–790.

Hunter R, Dayan AD & Wilson J (1972) Alzheimer's disease in one monozygotic twin. *Journal of Neurology, Neurosurgery and Psychiatry* **35**: 707–710.

Iseki E, Matsushita M, Kosaka K et al (1990) Morphological characteristics of senile plaques in familial Alzheimer's disease. *Acta Neuropathologica* **80:** 227–232.

Kang J, Lemaire HG, Unterbeck A et al (1987) The precursor of Alzheimer's disease amyloid A4 protein resembles a cell surface receptor. *Nature* **325:** 733–736.

Karlinsky H, Madrick E, Ridgley J et al (1991) A family with multiple instances of definite, probable and possible early-onset Alzheimer's disease. *British Journal of Psychiatry* **159:** 524–530.

Karlinsky H, Vaula MD, Haines JL et al (1992) Molecular and prospective phenotypic characterization of a pedigree with familial Alzheimer's disease and a missense mutation in codon 717 of the β-amyloid precursor protein gene. *Neurology* **42:** 1445–1459.

Kay DWK (1986) The genetics of Alzheimer's disease. *British Medical Bulletin* **42:** 19–23.

Kennedy AM, Newman S, McCaddon A et al (1992) Familial Alzheimer's Disease: A pedigree with a missense mutation in the Amyloid Precursor Protein gene (APP 717 valine to glycine). *Brain* (in press).

Kokmen E (1984) Dementia—Alzheimer type. *Mayo Clinic Proceedings* **59:** 35–42.

Landy PJ & Bain BJ (1970) Alzheimer's disease in siblings. *Medical Journal of Australia* **2:** 832–834.

Lantos PL, Luthert PJ, Hanger D et al (1992) Familial Alzheimer's disease with the amyloid precursor protein 717 mutation and sporadic Alzheimer's disease have the same cytoskeletal pathology. *Neuroscience Letters* **137:** 221–224.

Larsson T, Sjogren T & Jacobson G (1963) Senile dementia: a clinical sociomedical and genetic study. *Acta Psychiatrica Scandinavica* **39** (supplement I): 1–259.

Lauter H (1961) Genealogische Erhebungen in einer Familie mit Alzheimerscher Krankheit. *Arch Psychiatr Ges Neurol* **202:** 126–139.

Levy E, Carmen MD, Fernandez-Madrid IJ et al (1990) Mutation of the Alzheimer's disease amyloid gene in hereditary cerebral haemorrhage, Dutch type. *Science* **248:** 1124–1126.

Li G, Silverman JM & Mohs RC (1991) Clinical genetic studies of Alzheimer's disease. *Psychiatric Clinics of North America* **14:** 267–286.

Lowenberg K & Waggoner R (1934) Familial Organic Psychosis (Alzheimer's type). *Arch Neurol Psychiatr* **31:** 737–754.

Lua M (1920) Zur Kasuistik der Alzheimerschen Krankheit. *Z. Neurol Psych* **55:** 60–75.

Mackenzie IRA, McKelvie IA, Beyreuther K & Masters CL (1991) βA4 amyloid protein deposition in the cerebellum in Alzheimer's disease and Down's syndrome. *Dementia* **2:** 237–242.

McMenemey WH, Worster-Drought C, Flinch J & Williams HG (1939) Familial presenile dementia. Report of case with clinical and pathological features of Alzheimer's disease. *Journal of Neurology and Psychiatry* **2:** 293–302.

Mann DMA, Royston MC & Ravindra CR (1990) Some morphometric observations on the brains of patients with Down's syndrome: their relationship to age and dementia. *Journal of the Neurological Sciences* **99:** 153–164.

Mann DMA, Jones D, Snowden JS, Neary D & Hardy J (1992) Pathological changes in the brain of a patient with familial Alzheimer's disease having a missense mutation at codon 717 in the amyloid precursor protein gene. *Neuroscience Letters* **137:** 225–228.

Martin JJ, Gheuens J & Bruyland M (1991) Early onset Alzheimer's Disease in two large Belgian families. *Neurology* **41:** 62–68.

Maruyama K, Usami M, Yamao-Harigaya W, Tagawa K & Ishiura S (1991) Mutation of Glu[693] to Gln or Val[717] to Ile has no effect on the processing of Alzheimer amyloid precursor protein expressed in COS-1 cells by cDNA transfection. *Neuroscience Letters* **132:** 97–100.

Mayeux R, Sano M, Chen J, Tatemichi T & Stern Y (1991) Risk of dementia in first-degree relatives of patients with Alzheimer's disease. *Neurology* **29:** 538–539.

Mayeux R, Stern Y & Spanton S (1985) Heterogeneity in dementia of the Alzheimer's type: evidence of subgroups. *Neurology* **35:** 453–461.

Meggendorfer F (1925) Über familiengeschichtliche Untersuchungen bei arteriosklerotischer und seniler Demenz. *Zentralblatt für Neurologie und Psychiatrie* **40:** 359.

Mohs RC, Breitner JCS, Silverman JM & Davies KL (1987) Alzheimer's disease: morbid risk among first degree relatives approximates 50% by age 90. *Archives of General Psychiatry* **44:** 405–408.

Molsa PK, Marttila RJ & Rinne UK (1982) Epidemiology of dementia in a Finnish population. *Acta Neurologica Scandinavica* **65:** 541–552.

Mullan M, Crawford F, Axelman K, Houlden H et al (1992) A pathogenic mutation for probable Alzheimer's disease in the APP gene at the N-terminus of β-amyloid. *Nature Genetics* **1**: 345–347.

Mullan M, Tsuji S, Miki T et al (1992) Clinical and pathological comparison of Alzheimer's disease in pedigrees with the codon 717 Val→Ile mutation in the amyloid precursor protein gene. *Brain* (in press).

Murrell J, Farlow M, Bernardino G et al (1991) A mutation in the amyloid precursor protein associated with hereditary Alzheimer's disease. *Science* **254**: 97–98.

Nahman S & Rabinowicz TH (1963) Considérations sur un cas familial de maladie d'Alzheimer. *Encéphale* **4**: 366–381.

Naruse S et al (1991) Mis-sense mutation Val→Ile in exon 17 of amyloid precursor protein gene in Japanese familial Alzheimer's disease. *Lancet* **337**: 978–979.

Nee LR, Polinsky R & Eldridge R (1983) A family with histologically confirmed Alzheimer's disease. *Archives of Neurology* **40**: 203–208.

Nee LE, Eldridge R, Sunderland T et al (1987) Dementia of the Alzheimer type: clinical and family study of 22 twin pairs. *Neurology* **37**: 359–363.

Oliver C & Holland AJ (1986) Down's syndrome and Alzheimer's disease: a review. *Psychological Medicine* **16**: 307–322.

Oltersdorf T, Fritz LC, Schenk DB et al (1989) The secreted form of Alzheimer's amyloid precursor protein with the Kunitz domain is protease nexin-II. *Nature* **341**: 144–147.

Patel S (1989) A family with Alzheimer's disease. *British Journal of Psychiatry* **155**: 405–408.

Percy ME, Markovic VD, Crapper McLachlin DR et al (1991) Family with 22-derived marker chromosome and late-onset dementia of the Alzheimer type. I. Application of a new model for estimation of the risk of disease associated with the marker. *American Journal of Medical Genetics* **39**: 307–313.

Pericak-Vance MA, Bebout JL, Gaskell PC et al (1991) Linkage studies in familial Alzheimer's disease: evidence for chromosome 19 linkage. *American Journal of Human Genetics* **48**: 1034–1150.

Polinsky RJ, Noble H, Dichiro G et al (1987) Dominantly inherited Alzheimer's disease: cerebral glucose metabolism. *Journal of Neurology, Neurosurgery and Psychiatry* **50**: 752–757.

Pro JD, Sumi M & Smith CH (1979) Amyloid plaques in the cerebellum in presenile familial Alzheimer's disease. *Neurology* **29**: 538–539.

Quon D, Wang Y, Catalano RM et al (1991) Formation of beta-amyloid protein deposits in brains of transgenic mice. *Nature* **352**: 239–241.

Rainero I, Pinessi L, Bergamini L et al (1992) Sporadic and familial early-onset Alzheimer's disease: a comparison of the clinical features. *Neurology* **42** (supplement 3): 718.

Risse SC, Lampe TH, Bird TD et al (1990) Myoclonus, seizures and paratonia in Alzheimer's disease. *Alzheimer Disease and Associated Disorders* **4**: 217–225.

Rocca WA, Amaducci LA & Schoenberg BS (1986) Epidemiology of clinically diagnosed Alzheimer's disease. *Annals of Neurology* **19**: 415–424.

Rocca WA, Bonaiuto S, Lippi A et al (1990) Prevalence of clinically diagnosed Alzheimer's disease and other dementing disorders: a door to door survey in Appignano, Macerata Province, Italy. *Neurology* **40**: 626–631.

Ropper AH & Williams RS (1980) Relationship between plaques, tangles and dementia in Down's syndrome. *Neurology* **30**: 639–644.

Rossor MN (1991) Heterogeneity in Alzheimer's disease. 5th International Symposium of PRIT Alzheimer's disease, Jutendo, Japan. *Frontiers of Alzheimer Research*, pp 21–32. Amsterdam: Excerpta Medica, Elsevier.

Rossor MN, Kennedy A & Newman S (1992) Heterogeneity in Familial Alzheimer's disease (submitted Fondation Ipsen pour la Recherche Therapeutique Heterogeneity of Alzheimer's Disease pbs. Springer-Verlag).

Sadovnick AD, Tuokko H, Horton A, Baird PA & Beattie BL (1988) Familial Alzheimer's disease. *Canadian Journal of Neurological Sciences* **15**: 142–146.

Sadovnick AD, Irwin ME, Bird PA & Beattie BL (1989) Genetic studies on an Alzheimer clinic population. *Genetic Epidemiology* **6**: 633–643.

St George-Hyslop P, Tanzi R, Polinsky R et al (1987) The genetic defect causing familial Alzheimer's disease maps on chromosome 21. *Science* **235**: 885–890.

St George-Hyslop PH, Myers RH & Haines JL (1989) Familial Alzheimer's disease: progress and problems. *Neurobiology of Aging* **10**: 417–425.

St George-Hyslop PH, Haines JL, Farrer LA et al (1990) Genetic linkage studies suggest that Alzheimer's disease is not a single homogeneous disorder. *Nature* **347:** 194–197.

Scheele H (1933) Über ein Konkordantes Zweieiiges Zwillingspaar mit seniler Demenz. Ein Beitrag Zur Erbforschung bei der senilen Demenz. *Zeitschrift für Neurologie und Psychologie* **144:** 606–612.

Schellenberg GD, Bird TD, Wijsman EM et al (1988) Absence of linkage of chromosome 21q21 markers to familial Alzheimer's disease. *Science* **241:** 1507–1510.

Schottkey J (1932) Uber Prasenile Verblodungen. *Zeitschrift für Neurologie und Psychologie* **140:** 333–397.

Shalat SI, Seltzer B, Pidcock C & Baker EL (1987) Risk factors for Alzheimer's disease: a case control study. *Neurology* **37:** 1630–1633.

Sinex FM & Myers RH (1982) Alzheimer's disease, Down's syndrome, and aging: the genetic approach. *Annals of the New York Academy of Sciences* **396:** 3–13.

Sisodia SS, Koo EH, Beyreuther K, Unterbeck A & Price DL (1990) Evidence that β-amyloid protein in Alzheimer's disease is not derived by normal processing. *Science* **248:** 492–495.

Sjogren T (1952) A genetic study of morbus Alzheimer and morbus Pick. *Acta Psychiatrica et Neurologica Scandinavica* **82** (supplement 1): 8–51.

Sorbi S, Tesco G, Piersanti P et al (1992) Absence of APP gene mutation in early-onset familial Alzheimer's disease. *Neurology* **42** (supplement 3): 5675.

Struble RG, Polinsky RJ, Hedreen JC et al (1991) Hippocampal lesions in dominantly inherited Alzheimer's disease. *Journal of Neuropathology and Experimental Neurology* **50:** 82–94.

Sudarsky L, Myers RH & Walsh TM (1983) Huntington's disease in monozygotic twins reared apart. *Journal of Medical Genetics* **20:** 408–411.

Sumi SM, Bird TD, Nochlin D & Raskind MA (1992) Familial presenile dementia with psychosis associated with cortical neurofibrillary tangles and degeneration of the amygdala. *Neurology* **42:** 120–127.

Tanzi RE, Gusella JF, Watkins PC et al (1987) Amyloid beta protein gene: cDNA, MRMA distribution and genetic linkage near the Alzheimer locus. *Science* **235:** 880–884.

Timmers WF, Tagliavini F, Haan J & Frangione B (1990) Parenchymal preamyloid and amyloid deposits in the brains of patients with hereditary cerebral hemorrhage with amyloidosis—Dutch type. *Neuroscience Letters* **118:** 223–226.

Tzourio C, Alperovitch A, Maccario J & Dartigues J-F (1991) Is dementia of the Alzheimer type a purely genetic illness? A modelling approach. *Neuroepidemiology* **10:** 288–296.

Van Bogaert L, Maere M & Smeldt E (1940) Sur les formes familiales précoces de la maladie d'Alzheimer. *Monatsschrift für Psychiatrie und Neurologie* **102:** 249–301.

Van Broekhoven C, Genthe AM, Vandenberghe A et al (1987) Failure of familial Alzheimer's disease to segregate with the A4-amyloid gene in several European families. *Nature* **329:** 153–155.

Van Duijn CM, Clayton D, Chandra V et al (1991) Familial aggregation of Alzheimer's disease and related disorders: a collaborative re-analysis of case-control studies. *International Journal of Epidemiology* **20** (supplement 2): 513–520.

Wattendorff AR, Bots GTAM, Went LN & Endlz LJ (1982) Familial cerebral amyloid angiopathy presenting as recurrent cerebral hemorrhage. *Journal of the Neurological Sciences* **55:** 121–135.

Whalley LJ, Carothers AD, Collyer S et al (1982) A study of familial factors in Alzheimer's disease. *British Journal of Psychiatry* **140:** 249–256.

Yankner BA & Mesulam M-M (1991) β-amyloid and the pathogenesis of Alzheimer's disease. *New England Journal of Medicine* **325:** 1849–1857.

Zubenko GS, Huff FJ, Beyer J, Auerbach J & Teply I (1988) Familial risk of dementia associated with a biologic subtype of Alzheimer's disease. *Archives of General Psychiatry* **45:** 889–893.

4

Pick's disease

JEREMY BROWN

In 1892 Arnold Pick described the case of a 71-year-old man who presented with dementia and aphasia. Post-mortem examination revealed circumscribed temporal lobe atrophy. He published the case to illustrate that senile dementia could be caused by a localized temporal lobe atrophy, rather than necessarily by generalized atrophy, as Wernicke had suggested (Berrios, 1991). He described three more cases over the next 14 years, extending his observations to include atrophy of the frontal lobes with associated behavioural changes (Pick, 1906). He did not feel that he had described a new disease, an idea proposed much later. The major histopathological features of Pick's disease, namely argentophilic inclusions or Pick bodies and swollen chromatolytic neurones or Pick cells, were described by Alois Alzheimer of the rival Munich group in 1911, extending his demonstration of the importance of histopathology in the analysis of dementia.

Urechia and Milhalescu originally christened circumscribed lobar atrophy Spielmeyer's disease, Spielmeyer having described similar cases (Van Mansvelt, 1954), but Gans (1923) and Onari and Spatz (1926) first used the term Pick's disease (Berrios, 1991) and the following year Schneider popularized the concept and divided the development of the disease into three stages (Schneider, 1927, 1929). The first was characterized by disturbances of judgement and behaviour, the second by localized symptoms and the final stage by generalized dementia. Grünthal (1931) recognized the hereditary nature of some cases and single reports began to appear in the English literature. There has always been a vagueness in the criteria used in the diagnosis and ever since this time there has been a divergence between authors such as Sanders et al (1939), who emphasized the lobar atrophy, and authors who regard the presence of histopathological markers of paramount importance for the diagnosis. In the last 20 years there has been an increasing tendency to try to delineate neurodegenerative syndromes more accurately and a number of new diseases have been described which share features with Pick's disease, for example frontal lobe degeneration of non-Alzheimer type (FLD), corticobasal degeneration and hereditary dysphasic dementia. It seems possible that these and similar diseases were classified as forms of Pick's disease in the past. The classification of Pick's disease remains confused and there is still no consensus on the features needed for diagnosis. Some authors, e.g. Constantinidis (1985), have subdivided Pick's disease on clinical and neuropathological grounds, but without more

535
Copyright © 1992, by Baillière Tindall
All rights of reproduction in any form reserved

knowledge of the aetiology these divisions are difficult to justify as distinct nosological entities. The difficulties in the diagnosis and classification have contributed to its recent relative obscurity compared with Alzheimer's disease, Huntington's disease and prion dementia. Pick's disease and its variants are not uncommon and recent advances in imaging, neuropathology and molecular genetics should lead to major advances in our understanding of them in the next few years.

DEFINITION

Pick's disease is defined in the international classification of diseases (ICD-10) as: 'A progressive dementia commencing in middle life (usually between 50 and 60 years) characterized by slowly progressing changes in character and social deterioration leading to impairment of intellect, memory and language factors with apathy, euphoria and occasionally extrapyramidal phenomena. The neuropathological picture is one of selective atrophy of the frontal and temporal lobes without the occurrence of neuritic plaques and neurofibrillary tangles in excess of what is seen in normal aging. Early onset cases tend to exhibit a more malignant course. The social and behavioural manifestations often antedate frank memory impairment.' There are clear difficulties with this definition, for example the lack of precision and the avoidance of the relevance of histological features such as Pick cells and Pick bodies. At present the lack of knowledge of the aetiology of Pick's disease precludes accurate definition. This means that if sense is to be made of the publications on Pick's disease authors need to supply complete clinical and pathological data on their cases; unfortunately many papers fall short of this standard.

EPIDEMIOLOGY

The epidemiological data on Pick's disease are limited. The most common method of estimating the frequency is to compare it to Alzheimer's disease in a post-mortem series. The estimates have varied from one-fiftieth (Terry, 1976) to one-third (Heston, 1978) of the prevalence of Alzheimer's disease. This large variation could reflect differences in methodology, in particular differences in the definitions of Alzheimer's disease and Pick's disease, and neither confirms nor excludes geographical variation in the frequency of the disease. Two authors have used similar data to estimate absolute frequencies: Heston (1978) estimated the overall frequency of Pick's disease in Minnesota as 24 per 100 000, and Constantinidis (1985) estimated the frequency in Switzerland to be 30–60 per 100 000. Pick's disease has been described in many ethnic groups, including Chinese, Malay and South American (Moyano, 1932; Verhaart, 1936; Tong, 1990), but there have been no studies of the relative frequency of the disease in different ethnic groups.

Sjogren (1952) quotes a 2 : 1 female preponderance in Pick's disease based upon a large series from psychiatric hospitals. This may not be a valid measure, since women on average live longer than men and a woman is more likely to be the sole survivor of a partnership; this may predispose women to institutional care. Van Mansvelt (1954) reviewed 171 cases and found the female to male ratio to be 6:5. In familial cases there has been a slight male preponderance (Groen and Endtz, 1982), and overall the present evidence suggests that the age-matched sex incidence is approximately equal.

AETIOLOGY

A proportion of Pick's cases are familial. Groen and Endtz (1982) reviewed all cases of familial Pick's disease in the literature or known to them in which more than one generation were involved with pathological confirmation of the diagnosis. They list a total of 26 families. The mode of inheritance in all the large families described has been compatible with an autosomal dominant gene. There have been occasional reports of small families where the inheritance could be autosomal recessive (Constantinidis, 1985). The best characterized family is a Dutch one which was originally described in detail by Sanders and colleagues in 1939 and since reported twice more (Schenk, 1959; Groen and Endtz, 1982). A total of 25 cases have been described in six generations. The disease gene penetrance in this family appears to be close to 100%; the other families reported are too small to estimate penetrance. Collections of large families may overestimate the penetrance of disease genes because only families with apparent high penetrance will be selected. If the penetrance is low a late onset disease is unlikely to be recognized as familial.

The proportion of cases which are familial has been examined by several authors. Van Mansvelt (1954) in his review reported an affected relative in 27 out of 153 cases; however, in nearly half the cases he analysed no family details were supplied and rarely was the search for affected relatives exhaustive. Sjogren and co-workers (1952) and Heston (1978) both tried to trace affected relatives of a smaller number of probands. Sjogren found affected relatives in four out of 18 cases and Heston found secondary cases for six out of 11 probands. From these figures a reasonable estimate would be that between 20 and 50% of cases are familial. None of these authors has identified factors which correlate with inheritability, although Luers and Spatz (1957) suggested that patients with onset before the age of 40 years are more likely to have affected relatives.

The aetiology of the non-familial cases remains obscure. Constantinidis (1985) provided some experimental evidence for increased zinc deposition in Pick's disease and proposed a mechanism involving the neurotransmitter glutamate, but Ehmann et al (1984) failed to find any change in brain zinc levels. The latter group also measured concentrations of a number of other elements and found increased levels of iron, manganese, sodium, chloride and phosphate and reduced levels of chromium, caesium, rubidium and selenium. There have also been quantitative reports of abnormal brain gangliosides in Pick's disease (Scicutella and Davies, 1987).

Van Mansvelt (1954) reported that occasional cases of Pick's disease occurred after serious head trauma, which parallels similar observations in Alzheimer's disease (Roberts et al, 1991). The similarities between Pick bodies and bodies in cells undergoing axonal chromatolysis suggests a role for axonal damage in Pick's disease. Ramon y Cajal (1959) attempted to elucidate this by inducing Pick bodies experimentally by undercutting the cortex. Whether he was successful depends on which account you read (Schochet, 1968; Wisniewski et al, 1972). Following the demonstration that kuru and Creutzfeldt–Jakob disease were transmissible there have been at least eight unsuccessful attempts to transmit Pick's disease to laboratory animals (C. J. Gibbs quoted in Clark et al, 1986).

CLINICAL FEATURES

The youngest reported cases of Pick's disease (excluding occasional infantile encephalopathies with Pick bodies) are in the early twenties and the oldest one died aged 91 years (Moyano, 1932). The peak incidence is in the sixth decade (Van Mansvelt, 1954). The clinical features of very early onset Pick's disease (before the age of 40) are clinically and pathologically atypical and may represent a distinct disease (Munoz-Garcia and Ludwin, 1984); these cases are discussed later. The duration of the disease is difficult to estimate due to the insidious onset but the majority of affected individuals die between 3 and 15 years after onset. Bronchopneumonia is the most common cause of death (Van Mansvelt, 1954).

The division of the disease into three stages was popularized by Schneider (1929), although the lack of definite clinicopathological divisions renders it rather artificial. There is considerable variation in the clinical features of affected individuals of the large Dutch family which have the same genetic disease (Groen and Endtz, 1982), suggesting that even with a single aetiology there is variation in the phenotype. Two groups have found that the symptoms and signs in individuals are essentially dependent upon the macroscopic distribution of neuronal loss (Van Mansvelt, 1954; Tissot et al, 1985).

Analysis of the typical symptoms is difficult due to the heterogeneous nature of the disease. In addition there are a large number of reports in which the diagnosis was made at post-mortem and the clinical history assessed retrospectively. Sjogren et al (1952) noted that the frequency of signs is dependent on the stage of the disease at which the patient is assessed. If there are systematic differences between patient series with respect to the stage of the disease, then different authors will report markedly different frequencies of signs. The disease usually starts with personality change. The patient may become more withdrawn or disinhibited and extrovert. Of the 18 cases of Sjogren et al (1952), eight started with aspontaneity, five with mania and one with a paranoid reaction. Stereotyped movements and obsessional phenomena are frequent, for example compulsory walking routines. Gluttony and weight gain are also common, occurring in 33 of Van

Mansvelt's cases. There may be excessive alcohol intake (Groen and Endtz, 1982), which could lead to misdiagnosis as alcohol-related dementia.

Pick's original case was of selective temporal lobe atrophy and a number of authors have reported similar cases. Cummings and Duchen (1981) reported five patients with severe anterior temporal lobe atrophy and Pick cells. These patients showed a syndrome of reaching for any available object, compulsive mouthing of objects and dulling of affect. The authors pointed out parallels with the Kluver–Bucy syndrome in monkeys (Kluver and Bucy, 1939). Delusions and hallucinations are rare although cases misdiagnosed throughout their disease as schizophrenia have occurred. There is often a forensic history, either due to violence, aggression or shoplifting; Sjogren et al (1952) reported that five out of 13 of his series had 'ethical deficits'. Sexual problems are often mentioned and are presumably aggravated, if not caused, by disinhibition.

Speech problems are common, occurring in 129 of Van Mansvelt's cases (Van Mansvelt, 1954). If the disease is predominantly temporal there may be logorrhoea, but in the majority reduced spontaneous speech with anomia, perseveration and echolalia are seen. A proportion of patients become mute, particularly if they have predominantly frontal disease (Tissot et al, 1985). Sjogren et al (1952) reported a similar overall frequency of speech problems in Alzheimer's disease and Pick's disease.

Attentional problems were the most common clinical feature of Pick's disease in Van Mansvelt's series, occurring in almost 95% of assessed cases (Van Mansvelt, 1954). By contrast, the patient is orientated in time, person and place, at least in the early stages of the disease. In the Swedish series (Sjogren et al, 1952) spatial disorientation was rare in Pick's disease by contrast with Alzheimer's disease.

Extrapyramidal signs have been reported, particularly in young onset patients, and Tissot et al (1985) found that extrapyramidal signs were significantly more common with frontal lobe disease. Other movement disorders are rare, although chorea has been reported in two cases (Van Mansvelt, 1954). In the early stages of the disease Sjogren reported that tone changes were unusual. In the later stages of the disease, particularly if there is frontal lobe disease, pyramidal tract signs often develop (Tissot et al, 1985) and the patient may end with a spastic quadraparesis and contractures—*la paraplegie en flexion*. Gait tends to be affected late and its aetiology may be multifactorial, for example due to extrapyramidal dysfunction or a gait apraxia. Sjogren et al (1952) reported that there were no gait disturbances in their patients but gait disturbances occur in most series.

Mathematical and visuospatial skills are often well preserved and patients with advanced disease may score well compared with those with Alzheimer's disease on the mini-mental state examination (Folstein et al, 1975). Sjogren et al (1952) reported that 92% of their Pick's patients could perform serial 7s compared with only 44% of their Alzheimer's patients. Dyspraxia was only reported in 33 of the 171 cases reviewed by Van Mansvelt (1954), dysgraphia in 44 and dyslexia in 26. The Swedish group also reported a relatively low incidence of agraphia, apraxia and alexia compared with Alzheimer's disease patients (Sjogren et al, 1952).

Classical seizures are strikingly rare compared with Alzheimer's disease. Seven of the cases reviewed by Van Mansvelt (1954) had seizures and only in one of these was the diagnosis definite and the seizures frequent. A number of authors have reported hypotonic attacks with a reduction of consciousness (Van Mansvelt, 1954); the nature of these remains obscure but could be epileptic.

As the preceding account makes clear there are considerable differences between authors in the frequency of certain signs, e.g. gait disturbance. Whether this reflects variations in the frequency of subtypes of the disease in different geographical areas or methodological differences is unclear.

THE SCHENK DUTCH FAMILY

The probable heterogeneity of Pick's disease limits the value of general symptom reviews. The only large group of patients who definitely have the same disease are the Dutch family reported by Schenk, his collaborators and heirs (Sanders et al, 1939; Schenk, 1959; Groen and Endtz, 1982). It is therefore worth describing this family separately. Clinical details are available for 25 affected members. The age at onset in this family varies from 34 to 58 years and the reported duration of disease from 2 to 17 years. The youngest onset also has the longest duration of disease, suggesting a very early diagnosis in this case (otherwise the age range is 39–58 years and the duration 2–15 years). The symptoms and signs are varied, with no clear pattern. Common early symptoms include speech disturbance, behavioural and sexual problems, reduced personal hygiene, stealing, suicide, gluttony, euphoria and obsessive compulsive routines. In the later stages many become mute and develop mouthing behaviour. On examination some were found to have no abnormalities, others had a variety of focal signs, including orofacial dyskinesias, facial or lingual paralysis, unequal pupils, hemiplegia, increased tone and cogwheel rigidity. In the later stages of the disease pyramidal signs were frequent.

INVESTIGATIONS

Routine biochemical and haematological investigations are typically normal in Pick's disease. The CSF is usually normal although there may be a slight increase in protein. Computerized tomographic (CT) scanning can identify selective frontal and temporal lobe atrophy (Groen and Endtz, 1982). Groen and Endtz (1982) identified atrophy prior to the development of disease in one patient and suggested that the CT could be a presymptomatic test. CT scanning certainly aids the early diagnosis of selective lobar atrophy (Knopman et al, 1989), as does magnetic resonance imaging (MRI) with new generation scanners (Figure 1).

A useful investigation in Pick's disease is the electroencephalogram (EEG) which is typically normal, in contrast to Alzheimer's disease which shows slowing of the alpha rhythm (Gordon and Sim, 1967). Tissot et al

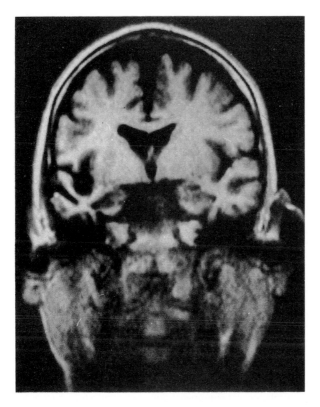

Figure 1. MRI scan of a case of Pick's disease, showing asymmetrical, predominantly temporal lobe atrophy.

(1985) reported that out of 21 EEG recordings on ten patients with Pick's disease only two were abnormal. In the large Dutch family the EEG was normal in 11 out of 13 cases (Groen and Endtz, 1982).

Regional cerebral blood flow studies show a selective reduction of blood flow in frontal and temporal regions in neuropathologically verified Pick's disease (Risberg and Gustafson, 1988). Positron emission tomography in three patients with biopsy proven Pick's disease showed a deficit in frontal lobe and temporal lobe metabolism in two patients; in a third, who presented with a dysphasia, the hypometabolism started in the left peri-sylvian region before extending to both frontal lobes (Salmon and Franck, 1989).

Neuropsychometry may highlight some of the difficulties in language and in other cognitive areas in Pick's disease; patients may show deficits in problem solving as tested, for example, on the Wisconsin card sorting test. One group assessing neuropsychological profiles retrospectively found the major discriminating factor between Pick's disease and Alzheimer's disease to be relative preservation of recent memory in the former (Knopman et al,

1989). Some very detailed neuropsychological assessments of patients with Pick's disease have been published (e.g. Warrington, 1975).

There have been a number of attempts to develop clinical criteria for the diagnosis of Alzheimer's disease, e.g. the National Institute of Neurological Disorders and Stroke (NINCDS) criteria (McKhann et al, 1984). These have concentrated on the distinction of Alzheimer's disease from vascular dementia rather than other neurodegenerative dementias such as Pick's disease. No such criteria have been developed for the other degenerative dementias, which often fulfil the NINCDS criteria for Alzheimer's disease. Nevertheless it is possible from reviewing the literature to suggest factors which favour the diagnosis of Pick's disease, although none are specific. Table 1 itemizes features which may contribute to a diagnosis of Pick's disease.

Table 1. Clinical features of Pick's disease.

Presentation with personality change
Attentional deficit
Preservation of spatial orientation with deficit in temporal orientation
Obsessive–compulsive behaviour
Gluttony, onset of excessive smoking or alcohol intake with illness
Lack of insight
Sexual disinhibition
Forensic history
Asymmetrical signs with a history of steadily progressive disease
Stereotypy
Suicide or parasuicide
Indiscriminate mouthing of objects
Absence of myoclonus and seizures
Preservation of calculation and visuospatial skills with relatively high score on the
    mini-mental test
Frontotemporal atrophy on CT or MRI scan
Normal alpha rhythm on EEG
Neuropsychometry showing frontal lobe deficits.
Positron emission tomography or single photon emission computerized tomography showing
    reduced frontal and/or temporal lobe blood flow or cerebral metabolism

NEUROPATHOLOGY

In Van Mansvelt's series (1954) the average weight of male brains was between 1100 and 1200 g and female brains between 900 and 1000 g, reflecting the tissue loss that occurs. This is selective and the classical gross appearance of Pick's disease is of well-circumscribed temporal and frontal lobe atrophy (Figures 2 and 3). The atrophy may be sufficiently severe to give the appearance of a knife-edge with a clear distinction between normal and abnormal cortex. In many cases, however, the atrophy is less well demarcated. The frontal atrophy is usually most severe at the pole or the orbital convolutions and the anterior part of the insula is often involved. Luers and Spatz (1957) recognized two main types of frontal lobe involvement, depending upon whether the medial surface or the frontal pole was more affected. The temporal atrophy affects the second and third temporal gyri and the anterior part of the first temporal gyrus, sparing the posterior two-thirds. The hippocampus is commonly but not invariably affected. If there is parietal atrophy it includes the angular or supramarginal gyri. In Van Mansvelt's review (1954), 94 had mixed atrophy; in 43 cases it was predominantly frontal and in 29 predominantly temporal, and he reported two cases with predominantly parietal atrophy. The frequent involvement of the hippocampus refutes the idea that the association areas are particularly

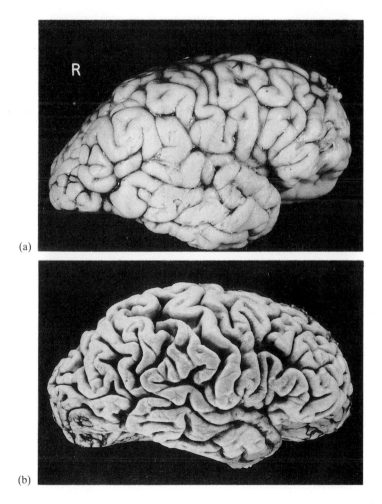

(a)

(b)

Figure 2. (a) Lateral view of normal right cerebral cortex. (b) Lateral view of right cerebral cortex in a patient with Pick's disease showing moderate atrophy of gyri and widening of sulci. The temporal lobe shows severe atrophy with relative sparing of the posterior third of the first temporal gyrus (source: Dr Clive Bruton and the Neuropathological department at Runwell Hospital, Wickford, Essex).

involved. The cortical atrophy is frequently asymmetrical. Van Mansvelt (1954) reviewed all the reported cases and found that of 184 cases in the literature, 117 had asymmetrical atrophy. In almost three-quarters of cases the left hemisphere was the more severely atrophied.

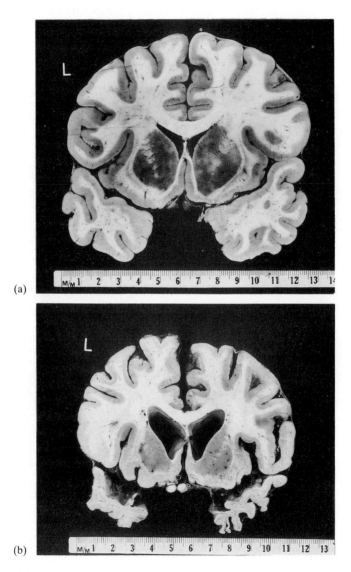

(a)

(b)

Figure 3. (a) Coronal slice at anterior striatal level, normal brain. (b) Coronal slice at anterior striatal level in a case of Pick's disease showing enlarged ventricles, gyral atrophy and widening of sulci. The anterior temporal lobe is severely affected showing virtual destruction of the normal gyral pattern (source: Dr Clive Bruton and the Neuropathological department at Runwell Hospital, Wickford, Essex).

Involvement of subcortical structures is very variable and can include the caudate nucleus, the thalamus, subthalamus, hypothalamus, mammillary bodies, putamen and substantia nigra. A clinicopathological study of 41 cases of Pick's disease (Kosaka et al, 1991) found the caudate was the most frequent part of the striatopallidonigral system to be affected, whilst the internal globus pallidus was the least. In total, 17 of the 41 cases had definite involvement of this system. In the substantia nigra the pars reticulata was more damaged than the pars compacta. The clinical factors which correlated with subcortical pathology were long duration of disease, being female and having predominantly frontal lobe disease. The last of these parallels the clinical correlation of frontal lobe disease and extrapyramidal signs (Tissot et al, 1985). The nucleus basalis of Meynert was involved in nine out of ten cases of Pick's disease studied by Mizukami and Kosaka (1989) but in only two of these was the cell loss and gliosis sufficient to suggest primary involvement of the nucleus as opposed to non-specific secondary changes; the anterior division of the nucleus was more severely affected. Cases with pyramidal tract (Kosaka et al, 1991) and locus coeruleus (Forno et al, 1989) disease have been described. A case with both olivopontocerebellar atrophy and striatonigral degeneration is exceptional (Horoupian and Dickson, 1991). The comparison of the patterns of atrophy between different members of one pedigree with the same disease allows a more precise estimation of the specificity of the changes to be assessed. All of the affected individuals in the large Dutch pedigree have shown marked lobar atrophy and, although the exact pattern of gyral atrophy is variable (Sanders et al, 1939), this does suggest that the pattern of atrophy is a useful marker of the disease.

Pick bodies (see Figure 3, Chapter 2) and Pick cells (Figure 4), the two hallmarks of Pick's disease, were first described by Alois Alzheimer (1911). He described three types of cells with:

1. Distinctive globular homogeneous argentophilic body, often containing lacunae.
2. A homogeneous argentophilic mass including the whole cytoplasm.
3. A tangled whorl of uniform, delicate fibrils.

The Pick cell is a neurone with swollen cytoplasm, which becomes homogeneous and weakly acidophilic, together with the disintegration of the Nissl substance. The nucleus is displaced laterally in the cell (Corsellis, 1976). Many authors have pointed out the similarities to cells undergoing axonal chromatolysis. Only a small minority of all described Pick's cases have both Pick cells and Pick bodies. Van Mansvelt (1954) reported that less than half the cases in his extensive review had swollen cells with or without Pick bodies. Escourolle, in his 1956 review, found Pick bodies in only 20% of all reported cases. Pick cells were more common and found in 110 cases out of a total of 192 (57%). Therefore Pick bodies and Pick cells are not sensitive indicators of the whole spectrum of reported Pick's disease.

One possible explanation for the lack of sensitivity of Pick cells and Pick bodies is that they are transitory phenomena and only seen in the early stages of Pick's disease. This has been proposed by a number of authors, although the idea originated with Schneider. However, there is no experimental evidence to support this theory and empirically it seems inadequate to explain why many reported cases contain neither Pick cells nor Pick bodies.

Argyrophilic inclusion bodies have been reported in a large number of other diseases, including encephalitis, disseminated encephalomyelitis, Hallervorden–Spatz disease, Binswanger's disease, lead poisoning, cachexia and vascular disease (Williams, 1935). It is possible that different neuropathologists have different thresholds for designating argyrophilic staining and Williams (1935) may have had a comparatively low threshold,

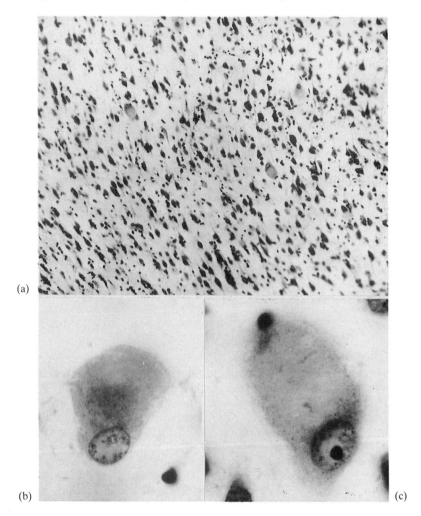

(a)

(b)   (c)

Figure 4. (a) Cresyl Violet Stain of neocortex in a case of Pick's disease showing neuronal loss, proliferation of glia and occasional Pick cells (× 150), (b) (× 1200), (c) Pick cells from the same section (× 1200) (source: Dr Clive Briton, etc.).

as suggested by Clark et al (1986). Nevertheless his basic assertion that argyrophilic inclusions are not specific to Pick's disease has not been seriously challenged; indeed the list of conditions in which they have been reported has lengthened to include, for example, Down's syndrome (Pogacar and Rubio, 1982).

The specificity of Pick cells in presenile dementia is undermined by reports of Pick-like cells in prion disease and Alzheimer's disease. Swollen neurones similar to Pick cells are often seen in Creutzfeldt–Jakob disease (Clark et al, 1986), and Pick bodies have been reported in experimentally induced kuru (Lampert et al, 1969). In addition there are a number of cases in which there is mixed Alzheimer's and Pick's pathology (Berlin, 1949; Smith and Lantos, 1983).

Clark et al (1986) noted similarities between what they describe as swollen chromatolytic cells and cells seen in a case of Lewy body dementia; however they could distinguish the haematoxylinophilic Pick bodies from eosinophilic Lewy bodies on haematoxylin and eosin staining. Forno et al (1989) compared Pick bodies in the locus coeruleus with Lewy bodies and could distinguish Pick bodies by their slight basophilia and lack of a halo on light microscopy.

Pick bodies are most numerous in the hippocampus in the majority of cases, particularly in the dentate gyrus and pyramidal cell layer (Ball, 1979). However many cases have more widespread Pick bodies involving neocortex, subcortical nuclei and even olfactory neurones (Yoshimura, 1988). They can be found in large or small neurones and are most common in upper cortical layers. Hansen et al (1988) found them in all cortical layers, although most numerous in layer 2. Brion et al (1973) noted Pick cells were more ballooned in the neocortex compared with the hippocampus. In a single case report Yoshimura (1989) found similarities in the pattern of distribution of Pick bodies to the classic pattern of neurofibrillary tangles in Alzheimer's disease. Hirano bodies and granulovacuolar degeneration are both non-specific features of Pick's disease.

There are two histological features which, although non-specific, occur in all cases of Pick's disease: neuronal loss and astrocytosis. The cell loss in Pick's disease is typically greatest in the three outer cortical layers (Corsellis, 1976). Hansen et al (1988) studied five Pick's disease brains from a much larger sample with Alzheimer's disease. These cases may be atypical in that they clinically resembled late onset Alzheimer's disease. The average age at death of 73 years is rather old for Pick's disease. They found a loss of large neurones in the frontal and temporal lobes similar in nature to that seen in Alzheimer's disease, but unlike Alzheimer's disease there was no cell loss in the inferior parietal lobule.

The white matter changes in Pick's disease are usually limited to demyelination and mild gliosis, the extent of these changes is, however, very variable and most authors consider them to be secondary to the cortical changes. The severe subcortical gliosis without the macroscopic or microscopic features of Pick's disease, first described by Neumann and Cohn (and originally termed Pick's disease type 2), is probably a separate entity.

Wechsler (1977) wrote a case report of a patient with Pick's disease.

Subsequent neuropathological analysis (Wechsler et al, 1982) noted the almost complete absence of dendritic spines on cortical pyramidal neurones (from frontal and temporal lobes) and a novel dendritic pattern using Golgi impregnation.

Electron microscopic studies of cells with Pick bodies show abnormalities in the cytoplasm with accumulation of filaments and tubules. There is no clear boundary between the Pick body and the remainder of the cytoplasm (Wisniewski et al, 1972). The detailed electron microscopic description of the tubules and filaments is somewhat variable: either 10–15 mm straight filaments or paired, twisted filaments (Rewcastle and Ball, 1968; Wisniewski et al, 1972; Schochet et al, 1968) described paired twisted filaments. Some authors have found both types of filament coexisting and this seems the most likely explanation (Murayama et al, 1990). Yoshimura (1989) described a different type of neurofibril in Pick bodies, with periodic constrictions as well as straight filaments.

The majority of reports do not identify specific differences ultrastructurally between swollen cells which do contain Pick bodies and swollen cells which do not (Wisniewski et al, 1972). One exception to this is Brion and colleagues (1973) who reported three types of distinct ultrastructural variants which they proposed were equivalent to Pick cells, 'half-ballooned cells' and Pick bodies. The Pick bodies consisted of straight neurofilaments and the Pick cells consisted of the larger neurotubules and altered mitochondria.

Recent advances in immunocytochemistry have also contributed to our understanding of Pick cells and Pick bodies. Ulrich et al (1987) compared the staining of Pick bodies and Alzheimer neurofibrillary tangles with a series of monoclonal antibodies to phosphorylated neurofilaments and found a similar but not identical pattern. Lowe et al (1988) showed that polyclonal antibodies raised against ubiquitin stained Pick bodies (as well as staining Lewy bodies and Alzheimer plaques and tangles). Murayama et al (1990) showed that antibodies to phosphorylated tau recognized both Pick bodies and Pick cells with a similar staining pattern and that anti-ubiquitin antibodies also recognized both of these features. In contrast to the intense staining of Pick bodies with anti-tau antibodies, Lewy bodies either fail to stain or just stain with a peripheral band; this can help distinguish the two (Forno et al, 1989). In summary, immunocytochemical studies have shown the presence of phosphorylated neurofilaments and ubiquitin in Pick bodies and Pick cells without elucidating their pathogenesis. These staining techniques have identified common elements between Pick bodies and other neuropathological bodies. The similarities between cells with and those without Pick bodies in immunocytological and ultrastructural studies suggest that they may not be a reliable basis for subdividing the disease.

NEUROCHEMISTRY

Neurochemical studies of Pick's disease have tended to assume that Pick's disease is a unified entity. However aetiological heterogeneity makes the interpretation of negative results difficult.

White et al (1977) and Yates et al (1980) first described neurochemical findings in Pick's disease. There has been general agreement that choline acetyltransferase (ChAT) activities in all brain regions are normal, in contrast to Alzheimer's disease, and that muscarinic receptor binding is diminished in those areas of the cortex affected by the disease (Hansen et al, 1988). One exception to this is the study of Wood et al (1983) in which the muscarinic receptor binding was found to be normal in their four patients. Yates et al (1980) reported that cortical activities of acetylcholinesterase and glutamic acid decarboxylase and concentrations of γ-aminobutyric acid (GABA) and dopamine were normal in the areas examined. These results suggest that cortical neuronal loss includes the intrinsic neocortical cholino-ceptive neurones. A more recent study (Kanazawa et al, 1988) reported on basal ganglia transmitter levels in four patients with Pick's disease. The authors found reduced GABA and substance P concentrations in the substantia nigra. The ChAT activity levels were reduced to a variable extent. The dopamine concentration in the striatum was reduced, in contrast to Huntington's disease where it is increased. Sparks and Markesbery (1991) reported new abnormalities, namely increased imipramine binding in the frontal pole and reduced 5-hydroxytryptamine (5HT) binding in various sites (but not the nucleus basalis of Meynert), in five cases of Pick's disease. They also report reduced choline acetyltransferase and acetylcholinesterase activities in the nucleus basalis of Meynert.

YOUNG ONSET PICK'S DISEASE

A number of authors have demonstrated that Pick's disease affecting the young adult (aged 20–40 years) is different from older onset disease. This view was first popularized by Luers and Spatz (1957) who noted that very young onset cases had an increased familial incidence, a short progressive clinical course and involvement of the caudate and other basal ganglia. There are certainly striking clinical features in some of these cases. One of the most famous Pick's families, first described by Lowenberg et al (1939) and later by Malamud and Waggoner (1943), is an example of this subtype.

The index case had onset at the age of 21 years. He was admitted at the age of 25 years with advanced mental deterioration and had a rapid downhill course. He ended with his left hand and arm held in flexion with tremors if his arm was straightened. He had constant muscular twitching of the entire body and face, more marked on the right. He died aged 27 years. His mother had developed a rapidly progressive dementia with seizures and visual loss and died aged 28 years. His brother, who developed the disease at 24 years of age, was studied by Malamud and Waggoner (1943). He was examined when he was 26 and had a festinant gait, rigidity and was mute. He later developed a rhythmic tremor of the right arm. Post-mortem examinations were performed on the two brothers and severe knife-edged frontal, temporal and parietal lobe atrophy and marked caudate atrophy were found. Microscopic examination revealed a severe loss of neurones with demyelination and gliosis. There were Pick cells in the affected cortex, caudate, amygdala and claustrum Pick bodies in the cortex and non-specific degeneration of the substantia nigra. Hori et al (1983) described a 31-year-old with a severe dementia and twitching of the left arm. He died aged 33 years and on pathological examination he had frontal atrophy with marked caudate atrophy and microscopic depigmentation of the substantia nigra. They reported no classic Pick bodies or cells.

More recently Munoz-Garcia and Ludwin (1984) described two cases with onset at age 29 and 30 years who had a more typical history of Pick's disease. They had frontotemporal atrophy with caudate atrophy, depigmentation of the substantia nigra and involvement of other subcortical nuclei. Pick bodies were scarce in the neocortex, absent from the hippocampus but common in subcortical nuclei. The authors comment that the argentophilic inclusions were dissimilar from their classic cases and proposed a subtype: the generalized variant of Pick's disease for these and similar cases. These young onset cases bear little resemblance to many other cases of Pick's disease except for the presence of Pick cells and bodies and it seems possible that they represent a separate disorder (or disorders).

PROGRESSIVE SUBCORTICAL GLIOSIS

Progressive subcortical gliosis was first described under the name Pick's disease type 2 by Neumann, but later reclassified separately (Neumann and Cohn, 1967). There have been a number of other case reports of similar patients. The generalized atrophy, absence of Pick cells and Pick bodies and severe subcortical gliosis all suggest that this is probably a separate disease with the gliosis as a primary pathology. There have been a number of intermediate cases which have been classified by a number of authors, as cases of Pick's disease (von Braunmuhl, 1928). Familial cases have also been described (Khoubesserian et al, 1985; Lanska et al, 1991).

DIFFERENTIAL DIAGNOSIS

There are a number of other neurodegenerative syndromes which show similarities to Pick's disease and there are potential areas of overlap between these. The lack of precise diagnostic criteria for Pick's disease compounds these problems. Frontal lobe degeneration of the non-Alzheimer type FLD is discussed in detail in Chapter 5. There are marked similarities in the clinical features of 'frontal lobe' Pick's disease and FLD. The proportion of familial cases compared to classical Pick's disease appears higher: about 50% of patients with FLD have a positive family history of dementia (Neary et al, 1988; Brun, 1987; Gustafson, 1987). The major distinction from Pick's disease is the absence of both Pick cells and Pick bodies microscopically (but, as noted previously, over half the reported cases of Pick's disease have neither Pick cells nor Pick bodies). There are a number of case reports in the literature which were identified as a type of Pick's disease but show similarities to FLD. A recent example of this is the four patients in et al, 1988; Brun, 1987; Gustafson, 1987). The major distinction from Pick's disease is the absence of both Pick cells and Pick bodies microscopically (but, as noted previously, over half the reported cases of Pick's disease have neither Pick cells nor Pick bodies). There are a number of case reports in the literature which were identified as a type of Pick's disease but show similarities to FLD. A recent example of this is the four patients in Constantinidis' subtype C2, although in these the gliosis may be more pronounced (Constantinidis, 1985). Both groups have reported (Gustafson, 1987; Neary et al, 1988) FLD to be relatively common, up to 20% of all presenile dementias. This may be due to regional clustering but it seems more likely that FLD represents a reasonably common but hitherto under-reported dementia.

Gydesen and co-workers (1987) reported a large family with a non-specific dementia with 15 affected members in three generations. The pattern of atrophy reported was variable but always included frontal lobe atrophy. Kim et al (1981) reported four siblings who also had a non-specific dementia with a predominantly frontal atrophy. There is no clear distinguishing feature from FLD in the description of these families, although the frontal preponderance may be less marked. The term Kraepelin's dementia has been used to describe non-specific familial dementia but is now little used (Schaumberg and Suzuki, 1968).

Corticobasal degeneration (see Chapter 10) was first described by Rebeiz et al (1968); since then, additional cases have been reported (Gibb et al, 1989; Sawle et al, 1991). The majority of cases present with an asymmetrical motor syndrome such as a focal dystonia or the alien limb syndrome. The disease is progressive and patients develop other features which can include a supranuclear gaze palsy, parkinsonism and mild cerebellar signs; some patients develop dementia. Pathological examination reveals frontoparietal atrophy with cortical cell loss, gliosis, Pick cells and corticobasal inclusion bodies in the substantia nigra. The described cases are a clearly distinct clinical and pathological entity. However Gibb et al (1989) have pointed out similarities between two cases previously described as Pick's disease and their cases of corticobasal degeneration, and it is possible that intermediate forms exist.

Morris et al (1984) described a family with a novel dementia affecting ten individuals in three generations. The disease presents with an insidious onset with memory deficits, dysphasia and behavioural changes. Bulimia and extrapyramidal features occur in most but not all individuals. Post-mortem examination revealed generalized atrophy affecting particularly the frontal and anterior temporal lobes. There was substantial nerve cell loss with spongiform degeneration and gliosis. There were no Pick cells or Pick bodies but neuritic plaques similar to those seen in Alzheimer's disease were found. The authors christened the disease hereditary dysphasic dementia. The macroscopic neuropathological appearance is reminiscent of Pick's disease and it is notable that the left side is predominantly affected, as it is in the majority of cases of asymmetrical Pick's disease. The presence of neuritic plaques in the absence of Pick cells and Pick bodies clearly distinguishes it from Pick's disease. The authors suggest that this disease cases of Pick's disease. Although modern opinion would place these as Alzheimer's disease, they represent an interesting subgroup.

Whilst it is not unusual for cases of Pick's disease to have a few plaques and tangles there are several reports of mixed Alzheimer's and Pick's pathology (e.g. Berlin, 1949; Smith and Lantos, 1983). Berlin's first case had focal anterior temporal and frontal atrophy. There were numerous Pick cells and Pick bodies but also numerous argentophilic plaques. The changes were most severe in the hippocampus. His second case had generalized atrophy with temporal accentuation. There were numerous Pick cells with extensive Alzheimer type changes and gliosis. There are two possible explanations for these and similar cases. The first is that Alzheimer's disease is sufficiently common (particularly in older patients) to occur in association with Pick's disease by chance. An alternative explanation is that either Pick's pathology or Alzheimer's pathology are not disease specific.

Mesulam (1982) reported a series of patients with progressive aphasia and focal cortical atrophy (see Chapter 6). A number of histopathological substrates may be associated with the syndrome of progressive aphasia, of which Pick bodies is one. Cole et al (1979) published an abstract in which they described a large family in which ten individuals suffered from a similar disorder. This was described by them as Pick's disease, although the pathology was non-specific.

Examination of a large family with the 144 bp insertion in the prion protein gene shows that there can be a wide clinical and pathological variation with prion disease (Collinge et al, 1992) including a patient with non-specific pathology (Collinge et al, 1990). However, despite the occurrence of Pick bodies and Pick cells in experimental and natural prion disease there have been no reports of a prion protein gene mutation causing typical neuropathologically verified Pick's disease.

There have been a number of reports of combined Pick's disease and motor neurone disease (e.g. Brion et al, 1982). The most striking of these is the family reported by Constantinidis (1987) with four affected members in two generations. The clinical and pathological features are a mixture of the two syndromes, with Pick cells but no Pick bodies.

CONCLUSIONS

Arnold Pick avoided many potential problems when he concentrated his pathological description of Pick's disease on macroscopic appearances. Reviewing the work of the intervening century it seems sensible to regard Pick's disease as a syndrome of lobar atrophy rather than a single disease. Pick cells and Pick bodies do not appear to be either sensitive or specific indicators of Pick's disease, although the possibility exists that they represent a subset of cases—the 'true' Pick's disease—more reliably. Van Mansvelt's thesis, published nearly 40 years ago, argued that the name Pick's disease should be changed to Pick's syndrome. There is now, I think, overwhelming evidence to support this view. The lack of a specific marker has led to frustration amongst clinicians, summarized by Sim and Bale (1973): 'To say that a patient with most of the clinical and laboratory features of non-Alzheimer's disease but with a positive histology for Pick's disease is suffering from Pick's disease, and that those with similar clinical and laboratory features are not, does not help in the elucidation of the various clinical varieties which go to make up the non-Alzheimer group of primary pre-senile dementias. If histological authority is to be maintained in the diagnosis of Pick's disease it should rest on a more secure clinico-pathological relationship. If a similar situation existed in cancer pathology where a 'positive' histology was found in only a small percentage of similar clinical syndromes, the histology would be discredited.'

Whilst this view is understandable it is a little unfair on neuropathologists; we do not expect a pathologist to be more than a guide to the cause of cirrhosis of the liver or a myopathy. What is lacking in the Pick's syndrome of diseases is knowledge of the aetiology of the diseases, not neuropathological skill.

In both Alzheimer's disease and prion disease the identification of an abnormal deposition of a protein provided the clue to the aetiology of the diseases, however no such protein has been found in Pick's disease. Moreover the probable heterogeneous nature of Pick's disease creates difficulties in its study. In the absence of specific clinical, investigational or pathological features it is only when studying the members of one family with a similar phenotype that one can be confident that one is studying a single disease. The identification of the causative gene in the familial form(s) of Pick's disease is the most direct way to unravel the pathogenesis of Pick's disease.

Van Mansvelt summarized his findings and the prospects for Pick's disease in 1954: 'We believe the genotype of the clinico-anatomical syndrome of Pick to be a highly pleomorphic one containing probably genes which play a part in other heredo-degenerative affections. If we want to trace the essential causes of this syndrome a very close co-operation between clinician, neuropathologist, biochemist and geneticist will be imperative.'

This statement still stands today. The major difference is that many of the tools needed to tackle the problems of Pick's syndrome have been developed and this work can now start.

REFERENCES

Alzheimer A (1911) Über eigenartige Krankheitsfalle des späteren Alters. *Zeitschrift für die Gesamte Neurologie und Psychiatrie* **4**: 356–385.
Ball MJ (1979) Topography of Pick inclusion bodies in hippocampi of demented patients. A quantitative study. *Journal of Neuropathology and Experimental Neurology* **38**: 614–620.
Berlin L (1949) Presenile sclerosis (Alzheimer's disease) with features resembling Pick's disease. *Archives of Neurology and Psychiatry* **61**: 369–384.
Berrios GE (1991) Other forms of dementia. In Berrios GE & Freeman HL (eds) *Alzheimer and the Dementias*, pp 89–99. London: Royal Society of Medicine. London.
Brion S, Mikol J & Psimaras A (1973) Recent findings in Pick's disease. In Zimmerman HM (ed.) *Progress in Neuropathology*, vol. 11, pp 421–452. New York and London: Grune and Stratton.

Brun A (1987) Frontal lobe degeneration of non-Alzheimer type. 1. Neuropathology. *Archives of Gerontology and Geriatrics* **6:** 193–208.

Clark AW, Manz HJ, White CL et al (1986) Cortical degeneration with swollen chromatolytic neurons: its relationship to Pick's disease. *Journal of Neuropathology and Experimental Neurology* **45:** 268–284.

Cole M, Wright D & Baker BD (1979) Familial aphasia due to Pick's disease. *Annals of Neurology* **6:** 58–179.

Collinge J, Owen F, Poulter M et al (1990) Prion dementia without characteristic pathology. *Lancet* **336:** 7–9.

Collinge J, Brown J, Hardy J et al (1992) Inherited prion disease with 144 base pair gene insertion. II: Clinical and pathological features. *Brain* **115:** 687–710.

Constantinidis J (1987) Family syndrome: association of Pick's disease and amyotrophic lateral sclerosis. *Encephale* **13:** 285–293.

Constantinidis J, Richard J & Tissot R (1985) Pick dementia: anatomoclinical correlations and pathophysiological considerations. *Interdisciplinary Topics in Gerontology* **19:** 72–97.

Corsellis JAN (1976) Pick's disease. In Blackwood W & Corseillis JAN (eds) *Greenfield's Neuropathology*, 3rd edn, pp 987–992. London: Edward Arnold.

Cummings JL & Duchen LW (1981) Kluver–Bucy syndrome in Pick's disease: clinical and pathologic correlations. *Neurology* **31:** 1415–1422.

Ehmann WD, Alauddin M, Hossain T & Markesbery WR (1984) Brain trace elements in Pick's disease. *Annals of Neurology* **15:** 102–104.

Escourolle R (1956) *La maladie de Pick. Etude critique d'ensemble et synthèse anatomo-clinique.* MD Thesis, Paris: Foulton.

Folstein MF, Folstein SE & McHugh PR (1975) 'Mini-mental state': a practical method of grading the cognitive state of patients for the clinician. *Journal of Psychiatric Research* **12:** 189–198.

Forno LS, Eng LF & Selkoe DJ (1989) Pick bodies in the locus coeruleus. *Acta Neuropathologica (Berlin)* **79:** 7–10.

Gans A (1923) Betrachtungen uber Art und Ausbreitung des krankhaften Prozesses in einem Fall von Pickscher Atrophie des Stirnhirns, *Zeitschrift für die Gesamte Neurologie und Psychiatrie* **80:** 10–28.

Gibb WRG, Luthert P & Marsden CD (1989) Corticobasal degeneration. *Brain* **112:** 1171–1192.

Gordon EB & Sim M (1967) The EEG in presenile dementia. *Journal of Neurology, Neurosurgery and Psychiatry* **30:** 285–291.

Groen JJ & Endtz LJ (1982) Hereditary Pick's disease: second re-examination of a large family and discussion of other hereditary cases, with particular reference to electroencephalography and computerized tomography. *Brain* **105:** 443–459.

Grünthal E (1931) Klinisch-genealogischer Nachweis von Erblichkeit bei Pickscher Krankheit. *Zeitschrift für die Gesamte Neurologie und Psychiatrie* **136:** 464.

Gustafson L (1987) Frontal lobe degeneration of non-Alzheimer type. II. Clinical picture and differential diagnosis. *Archives of Gerontology and Geriatrics* **6:** 209–223.

Gydesen S, Hagen S, Klinken L, Abelskov J & Sorensen SA (1987) Neuropsychiatric studies in a family with presenile dementia different from Alzheimer and Pick disease. *Acta Psychiatrica Scandinavica* **76:** 276–284.

Hansen LA, Deteresa R, Tobias H, Alford M & Terry RD (1988) Neocortical morphometry and cholinergic neurochemistry in Pick's disease. *American Journal of Pathology* **131:** 507–518.

Heston LL (1978) The clinical genetics of Pick's disease. *Acta Psychiatrica Scandinavica* **57:** 202–206.

Hori A, Volles E, Witzke R & Spaar FW (1983) Pick's disease of early onset with neurological symptomatology, rapid course and nigrostriatal degeneration. *Clinical Neuropathology* **2:** 8–15.

Horoupian DS & Dickson DW (1991) Striatonigral degeneration, olivopontocerebellar atrophy and 'atypical' Pick's disease. *Acta Neuropathologica (Berlin)* **81:** 287–295.

Kanazawa I, Kwak S, Sasaki H et al (1988) Studies on neurotransmitter markers of the basal ganglia in Pick's disease, with special reference to dopamine reduction. *Journal of the Neurological Sciences* **83:** 63–74.

Khoubesserian P, Davous P, Bianco C et al (1985) Familial dementia of the Neumann type (subcortical gliosis). *Revue Neurologique* **141:** 706–712.

Kim RC, Collins GH, Parisi JE et al (1981) Familial dementia of adult onset with pathological findings of a 'non-specific nature'. *Brain* **104**: 61–78.

Kluver H & Bucy P (1939) Preliminary analysis of functions of the temporal lobe in monkeys. *Archives of Neurology and Psychiatry* **42**: 979–1000.

Knopman DS, Christensen KJ, Schut LJ et al (1989) The spectrum of imaging and neuropsychological findings in Pick's disease. *Neurology* **39**: 362–368.

Kosaka K, Ikeda K, Kobayashi K & Mehraein P (1991) Striatopallidonigral degeneration in Pick's disease: a clinico-pathological study of 41 cases. *Journal of Neurology* **238**: 151–160.

Lampert PW, Earle KM, Gibbs CJ & Gajdusek DC (1969) Experimental kuru encephalopathy in chimpanzees and spider monkeys. *Journal of Neuropathology and Experimental Neurology* **28**: 353–368.

Lanska DJ, Currier RD, Cohen M et al (1991) Familial progressive subcortical gliosis. *Journal of Neuropathology and Experimental Neurology* **50**: 305.

Lowe J, Blanchard A, Morrell K et al (1988) Ubiquitin is a common factor in intermediate filament inclusion bodies of diverse type in man, including those of Parkinson's disease, Pick's disease and Alzheimer's disease, as well as Rosenthal fibres in cerebellar astrocytomas, cytoplasmic inclusion bodies in muscle and mallory bodies in alcoholic liver disease. *Journal of Pathology* **155**: 9–15.

Löwenberg K, Boyd DA & Salon DD (1939) Occurrence of Pick's disease in early adult years. *Archives of Neurology and Psychiatry* **41**: 1004–1020.

Luers T & Spatz H (1957) Picksche Krankheit (progressive umschriebene Grosshirnatrophie). In Lubarsch O, Henke F & Roessle R (eds) *Handbuch der Speziellen Pathologischen Anatomie und Histologie*, vol. 13, Nervensystem, part 1, pp 614–716. Berlin: Springer.

McKhann G, Drachman D, Folstein M et al (1984) Clinical diagnosis of Alzheimer's disease: report of the NINCDS–ADRDA Work Group under the auspices of the Department of Health and Human Services Task Force on Alzheimer's Disease. *Neurology* **34**: 939–944.

Malamud N & Waggoner RW (1943) Genealogic and clinicopathologic study of Pick's disease. *Archives of Neurology and Psychiatry* **50**: 288–303.

Mesulam M-M (1982) Slowly progressive aphasia without generalized dementia. *Annals of Neurology* **11**: 592–598.

Mizukami K & Kosaka K (1989) Neuropathological study on the nucleus basalis of Meynert in Pick's disease. *Acta Neuropathologica (Berlin)* **78**: 52–56.

Morris JC, Cole M, Banker B & Wright D (1984) Hereditary dysphasic dementia and the Pick–Alzheimer spectrum. *Annals of Neurology* **16**: 455–466.

Moyano BA (1932) I. Enfermedad de Alzheimer. II. Atrofiade Pick. *Archivos Argentinos de Neurologica* **7**: 231–286.

Munoz-Garcia D & Ludwin SK (1984) Classic and generalized variants of Pick's disease: a clinicopathological, ultrastructural and immunocytochemical comparative study. *Annals of Neurology* **16**: 467–480.

Murayama S, Mori H, Ihara Y & Tomonaga M (1990) Immunocytological and ultrastructural studies of Pick's disease. *Annals of Neurology* **27**: 394–405.

Neary D, Snowdon JS, Northen B & Goulding P (1988) Dementia of frontal lobe type. *Journal of Neurology, Neurosurgery and Psychiatry* **51**: 353–361.

Neumann MA & Cohn R (1967) Progressive subcortical gliosis, a rare form of presenile dementia. *Brain* **90**: 405–418.

Onari K & Spatz H (1926) Anatomische Beiträge zur Lehre von der Pickschen umschriebene-Grosshirnrinden-Atrophie ('Picksche Krankheit'). *Zeitschrift für die Gesamte Neurologie und Psychiatrie* **101**: 470–511.

Pick A (1892) Uber die Beziehungen der senilen Hirnatrophie zur aphasie. *Prager Medizinische Wochenschrift* **17**: 165–167.

Pick A (1906) Uber einen weiteren Symptomencomplex im Rahmen der Dementia Senilis, bedingt durch umschriebene starkere Hirnatrophie (gemischte Apraxie). *Monatsschrift für Psychiatrie und Neurologie* **19**: 97–108.

Pogacar S & Rubio A (1982) Morphological features of Pick's disease and atypical Alzheimer's disease in Down's syndrome. *Acta Neuropathologica* **58**: 249–254.

Ramon y Cajal S (1959) In May RM (ed.) *Degeneration and Regeneration of the Nervous System*, vol. 2, p. 563. New York: Hafner.

Rebeiz JJ, Kolodny EH, Whitehouse PJ & Price DL (1968) Corticodentatonigral degeneration with neuronal achromasia. *Archives of Neurology* **18**: 20–33.

Rewcastle NB & Ball MJ (1968) Electron microscopic structure of the 'inclusion bodies' in Pick's disease. *Neurology* **18:** 1205–1213.

Risberg J & Gustafson L (1988) Regional cerebral blood flow in psychiatric disorders. In Knezevic S, Maximilian VA, Mubrin Z et al (eds) *Handbook of Regional Blood Flow.* New Jersey: Lawrence Erlbaum Associates.

Roberts GW, Gentleman SM, Lynch A & Graham DI (1991) Beta amyloid protein deposition in brain after head trauma. *Lancet* **338:** 1422–1423.

Salmon E & Franck G (1989) Positron emission tomographic study in Alzheimer's disease and Pick's disease. *Archives of Gerontology and Geriatrics* **1** (supplement): 241–247.

Sanders J, Schenk VWD & van Veen P (1939) *A Family with Pick's Disease.* Amsterdam: Koninkiljke Nederlandsche Akademie van Wetenschappen.

Sawle GV, Brooks DJ, Marsden CD & Frackowiak RSJ (1991) Corticobasal degeneration. A unique pattern of regional cortical oxygen hypermetabolism and striatal fluorodopa uptake demonstrated by positron emission tomography. *Brain* **114:** 541–556.

Schaumberg HH & Suzuki K (1968) Non-specific familial presenile dementia. *Journal of Neurology, Neurosurgery and Psychiatry* **31:** 479–486.

Schenk VWD (1959) Re-examination of a family with Pick's disease. *Annals of Human Genetics* **23:** 325–333.

Schneider C (1927) Uber Picksche Krankheit. *Monatsschrift für Psychiatrie und Neurologie* **65:** 230–275.

Schneider C (1929) Weitere Beitrage zur Lehre von der Pickschen Krankheit. *Zeitschrift für die Gesamte Neurologie und Psychiatrie* **120:** 340–384.

Schochet SS, Lampert PW & Lindenburg R (1968) Fine structure of Pick and Hirano bodies in a case of Pick's disease. *Acta Neuropathologica (Berlin)* **11:** 330–337.

Scicutella A & Davies P (1987) Marked loss of cerebral galactolipids in Pick's disease. *Annals of Neurology* **22:** 606–609.

Sim M & Bale RN (1973) Familial presenile dementia: the relevance of a histological diagnosis of Pick's disease. *British Journal of Psychiatry* **122:** 671–673.

Sjogren T, Sjogren H & Lindgren AGH (1952) Morbus Alzheimer and morbus Pick; a genetic, clinical and patho-anatomical study. *Acta Psychiatrica et Neurologica Scandinavica. Supplement* **82:** 1–152.

Sparks DL & Markesbery WR (1991) Altered serotinergic and cholinergic synaptic markers in Pick's disease. *Archives of Neurology* **48:** 796–799.

Smith DA & Lantos PL (1983) A case of combined Pick's disease and Alzheimer's disease. *Journal of Neurology, Neurosurgery and Psychiatry* **46:** 675–677.

Terry RD (1976) Dementia, a brief and selective review. *Archives of Neurology* **33:** 1–4.

Tissot R, Constantinidis J & Richard J (1985) Pick's Disease. In Fredericks JAM (ed.) *Handbook of Clinical Neurology*, vol. 2, no. 46, pp. 233–246. Amsterdam: Elsevier.

Tong Q (1990) Aetiology and pathology of 71 dementia patients during presenile and senile periods. *Chung-Hua I Hsueh Tsa Chih (Chinese Medical Journal)* **70:** 431–433.

Ulrich J, Haugh M, Anderton BA et al (1987) Alzheimer dementia and Pick's disease: Neurofibrillary tangles and Pick bodies are associated with identical phosphorylated neurofilament epitopes. *Acta Neuropathologica* **73:** 240–246.

Van Mansvelt J (1954) *Pick's Disease: A Syndrome of Lobar Cerebral Atrophy, Its Clinico-Anatomical and Histopathological Types.* Enschede: Loeff.

Verhaart WJC (1936) Über das Vorkommen der Pickschen Krankheit von Alzheimer bei den Malaien und Chinesen in Niederlandisch-ost-Indien. *Mededelingen van Dienst der Volksgezondheid in Nederlandisch-Indie* **25:** 341–345.

Von Braunmuhl A (1928) Zur Histopathologie der umschriebenen Grosshirnatrophie (Picksche Krankheit). *Virchows Archiv für Pathologische Anatomie und Physiologie und für Klinische Medizin* **270:** 448–486.

Warrington EK (1975) The selective impairment of semantic memory. *Quarterly Journal of Experimental Psychology* **27:** 635–657.

Wechsler AF (1977) Presenile dementia presenting as aphasia. *Journal of Neurology, Neurosurgery and Psychiatry* **40:** 303–305.

Wechsler AF, Verity MA, Rosenschein S et al (1982) Pick's disease: a clinical, computerized tomographic and histologic study with Golgi impregnation observations. *Archives of Neurology* **39:** 287–290.

White P, Goodhart M, Keet JP et al (1977) Neocortical cholinergic neurons in elderly people. *Lancet* **i**: 668–670.

Williams HW (1935) The peculiar cells of Pick's disease: their pathogenesis and distribution in disease. *Archives of Neurology and Psychiatry* **34**: 508–519.

Wisniewski HM, Coblentz JM & Terry RD (1972) Pick's disease: a clinical and ultrastructural study. *Archives of Neurology* **26**: 97–108.

Wood PL, Etienne P, Lal S et al (1983) A post mortem comparison of the cortical cholinergic system in Alzheimer's disease and Pick's disease. *Journal of Neurological Sciences* **62**: 211–217.

Yates CM, Simpson J, Maloney AFJ & Gordon A (1980) Neurochemical observations in a case of Pick's disease. *Journal of Neurological Sciences* **48**: 257–263.

Yoshimura N (1988) Olfactory bulb involvement in Pick's disease. *Acta Neuropathologica (Berlin)* **77**: 202–205.

Yoshimura N (1989) Topography of Pick body distribution in Pick's disease: a contribution to understanding the relationship between Pick's and Alzheimer's disease. *Clinical Neuropathology* **8**: 1–6.

5

Frontal lobe degeneration of non-Alzheimer type

LARS GUSTAFSON
ARNE BRUN
ULLA PASSANT

Epidemiological studies show that the majority of organic dementias are caused by Alzheimer's disease (AD), cerebrovascular disease or the combination of these two. Since a precise diagnosis requires pathological examination of the brain, the prevalence of less common primary degenerative dementia is mainly unknown or underestimated. In our long-term prospective study of dementing illnesses several hundred cases have accumulated. They have been studied from a psychiatric, neurological, neuroradiological, neurophysiological, neurochemical and neuropathological point of view. A total of 470 patients have so far (December 1991) been studied longitudinally until death. In about 350 (75%) cases detailed neuropathological investigations have been obtained. The primary degenerative dementia group was dominated by AD and by non-Alzheimer dementias with frontotemporal cortical degeneration. Alzheimer's disease accounted for about 50% of early as well as late onset dementia and frontotemporal cortical degeneration was diagnosed in about 12% of our first 150 deceased cases dominated by early onset dementia (Brun, 1987).

The distribution of cortical degeneration in the frontotemporal cortical degeneration group deviated clearly from the majority of AD cases, as did the histopathology. There was a frontal or frontotemporal and anterior cingulate gyrus predominance of the cortical damage (Brun and Gustafson, 1978; Brun, 1987), a pattern almost inverse to the mainly temporoparietal and posterior cingulate gyrus involvement in AD (Brun and Gustafson, 1976). Surprisingly, only four of the first 20 frontotemporal cortical degeneration cases had Pick's disease, which is however in accordance with the frequency of 2–3% found in most series. Sixteen cases lacking Pick or Alzheimer features were, after some hesitation, presented as a separate clinicopathological entity. We suggested the designation 'frontal lobe degeneration of non-Alzheimer type' (FLD) and neuropathological, clinical, neuropsychological and regional cerebral blood flow (rCBF) findings were presented at the Non-Alzheimer Frontal Lobe Dementia meeting in Lund in 1986 (Brun, 1987; Gustafson, 1987; Risberg, 1987; Englund and Brun, 1987; Johanson and Hagberg, 1989). Other research groups are working with similar clinical materials, and a large study of 'dementia of frontal lobe type' has been published by Neary and his colleagues in Manchester.

Neary et al (1988) presented clinical findings in seven patients with primary degenerative dementia of frontal lobe type without AD or vascular brain lesions. All patients had single photon emission computerized tomography (SPECT) evidence of anterior hemisphere damage. During a 2 year period 26 patients were diagnosed as 'dementia of frontal lobe type'. Eleven patients were female and 15 were male. A family history of dementia in a first-degree relative was recorded in 46% of the cases. The mean age at onset of symptoms of dementia was 54 ± 6.7 years (range 42–65 years). Neary et al described a clinical picture characterized by early and progressive changes in personality, with inappropriate and disinhibited behaviour, lack of insight and stereotyped speech, while spatial ability was better preserved. There was a striking similarity between the clinical picture, electroencephalography (EEG) and SPECT results in these patients and the findings in our FLD cases.

The relationship between FLD and Pick's disease is still an open question in spite of certain important clinical and pathological similarities. The vast literature on the variability of clinical and histopathological findings in Pick's disease has in many ways anticipated clinical and pathological questions regarding frontal lobe dementia in a wider sense. Constantinidis et al (1974) reported lobar atrophy without neuronal swellings and argyrophilic inclusions in one-third of a 'typical Pick material'. The clinical picture in these cases ($n = 12$) with moria or pathological joking, bipolar mood changes, bulimia and the PES (palilalia, echolalia, stereotyped activity) syndrome but less extrapyramidal signs show similarity to our FLD cases. A general conclusion in the study was that clinical differences in dementia are mainly due to the localization of brain damage and are not explained by the structural differences. This is in agreement with the difficulties encountered in the clinical differentiation between FLD and Pick's disease (Gustafson, 1987). The distinction has to be confirmed with neuropathological examination and genetic evidence. To our knowledge FLD and Pick's have not been diagnosed in the same family.

Clark et al (1986) found 70 cases with AD and 22 cases with primary degenerative dementia without Alzheimer pathology in a consecutive autopsy series. The majority of these cases showed frontal and/or temporal cortical atrophy. The pathological diagnosis was Pick's disease in six cases, cortical degeneration with frontal accentuation and motor neurone disease in two cases, hippocampal and temporal lobe sclerosis in three cases (in two cases with moderate or marked frontal atrophy), and non-specific degeneration or other disorders in the remaining seven cases. Thus non-Alzheimer frontal lobe pathology was common among the primary degenerative dementia cases.

Knopman et al (1990) described 14 cases with a dementing illness termed 'dementia lacking distinctive histology', selected from 460 dementia patients referred to a brain bank for brain autopsy between 1980 and 1986. The minimum criteria for diagnosis were: (1) frontal and temporal or parietal neocortical cell loss and astrocytosis; (2) subcortical cell loss and astrocytosis involving at least the substantia nigra; and (3) absence of or rare senile plaques and neurofibrillary tangles and no Pick or Lewy bodies. These cases comprised 10% of the brain bank patients below 70 years of age, and 3% of all demented patients referred to the bank. By comparison, 6.8% of cases under age 70 years at death and 3% of all cases suffered from Pick's disease, and Lewy body disease was diagnosed in 5.6% of all cases, mostly over 70 years at death. Personality changes with early loss of insight, mood changes and emotional lability with inappropriate laughing and/or crying were frequently reported. The changes of personality and behaviour sometimes overshadowed the progressive cognitive failure, although memory failure, dyscalculia and language and speech disturbances were often reported. Motor disturbances were not prominent, but later on most cases developed rigidity, masked facies, gait disturbance, dysgraphia, dysarthria and even anarthria. Speech disturbances such as logorrhoea, echolalia, palilalia and mutism were also reported. These patients thus fall within the same clinical framework as FLD. The first symptoms of the cases described by Knopman et al (1990) appeared before 70 years of age. The course was comparatively rapid, with death within 5 years in five cases, in three of these with indications of motor neurone loss.

Most reports on dementia of frontal lobe type present only few cases with a complete clinical and pathological report. Kim et al (1981) described a family with four or possibly five siblings of both sexes affected by progressive dementia and cerebral atrophy of non-specific type with frontal predominance. Changes of personality, tearfulness, reduced verbal fluency, loss of recent memory, and dyscalculia were characteristic features and all cases eventually developed gait disturbance and mutism. The cortical involvement was, however, more widespread than in FLD in general and also involved the dorsomedial thalamic nucleus and the hippocampus.

It is difficult to estimate the true prevalence of FLD in an unselected dementia population. Neary (1990) drew the conclusion that as many as 20% of patients with presenile dementia suffer from FLD. A survey of our own data from 470 deceased dementia cases showed that 54 (11%) were diagnosed clinically as suffering from FLD or Pick's disease. Among 349 cases with full neuropathological examination, five cases (1.4%) had Pick's disease and 28 cases (8%) were diagnosed as FLD, in two cases in combination with motor neurone disease. We have at present more than 40 patients in our longitudinal study who are diagnosed clinically and with brain imaging methods.

A connection between dementia of frontal lobe type and amyotrophic lateral sclerosis (ALS) has been shown in several studies (Wikström et al, 1982; Mitsuyama, 1985; Morita et al, 1987). Personality changes and language dysfunction may appear early in ALS-dementia, offering an interesting differential diagnostic alternative to FLD, especially since the histopathological changes are of a similar type and distribution.

NEUROPATHOLOGY

The neuropathology of FLD has been analysed with subserial whole brain coronal sectioning, allowing extensive mapping of brain changes with respect to topography, severity and type, together with exclusion of other possible concomitant disorders (Brun, 1987). The pathological changes have also been validated against extensive neuropsychiatric and neuro-physiological investigations, which were repeated during the course of the disease.

On macroscopic examination the exterior as well as the brain slices were often unremarkable or showed at most a mild and never a circumscribed or severe cortical atrophy; brain weight was either normal or slightly reduced. A right–left asymmetry was observed in a few cases. Gross changes were never noted in the striate body, thalamus, amygdaloid nucleus or hippo-campus. Cases like these would probably have been dismissed as normal if lacking a well-documented clinical history of dementia.

Microscopical changes were virtually limited to the superior half of the cortex, laminae II and III showing a mild loss of neurones, with slight gliosis and microcavitation in laminae I–III. These changes were most severe in the frontal lobe convexity cortex and, when more advanced, also in the basal frontal gyri. In the majority of cases the degeneration also involved the anterior one-third of the temporal lobe, where the changes were often mild, and in some cases absent. These changes also involved the insula and anterior half of the cingulate gyrus, but in a few cases were found in the sensory motor area, and rarely in the parietal and occipital lobes. The amygdala, hippocampus, the nucleus basalis of Meynert, the globus pallidus and thalamus revealed these changes only occasionally and then slightly in the large majority of cases. The striate body showed either none or slight changes in most cases but moderately severe changes in a few.

This topographic pattern is supplemented by the absence of senile plaques and neurofibrillary tangles, with the exception of occasional changes in older cases. There were no Pick cells or inclusions including Lewy bodies and only occasional blood vessels with amyloid angiopathy, and again in older cases. There was thus no Alzheimer encephalopathy but in about half of the cases a few or a moderate number of diffuse deposits were shown by β-amyloid antibodies and Campbell's method. Dystrophic neurites in small numbers were found in a few cases with Gallyas' method but anti-ubiquitin immuno-histochemistry revealed no inclusions. These diffuse deposits are sometimes considered as possible forerunners of senile plaques but seem to be non-specific, since they are found in a variety of conditions, including normal ageing, without an increase of senile plaques beyond what is normal for old age. The substantia nigra was normal in the majority of cases but showed a mild to moderate loss of neurones in a few. The cerebellar cortex showed a slight loss of Purkinje cells, which, when prominent (in two cases), was combined with a slight loss of neurones in the inferior olive. In two cases there was a mild loss of spinal anterior horn neurones but no changes in the motor cortex. Prion protein could not be shown with anti-prion protein immunohistochemistry (kindly supplied by Dr S. Prusiner), whereas the method was positive in the Gerstmann–Sträussler–Scheinker syndrome and Creutzfeldt–Jakob disease.

In parallel with the distribution of the grey matter changes, the white matter exhibited a mild loss of myelin and slight astrocytic gliosis which, in a few cases, were also present in the occipital deep white matter (Englund and Brun, 1987). These changes may be connected with the neuronal loss. Alternatively, they may be independent and related to a mild fibrohyaline sclerosis of the penetrating arterioli and, as such, represent mild incomplete white matter infarction. The changes were on the whole inconspicuous and never accompanied by gliosis of the thalamus or inferior olives, as in progressive subcortical gliosis. Moreover, by contrast with progressive subcortical gliosis, there was only slight involvement of the deep cortical laminae.

Considering the clinical similarities between these cases and those of Pick's disease (see Chapter 4), it should be emphasized that the cortical atrophy in FLD was neither of the knife-blade type nor circumscribed, and furthermore did not selectively involve frontobasal regions or the striate body. In addition, neither ballooned neurones nor Pick bodies were seen. However, the latter may, according to Constantinidis (1974), be missing in a proportion of Pick cases and so a relationship between FLD and Pick's disease can still exist, depending upon the diagnostic criteria used. However, Pick cases, according to conventional diagnostic criteria, only make up a few per cent of our material.

Similarities also exist between FLD and ALS with dementia, with similar frontal cortical changes described (see Chapter 7) and two cases of ALS-dementia were found in our series. In addition to the cases of a condition identical with or closely similar to FLD (Neary et al, 1988), Neary et al (1990) have described further cases of ALS with dementia, lobar sclerosis or progressive language disorder due to lobar atrophy (Snowden et al, 1991). The latter had asymmetric lobar, mainly frontal cortical atrophy, with a histopathological overlap with FLD, and thus probably expands the family of disorders belonging to this group. Snowden et al (1989) also described a semantic dementia with circumscribed cerebral atrophy, histopathologically similar to FLD, and without Alzheimer pathology, although differences in distribution and circumscription of changes were more reminiscent of Pick's disease.

The cases described by Knopman et al (1990), under the heading of 'dementia lacking distinctive histologic features' (see above), involved microvaculation and gliosis but of a slightly different nature and location, with prominent changes in structures not usually afflicted in FLD, such as the hippocampal formation, thalamus and substantia nigra.

Green et al (1990), under the heading of progressive aphasia, reported a case without Alzheimer pathology but with changes similar to those in FLD, although with some differences. Clark et al (1986) included a case of primary degenerative dementia without Alzheimer pathology in a group of 'few or no specific abnormalities', again with a frontal predominance and with a possible relationship to FLD.

Prion disease has also been implicated in dementia without characteristic pathology (Collinge et al, 1990). In one case from the family with a 144 bp insert in the prion protein gene reported pathologically there were none of the changes described in FLD, although another case from the same family had a form of Creutzfeldt–Jakob disease, indicating a spectrum of changes from none to overt pathology (see Chapter 8). As stated above, our FLD cases were negative for antiprion protein immunohistochemistry, which revealed no positive amyloid plaques; diffuse prion staining may be more difficult to exclude but at present a prion aetiology appears less likely for FLD, considering the uniform though non-specific pathology found in the 26 cases of our original material. Clinically, our material of frontal dementia also included a few examples of Creutzfeldt–Jakob disease with a predominantly frontal involvement, but histopathologically clearly different from FLD, and these cases were prion protein positive (Brun, 1991).

In a survey of frontal and Alzheimer dementias Brion et al (1991) pointed out the possibility of using the glial reaction as shown by the glial fibrillary acidic protein (GFAP) method as a distinguishing marker between the various forms, including many of those listed in Table 1, although not

Table 1. Organic dementia with frontal features.

FLD and closely allied conditions
  Frontal lobe degeneration of non-Alzheimer type (FLD)
  ALS with frontal dementia
  Pick's disease
  Progressive language disorder due to lobar atrophy, semantic
    dementia, progressive aphasia, etc
  Dementia lacking distinctive histological features (some cases)

Other clinically similar disorders
  Progressive subcortical gliosis
  Rare familial forms (e.g. Kim et al, 1981)
  Prion dementia without characteristic pathology
  Creutzfeldt–Jakob disease with frontal emphasis
  Alzheimer's disease with frontal emphasis
  Progressive supranuclear palsy
  Selective incomplete white matter infarction
  Binswanger's disease—multi-infarct dementia with frontal emphasis
  Bilateral thalamic infarcts

specifically FLD. The difference between progressive subcortical gliosis and ALS would be more a matter of distribution of glial reaction, which itself is influenced by the duration of the disorder evoking a glial reaction.

The cases described by Kim et al (1981) belong to the group of non-specific, often mainly frontal dementias but the cortical pathology was more widespread and included the thalamus and hippocampus.

Other disorders such as AD with a frontal predominance, selective incomplete white matter infarction, which often predominates frontally, and Binswanger's disease with mainly frontal white matter widespread incomplete infarctions around small lacunae may clinically appear as FLD (Brun and Gustafson, 1991). Other disorders like bilateral thalamic infarcts and progressive supranuclear palsy may also show clinical similarities with

FLD, however they clearly differ neuropathologically. In many of these conditions further neuropsychiatric details will unveil the correct diagnosis.

From a neuropathological point of view FLD, as defined by Brun (1987) as one form of frontal dementia, can still be delineated from the majority of cases described under headings such as unspecific or uncharacteristic pathology. These cases show greater inhomogeneity than the FLD group, even if some cases may in fact represent true FLD. Other structurally related disorders may be ALS with dementia, lobar atrophy with progressive aphasia and Pick's disease, whereas many of the other forms show greater clinical than structural similarities (Table 1). FLD is thus by far the largest group, accounting for about 10% of our organic dementias, and with a consistent neuropathology both from a structural and topographic point of view.

NEUROCHEMISTRY

Little is known about neurochemical changes in FLD. The cortical regions involved in FLD have important connections with the dorsomedial thalamic nucleus and with ascending monoaminergic neurone systems (Lindvall and Björklund, 1983). The possibility of a transmitter failure might be supported by the Shy–Drager-like syndrome in one FLD case, and orthostatic hypotension in several other cases (Gustafson, 1987). Nigrostriatal dopamine deficiency has been reported in dementia combined with parkinsonism and motor neurone disease, in non-specific frontal cortical degeneration (Gilbert et al, 1988) and in Pick's disease (Kanazawa et al, 1988). Normal choline acetyltransferase (ChAT) activities in the brain were reported in the 'dementia lacking distinctive histology' group of Knopman et al (1990) and in frontal lobe degeneration with motor neurone disease (Clark et al, 1986). Minthon et al (1990a), analysing cerebrospinal fluid (CSF) levels of neuropeptide Y-like immunoactivity (NPY-LI) found significantly lower NPY-LI levels in AD than in cases of frontotemporal degeneration and in normals. The difference was largest between frontotemporal degeneration and AD, indicating a different involvement of NPY neurones. Several studies have documented reduced concentration of somatostatin-like immunoreactivity in the brain and in CSF in AD. Minthon et al (1991), confirming these results, also showed reduced CSF levels of somatostatin in frontotemporal degeneration compared with controls. There was no significant correlation between somatostatin-like immunoreactivity and duration of illness, indicating an early involvement of cortical somatostatin neurones in both AD and FLD. The delta-sleep-inducing-peptide (DSIP) (Minthon et al, 1990b) was slightly reduced in CSF from patients with AD and slightly increased in frontotemporal degeneration, with a wide range in the latter group. The differences between AD and frontotemporal degeneration in peptide expression might be related to differences in localization of the disease process or in the sequence in which different neurones are affected. Hopefully, CSF peptide analysis might improve the understanding and differential diagnoses of the primary degenerative dementias.

BRAIN IMAGING IN FLD

Computed tomography (CT) and magnetic resonance imaging (MRI) techniques are widely used for diagnosis of organic brain damage and diseases. Cortical atrophy with or without focal accentuation has been reported in degenerative dementia but very often the changes are non-specific, with an important overlap between normals and demented subjects

REPEATED RCBF MEASUREMENTS IN A PATIENT WITH TENTATIVE FLD

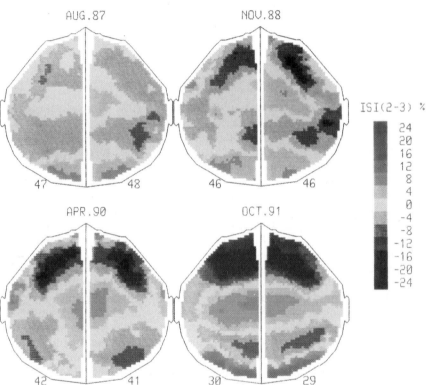

Figure 1. Topographic illustrations of cortical blood flow (vertex view), in a female patient with FLD. The frontal pole is shown at the top and the occipital pole at the bottom. The colours represent flow distribution values (ISI) (regional values as percentage of the hemispheric mean) as defined by the key on the right. These illustrations show a very clear and progressive decline of frontal blood flow. 1986: Age 61 years, poor concentration, anxious, apathetic and failed at work. 1987: Lack of insight, perseveration, moderate amnesia but preserved orientation. In August the CBF level was normal, but the flow distribution was pathological with a relative flow decrease in the frontal cortex. 1988: Emotional unconcern and social neglect. In November, CBF was unchanged, but an accentuation of the regional frontal flow decrease was seen. 1990: Restlessness, memory failure and semimutism. In April CBF was decreased by 11% with an additional accentuation of the frontal flow pathology. 1991: Mutism, amimia, aggressiveness, hyperphagia, auditory hallucinations, still capable of writing her name and date of birth. Further decrease to clearly subnormal CBF levels with a pronounced frontal flow pathology.

(Creasey et al, 1986). The differentiation between vascular and primary degenerative changes is also difficult. CT and MRI may show white matter low attenuation in vascular dementia but also frequently in AD, due to the presence of selective incomplete white matter infarctions in about two-thirds of AD patients (Brun and Englund, 1986). The recognition of vascular lesions is of great clinical importance, since frontal grey and white matter lesions, as well as subcortical strategic infarcts, may cause dementia with frontal lobe clinical features (Brun and Gustafson, 1991; Miller et al, 1991a). CT and MRI may, however, contribute to the differentiation between AD and frontotemporal degeneration based on the anterior–posterior gradient of the atrophic changes. CT and MRI findings in 14 patients with AD (mean age 64 years) and nine frontotemporal degeneration cases (mean age 61 years) showed cortical atrophy in all AD cases, with parietal predominance in eight cases and frontal predominance in one case only (Gustafson et al, 1989). Seven out of the nine frontotemporal degeneration cases showed cortical atrophy, with a frontal accentuation in four cases and postcentral predominance in one case. CT and MRI revealed white matter changes in eight AD cases and four frontotemporal degeneration cases. Regional cerebral blood flow (rCBF) was measured in 23 degenerative dementia cases with the non-invasive ^{133}Xe inhalation technique (Risberg et al, 1990) and showed the characteristic frontal flow pathology in all frontotemporal degeneration cases and temporoparietal accentuation of the flow decrease in all AD cases. Other studies have shown less conclusive CT and MRI findings in dementia of frontal lobe type (Knopman et al, 1989, 1990; Miller et al, 1991b).

We have reasons to believe that functional brain imaging such as rCBF and SPECT are sensitive to the brain dysfunction at an early stage of degenerative dementia. Data from our longitudinal study have shown excellent agreement between rCBF and the pattern of cortical degeneration (Gustafson et al, 1977; Risberg et al, 1990). Temporoparietal flow pathology is found early in AD and contrasts strongly with the flow abnormalities in frontotemporal areas in FLD and Pick's disease (Gustafson et al, 1985; Risberg, 1987). Repeated rCBF measurements in patients with FLD and Pick's disease have shown progress of the flow pathology in prefrontal areas (Risberg, 1987; Gustafson et al, 1990). However, AD patients with marked frontal lobe symptoms and pathology showed low frontal as well as low parietal flow values. Frontal rCBF was also reduced in two cases with Creutzfeldt–Jakob disease with frontal lobe degeneration, while fluctuating hypofrontality was found in a patient with thalamic infarcts (Risberg, 1987). Frontal rCBF pathology might be found in different types of organic dementia, usually in good agreement with the frontal lobe symptom pattern (Brun and Gustafson, 1991). The clinical usefulness of rCBF for diagnosis and follow-up of dementia is illustrated in Figure 1.

Brain imaging techniques such as positron emission tomography (PET) and SPECT have confirmed the patterns of cortical hypometabolism shown with rCBF measurements. These three-dimensional techniques give additional information about the white matter and subcortical structures (Friedland et al, 1983; Tyrrell et al, 1990). Chase et al (1987) used PET to differentiate between dementia with anterior and posterior types of cortical degeneration. SPECT studies have also shown frontal and temporal hypoperfusion in FLD, with relative sparing of parietal and occipital blood flow (Jagust et al, 1989; Kitamura et al, 1990; Miller et al, 1991b). Jagust et al (1989) found diminished perfusion in orbitofrontal, dorsolateral frontal and temporal cortex in FLD patients compared with controls, while AD patients showed low perfusion in the temporal and parietal cortex. Frontal lobe hypometabolism has also been shown with PET in patients with progressive supranuclear palsy by D'Antona et al (1985) and Goffinet et al (1989), and in patients with Pick's disease (Kamo et al, 1987).

The differential diagnosis between early stages of FLD and Huntington's disease may be difficult when personality changes and psychotic features dominate the clinical picture. However CT scan and MRI may show a gradual loss of the heads of the caudate nuclei and PET may be an early predictor of the development of the disease (Mazziotta, 1989). Kuhl et al (1982) found a metabolic decrease in frontal relative to parietal cortex in Huntington patients with a duration of disease of more than 6 years.

ELECTROPHYSIOLOGY

Patients with frontotemporal dementia often have a normal or only mildly abnormal EEG, which may remain so even when the signs of dementia are marked (Johannesson et al, 1977). By contrast, the proportion of abnormal EEGs approaches 100% in neuropathologically verified AD cases. In Down's syndrome dementia, the EEG pathology appears at the same time as the first symptoms of dementia (Johanson et al, 1991). Recent studies indicate that the distribution of somatosensory-evoked potentials in AD is different from other organic dementias and from normals (Maurer et al, 1988). The use of topographic displays of frequency analysed EEG seems to re-establish the EEG technique as an important tool for diagnosis and evaluation of treatment in dementia. In a pilot study Rosén et al (1992) investigated somatosensory evoked potentials in patients with AD, frontotemporal degeneration and multi-infarct dementia. The frontotemporal degeneration cases showed only a moderate delay of the precentral N30 component, while the AD group showed an enhanced N20–P25 wave of normal latency, followed by a pathologically delayed parietal P45 response. Other studies have confirmed the high prevalence of normal EEGs in dementia of frontal lobe type (Neary et al, 1988; Knopman et al, 1990), in contrast to the common EEG pathology in AD and Creutzfeldt–Jakob disease. Sleep studies have supplied EEG criteria that might help to discriminate AD from Pick's disease and other dementias and from normal patients (Blois et al, 1989).

CLINICAL FEATURES

The following description is based mainly on clinical observations of patients in whom the FLD diagnosis has been confirmed by a detailed post-mortem examination. Clinical findings in patients followed for several years until death but lacking post-mortem confirmation and patients still alive are also considered. The FLD diagnosis was strongly supported by functional and/or structural brain imaging.

FLD is a progressive brain disease with its early manifestations in the presenium. The mean age at onset in our FLD material was 56 ± 7.6 years (range 45–70 years) and the total duration of the illness had a wide range of 3 to 17 years (mean 8.1 ± 3.4 years). The duration is somewhat shorter than in Pick's disease 10.5 ± 6 years (range 4–17 years) and presenile AD 10.6 ± 3 years (range 5–16 years) in the long-term study. This is in accordance with the age characteristics in other studies (Neary et al, 1988; Knopman et al, 1990).

The clinical manifestations usually start insidiously and develop slowly. The early stage is dominated by changes and deterioration of personality, behaviour and speech, and less by cognitive deterioration, although memory failure and lack of concentration are almost always found. The constellation of symptoms and impairments indicates a frontal lobe and/or temporal lobe dysfunction at this early stage of the disease. The most common features are presented in Table 2.

In FLD, changes of emotional and behavioural characteristics are always present and may stand out as non-specific manifestations and be difficult to interpret as expressions of an organic brain disease. Other explanations such as a reaction to external problems or family affairs may be suggested, especially by people lacking previous knowledge of the patient. However,

Table 2. Clinical findings in frontal lobe degeneration of non-Alzheimer type.

Insidious onset and slow progression

Changes of personality
    Disinhibition—social neglect
    Blunting of emotions
    Lack of insight and judgement
    Irritability—restlessness
    Anxiety—euphoria
    Apathy

Dissolution of language
    Progressively reduced speech
    Stereotyped phrases
    Echolalia
    Mutism—amimia

Depressive episodes
Hypochondriasis—symptoms of pain
Deceptions—delusions

Changes of oral/dietary behaviour
Stereotyped behaviour

Memory, receptive speech and spatial functions comparatively spared
Dyscalculia
Intermittent dyspraxia
Epileptic seizures less common
Syncopal attacks

even for close relatives it may be difficult to decide when the first signs of the dementing disease appeared and therefore its duration may easily be underestimated.

Signs of disinhibition, lack of judgement, emotional unconcern and lack of insight into ill-health are found early in FLD. The impaired control and modulation of emotions are seen as tearfulness, inadequate smiling and spells of crying and laughing, later developing into hypomimia.

The early emotional changes in FLD are often described as shallowness, bluntness and lack of insight and its consequences. The patient becomes self-centred, less concerned about family and friends, who often describe the patient as uninterested and emotionally cold. The emotional tuning may be that of euphoria or moria (pathological joking), sometimes combined with inappropriate talkativeness and confabulation, but true Witzelsucht or pathological punning is rare. Stereotyped smiling and giggling, when present, seem less related to elated mood than to impaired control of emotional expression. The patient's emotional changes and unpredictable behaviour may easily lead to conflicts with, and even rejection from, the family and society, at least as long as no reasonable explanation is offered. One consequence of the diagnostic process is the opportunity to explain and understand the patient's strange behaviour. It is important to relieve the pressure on the family by psychological and social support, legal advice and, when necessary, hospital care for diagnosis and treatment of the patient. The severe strain will easily cause mental ill health among relatives, economic problems and even divorce and suicide in the family. Complications of this type are uncommon in families with an Alzheimer patient.

Craving for affection and sexual contact may become more frequent and easily provoked. Usually the expressions of sexual disinhibition are rather childish and innocent and possible to divert. Other signs of disinhibition such as irritability and explosive temper may cause conflicts and quarrels and even provoke acts of violence. Unrestrained behaviour, such as impulse buying, gambling and shoplifting, have led to social and economic crises.

Restlessness and an irresistible impulse to explore the environment are often observed at interview. The patient stands up, moves around, touches and tries to use various objects on sight. This behaviour shows important similarities to the 'hypermetamorphosis' or distractibility of the Klüver–Bucy syndrome, especially when oral exploration is used. This 'utilization behaviour' in patients with focal lesions in the frontal lobes has been described by Lhermitte et al (1986). The other components of the Klüver–Bucy syndrome in man (Pilleri, 1966), disinhibited oral behaviour and blunting of drive and emotions, are also prevalent in FLD. Changes of oral/dietary behaviour, such as excessive smoking, drinking, and eating with preference for special foods, were observed in about 30% of our FLD cases. The Klüver–Bucy syndrome in AD is usually less complete than in FLD, supporting the suggestion that frontal as well as temporal lobe involvement is needed to produce the syndrome in man (Brun and Gustafson, 1976).

Two serious consequences of disinhibition and lack of judgement in FLD are traffic accidents and changes of drinking behaviour, the latter also considered a change of oral/dietary behaviour. FLD patients may continue to drive their cars after clinical onset of the dementia. Although still driving on the correct side of the road, they tend to be inattentive and careless. They may exceed speed limits, neglect traffic lights and overtake dangerously. FLD patients usually remember these events and agree that their driving has changed lately, which does not mean that they judge their behaviour to be strange or to indicate ill health. By contrast the typical AD patient is more self-critical, anxiously aware of difficulties in driving. The left–right insecurity in AD is easily revealed in Sweden since most elderly people learned to drive before 1967, when Sweden changed to right-hand traffic. In addition, FLD patients may display more direct errors or difficulties in handling the driving situation. This might be an expression of the 'inter-mittent dyspraxia' described in FLD and Pick's disease (Mallison, 1947). Changes of drinking behaviour were reported in several patients with FLD. Patients who previously had a normal alcohol consumption started to drink more frequently and in larger quantities than before. In some cases alcohol was probably used to reduce anxiety or depressed mood. The tendency to pathological drinking could often be controlled by a firm attitude from the relatives.

The emotional changes in FLD can be difficult to differentiate from affective disorders. Elated mood, especially when associated with voluble speech and signs of disinhibition, may be mistaken for a hypomanic or manic state. Restlessness and agitation might also give a strong impression of anxiety and, when coupled to deceptions and delusions, might lead to the diagnosis of schizophrenia. FLD patients may sometimes describe, mostly short-lasting, deep depressions with suicidal thoughts. Slowly developing apathy and social withdrawal in combination with sparse mimical movements and reduced speech may be misdiagnosed as a non-organic major depression. None of our verified cases committed suicide, although suicide was suspected in one verified case and in one additional case lacking neuropathology.

Most patients with FLD denied any awareness of an illness and saw very little reason for a medical examination. In spite of this, several patients asked for medical examination and treatment, complaining of various somatic symptoms, such as pain, combined with bizarre hypochondriacal ideas. In some cases the hypochondriasis was considered secondary to hallucinations or perceptual distortions.

Sensory deceptions (hallucinations and illusions) and delusions have been described in AD and Pick's disease, although the reported frequencies vary markedly between studies (Eiden and Lechner, 1950; Van Mansvelt, 1954; Burns et al, 1990). In our longitudinal study hallucinations and delusions were reported in about 20% of FLD and early onset AD cases and in 50% of the late onset AD group. In FLD hallucinations and delusions showed important clinical variability. The psychotic traits often gave the impression of functional psychosis, with schizophrenia as an early tentative diagnosis (Gustafson, 1987; Neary et al, 1988; Knopman et al, 1990). This mis-interpretation is likely when there is a combination of personality changes, delusions and language dysfunction of frontal lobe type. In FLD the psychotic symptoms are often bizarre and badly controlled. The combination with other frontal lobe symptoms makes it difficult to support and treat these patients with traditional psychological and pharmacological techniques. Due to communication problems the recognition of psychotic symptoms is often difficult. The association between psychosis and frontal lobe damage has also been described in AD and vascular dementia with degeneration and ischaemic white matter lesions in the frontal lobes (Brun and Gustafson, 1991; Miller et al, 1991a). Visual, auditory and tactile hallucinations are reported in FLD as well as in AD. Sensory distortions, especially hyperaesthesia, previously reported in Pick's disease were found in about 30% of the FLD group and in 10% of the AD cases (Gustafson and Risberg, 1992). The pain was more severe and long lasting in the FLD group. In two cases it was associated with bizarre hypochondriasis with psychotic features. The psychotic symptoms in primary degenerative dementia seem to be related to the localization of the disease process, although the premorbid personality remains an important factor. In FLD the psychotic symptoms give the impression of functional psychosis, while in AD with early onset the symptoms are related more to the general cognitive failure with dysgnosia and visuospatial dysfunction (Gustafson and Risberg, 1992).

In our patients with FLD the premorbid personality was judged to be fairly normal. However, nervousness and anxiety were sometimes reported. Five of our 16 FLD cases had psychotic episodes, mostly of a paranoid aggressive type or with hypochondriasis. One of the psychotic cases and two others manifested severe acts of easily provoked violence. Compulsive behaviour, seen as obsessional concern about daily routines such as washing, locking doors, physical training or walking following a strict pattern, was observed in four cases. The intensity of such repetitive behaviour was almost psychotic at times. According to Luria (1973), massive bilateral lesions of the frontal lobes may cause such perseverative and stereotyped behaviour. This has also been reported in patients with frontal and caudate-frontal lesions (Seibyl et al, 1989; Tonkonogy and Barreira, 1989). As described by Eiden and Lechner (1950), when analysing psychotic reactions in Pick's disease and AD, the possibility of brain atrophic disease must always be considered in atypical psychoses starting in the presenium and in late life.

Dissolution of language

A typical feature of dementia with predominant frontotemporal degeneration is progressive loss of expressive speech, which in Pick's disease has been described as 'dissolution du langage' or 'Sprachverödung' (Delay et al, 1944; Van Mansfeldt, 1954; Escourolle, 1958). It usually starts as verbal aspontaneity with amnesic dysphasia, stereotyped comments and frequent repetitions of a limited number of set phrases. During the early stage of the disease there may be a period of increased, unrestrained talking and singing, sometimes in combination with confabulation. Imitating behaviour, especially echolalia, was found in about 25% of the post-mortem verified FLD cases, rising to almost 50% in a more recent sample of FLD cases. According to Lhermitte (1986), echo phenomena and utilization behaviour belong to the 'environmental dependency syndrome' in patients with frontal lobe lesions. The FLD patient may also lose his normal pitch of voice and talk in an unmodulated inadequately high tone. This symptom is similar to the verbal mannerisms associated with schizophrenic processes. The language dysfunction is thus dominated by a dynamic, expressive failure rather than by a receptive one. The handwriting may change in various ways, such as the magnitude and type of letters, speed of writing, misspellings and stereotypes. These disturbances are usually unlike the dysgraphia in AD. This type of progressive dysphasia has been described in a consistent way by different research groups (Neary et al, 1988; Knopman et al, 1990; Snowden et al, 1991). The expressive dysphasia in FLD with dysregulation of initiation, sequencing and rhythm is in accordance with the consistent degeneration of premotor cortex and sometimes also of Broca's area.

The symptom constellation of palilalia, echolalia, mutism and amimia (PEMA syndrome of Guiraud) is typical of FLD and rare in AD. The progressive disappearance of verbal as well as non-verbal communication makes it extremely difficult to evaluate to what extent the FLD patient perceives and understands what is said. However, even at an advanced stage of the disease the mute and amimic patient seems capable of some understanding and recognition.

All patients with progressive dysphasia do not necessarily develop dementia (Mesulam, 1982; Tyrrell et al, 1990) (see Chapter 6), although generalized cognitive impairment, usually dementia of non-Alzheimer type, often develops eventually (Green et al, 1990).

Cognitive symptoms and neuropsychological testing

In FLD, cognitive symptoms appear early, although often overshadowed by emotional and conative disturbances. However, the evaluation must be judged against the patient's premorbid mental capacity. Reduced recent memory and increased distractibility are common findings and remote memory is also disturbed, although to a lesser extent than in AD. Temporal and spatial orientation is usually preserved for a long time, although often difficult to evaluate by traditional methods. The cognitive functions are difficult to evaluate for several reasons, such as the patient's emotional changes and speech dysfunction. Surprisingly, dyscalculia is often mentioned as an early symptom, as well as misspelling as an expression of sequential language dysfunction.

In our experience neuropsychological testing can be used for the early recognition of FLD and to distinguish it from other dementias, normal ageing and non-organic mental disease. For diagnostic purposes it is important to rely not only on quantitative measures but also on systematic observation and recording of the patient's behaviour in the test situation (Hagberg, 1987).

Johanson and Hagberg (1989) reported test results from 16 FLD cases and four cases with Pick's disease. All FLD patients showed memory disturbances, although verbal and spatial memory were within the normal range in six patients. These patients showed the best preserved hippocampal structures at autopsy. By contrast, patients of similar age with post-mortem verified AD ($n = 20$) showed severely impaired verbal and spatial memory. All 13 testable FLD patients were able to copy simple geometrical figures, in contrast to a more general failure among AD patients. The systematic evaluation of behaviour qualities, such as cooperation, self-criticism, distractibility, flight reactions and strategy, in the test situation strongly contributed to the differentiation from AD. 'Rotation', a turning of test items (blocks or drawn figures) in 45–180° deviation from the presented pattern was significantly more common in AD than in FLD. Dysphasia was examined according to Eisenson (1954), with additional evaluation of speech characteristics such as logorrhoea, echolalia, stereotyped speech, verbal perseveration, dysgraphia and dyscalculia. On the first test 12 out of 16 FLD patients showed expressive dysphasia, while only two out of 11 patients tested in this respect demonstrated receptive dysphasia. Three out of four patients with Pick's disease showed both expressive and receptive dysphasia at the time. Stereotypy of speech was observed in nine and echolalia in four of the FLD cases. Four out of nine FLD patients and two of three Pick cases displayed dyscalculia. Receptive dysphasia was rather uncommon and difficulty in understanding instructions, which is common in AD even early in the disease, was only found in two out of 11 FLD patients.

The early test profile in degenerative dementia of frontal lobe type is characterized by slow verbal production and relatively intact reasoning and memory, while intellectual and motoric speed are reduced. By contrast, the early Alzheimer patient shows a relatively intact verbal ability and a simultaneous impairment of reasoning ability, verbal and spatial memory dysfunction, dysphasia and dyspraxia. AD cases with a later onset show a less consistent test profile with a more marked verbal memory dysfunction.

The Meta-Contrast-Technique (MCT), a percept generation technique, has also been used to differentiate between dementias (Johanson et al, 1990). FLD patients showed the lowest liminal values of recognition close to the results of the normal reference group, and significantly different from the high liminal values in AD. Signs of moderate and severe anxiety were most frequent among patients with AD, and 'projective signs' were more common among the FLD patients. These studies help to elucidate the perceptual disturbances and emotional adaption in dementia which arise with different localizations of the disease process.

Elfgren et al (1991) have recently compared the test profiles in 12 patients with the clinical diagnosis of FLD (mean age 60 years, range 50–76) and 12 patients diagnosed as AD (mean age 59 years, range 45–74). The mean hemispheric CBF values in the two patient groups were identical and slightly reduced compared with age matched controls. rCBF was, however, significantly lower in the temporoparietal cortex in AD and significantly lower in the frontal cortex in the FLD group. There were significantly lower scores of verbal ability in the FLD group and significantly lower visuospatial ability and spatial memory in the AD group. Moreover, there was a significant positive correlation between verbal ability and rCBF in frontotemporal and superior frontal regions, and significant correlations between performance in spatial memory and visuospatial ability and rCBF in the temporoparietal cortex.

Neary et al (1988) also showed better preserved spatial orientation and practical abilities in dementias of frontal lobe type, although the performance was disturbed by the patients' lack of strategy and self-criticism. The patients were typically well oriented in place and time yet performed poorly on formal tests of memory, interpreted as being due to impaired strategy. Reduced verbal fluency with concrete and stereotyped language was a consistent finding, as was comparatively preserved verbal understanding. Other tests sensitive to frontal lobe dysfunction, such as the Wisconsin card sorting test (Nelson, 1976), might be useful for recognition of FLD (Neary et al, 1990).

Knopman et al (1990) reported neuropsychometric findings in five of their 14 patients in the 'dementia without distinctive histology' group. All five patients showed impaired recent memory but retention was greater than expected in at least two cases, especially compared with individuals with AD. Executive or frontal lobe-based functions such as Porteus maze, trail-making and word fluency were severely affected in four out of five tested cases.

Non-neurological features

Pathological somatic findings were few in our autopsy-verified FLD cases. A relatively high frequency of syncopal attacks have been reported in Pick's disease in several studies (Stertz, 1926; Mallison, 1947). Therefore our observations of low mean blood pressure (103 ± 9.7 mmHg) and a tendency to orthostatic reactions in FLD may be of special interest. The question remains whether this somatic feature is primary or secondary to the degenerative brain disease.

Neurological features such as fascicular twitchings, muscular wasting, dysarthria and dysphagia may sometimes develop in patients with Pick's disease (Wikström et al, 1982; Mitsuyama, 1985) and FLD. The pathological changes in FLD and ALS are in certain respects similar (see Chapters 2 and 7). Morita et al (1987) in a review of 34 Japanese ALS cases reported early character changes in about 70%. Four autopsy verified ALS–dementia cases showed diffuse brain atrophy with frontotemporal accentuation on CT, and almost normal EEG. Two of our FLD cases reported in 1987 showed fascicular twitchings but no muscular atrophy or hyperactive reflexes. The clinical course was rapidly progressive in one case and slowly deteriorating in the other.

Neary et al (1990) reported four cases of rapidly progressive dementia and motor neurone disease with a striking clinical, and in two cases neuropathological similarity to FLD. The nosological classification of the ALS–dementia complex is unsettled, although it seems justified to classify a majority as primary degenerative dementia with frontotemporal predominance, as suggested in the Swedish consensus on classification of dementia (Wallin, 1990). The relationship is further indicated by the high frequency of normal EEG and frontotemporal atrophy on brain imaging in these cases.

Differential diagnosis

The clinical differences between FLD and AD and cerebrovascular dementia have been analysed in detail elsewhere (Gustafson, 1987; Gustafson et al, 1990). It seems justified to conclude that it is possible to separate these dementias based on well-defined clinical criteria and functional and structural brain imaging techniques. Certain neurological features may, however, contribute to the differentiation between FLD and AD, for example generalized epileptic seizures, myoclonus and logoclonia are more common in AD than in FLD. The clinical differentiation from two additional dementing illnesses with frontal accentuation will be touched upon briefly. The progressive subcortical gliosis described by Neumann (1949) and Neumann and Cohn (1967) was first considered a variant of Pick's disease but now holds its own nosological position. In 1987, Verity and Wechsler reported two additional cases of progressive subcortical gliosis with a duration of 3 years in one case and 16 months in the other. The clinical picture was characterized by early loss of word comprehension, dysgraphia and disorientation. Verity and Wechsler did not support the suggestion by Masse et al (1981) that progressive subcortical gliosis and Kraepelin's disease are the same clinical and neuropathological entity. Masse et al based this suggestion on a review of publications on 12 cases with progressive subcortical gliosis and 11 cases with Kraepelin's disease. They concluded that stereotyped behaviour, disorders of orientation and various neuro-logical problems were observed in both groups. Psychotic depressive reactions were, however, more common in Kraepelin's disease, and dementia a more consistent finding in progressive subcortical gliosis. Masse et al added one case of progressive subcortical gliosis with clinical similarities to FLD. The patient had a progressive dementia starting with anxiousness, tearfulness, expressive dysphasia, stereotyped writing, unsteady gait, psychomotor slowing and drop attacks without unconscious-ness. Mood changes with periods of euphoria and bulimia, hypochondriasis and symptoms of pain were also observed. The post-mortem investigation showed subcortical gliosis with slight frontal atrophy.

AETIOLOGY

The aetiology of FLD and its relationship to Pick's disease are unknown. In both diseases there is strong evidence for genetic factors, with a positive family history reported in about 50% of patients with Pick's disease (Sjögren et al, 1952; Van Mansvelt, 1954; Heston, 1978; Groen and Endtz, 1982) and FLD (Gustafson, 1987; Neary et al, 1988; Knopman et al, 1990). The similarity between neuropathological and clinical findings in FLD and ALS with and without dementia has been pointed out by several authors and the possibility of environmental factors as precipitating causes cooperating with genetic predisposition has been mentioned. The possibility that some cases are due to prion disease has been considered (Collinge et al, 1990). We will briefly describe a family with several generations affected by frontal lobe

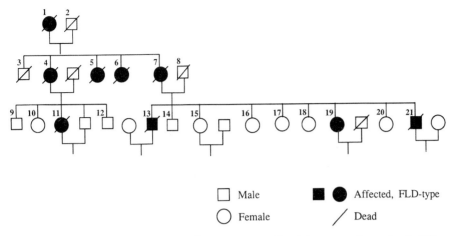

Figure 2. Pedigree of family with FLD. *Short case reports: Case 1*. Late onset dementia, died 88 years. Stroke? *Case 2*. Died 49 years. Cardiac disease. *Case 4*. Presenile dementia with onset at 57 years. Died 69 years. Restless, disinhibited, lack of insight, preserved spatial orientation, logorrhoea, later echolalia, mutism and amimia. *Case 5*. Died 70 years. Stroke? Clinical picture similar to case 7. *Case 6*. Slowly progressive dementia of frontal lobe type. Terminal stroke, age 86 years. *Case 7*. Onset at 55 years. Died 61 years. Personality change, quarrelsome, social neglect, lack of insight, preserved orientation, auditory hallucinations, tearfulness, suicidal thoughts, increased verbal productivity with stereotyped phrases, subsequently agitation, hyperorality, echolalia, apathy and bulimia. *Case 11*. Onset at 50 years. Died 55 years. Emotional unconcern, restless, verbal stereotypes and confabulations. Memory and spatial functions were preserved. Visual hallucinations with erotic paranoia, and subsequently aggressiveness, echolalia, mutism and amimia. Hyperorality and sudden death from aspiration. Early EEG was normal. Neuropathology: FLD. *Case 13*. Onset at 46 years. Died 61 years. Tearfulness, suspiciousness, suicidal thoughts, disinhibited, sexually offensive behaviour and had several traffic accidents. Increased alcohol consumption, stereotyped phrases and behaviour. Subsequently echolalia, mutism and amimia. Early EEG was normal. Neuropathology FLD. *Case 19*. Onset at 52 years. Untidy, disinhibited, restless, social neglect, stereotyped phrases and later echolalia. Preserved spatial and temporal orientation. Oral tendencies with hyperphagia, subsequently mutism and stereotyped movements. At present bedridden and mute. Early EEG was normal. rCBF and SPECT showed severe frontal lobe pathology. *Case 21*. Onset at 43 years. Died 60 years. Personality changes with apathy and emotional unconcern. Later restlessness, lack of insight, increased alcohol consumption, explosive temper, impulsive economic transactions, visual and tactile hallucinations. Preserved orientation in time and space. Stereotyped phrases, later echolalia, mutism and amimia. EEG 1 year before death was pathological. rCBF and SPECT showed severe frontal pathology. Neuropathology: FLD.

type of dementia which in three patients has been verified at post mortem as typical FLD (Figure 2). The clinical and pathological similarities between the dementia cases in this family are impressive.

FLD is, in our experience, the second most common primary degenerative dementia with a consistent pathology and a characteristic clinical picture. This conclusion is based on large samples of patients with post-mortem verified diagnoses and living patients followed in a longitudinal study. The clinical picture dominated by personality changes and progressive dynamic aphasia in combination with comparatively spared memory and spatial functions is in good agreement with the consistent distribution and type of cortical degeneration. Early clinical diagnosis can be reached in a majority of cases by systematic clinical evaluation in combination with functional brain imaging. It is likely that many of the cases described by others (Clark et al, 1986; Neary et al, 1988, 1990; Knopman et al, 1990) belong to this group, perhaps with a larger variability of pathology than originally defined by us for the FLD group.

SUMMARY

In a longitudinal prospective study of dementias, several hundred cases have been examined from a clinical, brain imaging, neurochemical and neuro-pathological point of view. Frontal lobe degeneration of non-Alzheimer type (FLD) was the second most common primary degenerative dementia found in about 10% of the material. FLD has a consistent pathology and a characteristic clinical picture, which have been described by several independent research groups. The cortical degeneration mainly involves frontal or frontotemporal grey matter, without the circumscribed or knife-blade atrophy seen in Pick's disease. The degeneration involves predominantly frontal areas, including the insula and cingulate gyrus in its anterior parts. The striate body is normal or only slightly altered. The pathological changes are non-specific, with neuronal loss, slight gliosis and spongiosis but none or few senile plaques, tangles, congophilic vessels or Pick cells. Pathological changes are in some respects similar to those in amyotrophic lateral sclerosis. FLD is a slowly progressive dementia with personality changes, lack of insight, disinhibition, stereotypy and later apathy. There is also progressive dynamic aphasia which ends in mutism and amimia. Memory, spatial ability and receptive language functions are comparatively spared. Psychotic symptoms, emotional reactions, hypochondriasis and a Klüver–Bucy-like syndrome are sometimes observed. Electroencephalography is normal, at least during the early stage, while functional brain imaging such as regional cerebral blood flow reflects the frontal pathology. It is possible to achieve early diagnosis and differentiation from Alzheimer's disease and cerebrovascular dementia by clinical examination with neuropsychological assessment supported by brain imaging, and in the future probably various biological markers. The aetiology is unknown but there is a positive family history for dementia of similar type in about 50% of post-mortem verified cases.

Acknowledgements

This study was supported by the Swedish Medical Research Council (Grant No. 3950) and the Greta and Johan Kock Foundation. We are grateful to Jarl Risberg for analysis of rCBF data, to Aniko Wolf and Siv Karlsson for the illustrations and to Anette Welin for secretarial aid.

REFERENCES

Blois R, Gailland J-M & Richard J (1989) Clinical and sleep EEG finding. In Hovaguimian T, Henderson S, Khachaturian Z & Orley J (eds) *The Classification and Diagnosis of Alzheimer Disease, An International Perspective*, pp 145–151. Toronto: Hogrefe & Huber.

Brion S, Plas J, Masse G & Jeanneau A (1991) Clinico-pathological studies in frontal non-Alzheimer dementias. In Racagni G, Brunello N & Fukuda P (eds) *Biological Psychiatry*, vol. 2, pp 128–130. Amsterdam: Elsevier.

Brun A (1987) Frontal lobe degeneration of non-Alzheimer type. I. Neuropathology. *Archives of Gerontology and Geriatrics* **6**: 193–208.

Brun A (1991) Dementia of frontal lobe type. In Racagni G, Brunello N & Fukuda P (eds) *Biological Psychiatry*, vol. 2, pp 127–128. Amsterdam: Elsevier.

Brun A & Englund E (1986) A white matter disorder in dementia of the Alzheimer type: a pathoanatomical study. *Annals of Neurology* **19**: 253–262.

Brun A & Gustafson L (1976) Distribution of cerebral degeneration in Alzheimer's disease. A clinico-pathological study. *Archiv für Psychiatrie und Nervenkrankheiten* **223**: 15–33.

Brun A & Gustafson L (1978) Limbic lobe involvement in presenile dementia. *Archiv für Psychiatrie und Nervenkrankheiten* **226**: 79–93.

Brun A & Gustafson L (1991) Psychopathology and frontal lobe involvement in organic dementia. In Iqbal K, McLachlan DRC, Winblad B et al (eds) *Alzheimer's Disease: Basic Mechanism, Diagnosis and Therapeutic Strategies*, pp 27–33. London: Wiley.

Burns A, Jacoby R & Levy R (1990) Psychiatric phenomena in Alzheimer's disease. I: disorders of thought content. *British Journal of Psychiatry* **157**: 72–76.

Chase TN, Burrows GH & Mohr E (1987) Cortical glycose utilization patterns in primary degenerative dementias of the anterior and posterior type. *Archives of Gerontology and Geriatrics* **6**: 289–297.

Clark AW, White III CL, Manz HJ et al (1986) Primary degenerative dementia without Alzheimer pathology. *Canadian Journal of Neurological Sciences* **13**: 462–470.

Collinge J, Owen F, Poulter M et al (1990) Prion dementia without characteristic pathology. *Lancet* **336**: 7–9.

Constantinidis J, Richard J & Tissot R (1974) Pick's disease. Histological and clinical correlations. *European Neurology* **11**: 208–217.

Creasey H, Schwartz M, Frederickson H et al (1986) Quantitative computed tomography in dementia of the Alzheimer type. *Neurology* **36**: 1563–1568.

D'Antona R, Baron JC, Samson Y et al (1985) Subcortical dementia. *Brain* **108**: 785–799.

Delay J, Neveu P & Desclaux P (1944) Les dissolutions du langage dans la maladie de Pick. *Revue Neurologique* **76**: 37–38.

Eiden H-F & Lechner H (1950) Über psychotische Zustandsbilder bei der Pickschen und Alzheimerschen Krankheit. *Archiv für Psychiatrie und Zeitschrift Neurologie* **184**: 393–412.

Eisenson J (1954) *Manual for the Examination of Aphasia and Related Disturbances*. New York: Psychological Corporation.

Elfgren C, Gustafson L, Johanson A et al (1991) Cognitive function in dementia of Alzheimer type and in frontal lobe dementia related to regional cerebral blood flow. *Journal of Cerebral Blood Flow and Metabolism* **11** (supplement 2): 176.

Englund E & Brun A (1987) Frontal lobe degeneration of non-Alzheimer type. IV. White matter changes. *Archives of Gerontology and Geriatrics* **6**: 235–243.

Escourolle R (1958) *La Maladie de Pick. Étude Critique d'Ensemble et Synthèse Anatomo-clinique*. Paris: Foulon.

Friedland RP, Buldinger TF, Ganz E et al (1983) Regional cerebral metabolic alterations in dementia of the Alzheimer type. *Journal of Computer Assisted Tomography* **7**: 590–598.

Gilbert JJ, Kish SJ, Chan L-J et al (1988) Dementia, Parkinsonism, and motor neurone disease: neurochemical and neuropathological correlates. *Neurology* **24**: 688–691.

Goffinet AM, De Volder AG, Gillian C et al (1989) Positron tomography demonstrates frontal lobe hypometabolism in progressive supranuclear palsy. *Annals of Neurology* **25**: 131–139.

Green J, Morris JC, Sandson J, McKeel DW & Miller JW (1990) Progressive aphasia: a precursor of global dementia? *Neurology* **40**: 423–429.

Groen JJ & Endtz LJ (1982) Hereditary Pick's disease. *Brain* **105**: 443–459.

Gustafson L (1987) Frontal lobe degeneration of non-Alzheimer type. II. Clinical picture and differential diagnosis. *Archives of Gerontology and Geriatrics* **6**: 209–223.

Gustafson L, Brun A, Cronquist S et al (1989) Regional Cerebral Blood Flow, MRI, and BEAM in Alzheimer's disease. *Journal of Cerebral Blood Flow and Metabolism* **9** (supplement 7): 513.

Gustafson L, Brun A, Franck-Holmkvist A & Risberg J (1985) Regional cerebral blood flow in degenerative frontal lobe dementia of non-Alzheimer type. *Journal of Cerebral Blood Flow and Metabolism* **5**: 141–142.

Gustafson L, Brun A & Ingvar DH (1977) Presenile dementia: clinical symptoms, pathoanatomical findings and cerebral blood flow. In Meyer JS, Lechner H & Reivich M (eds) *Cerebral Vascular Disease*, pp 5–9. Amsterdam: Excerpta Medica.

Gustafson L, Brun A, Johanson A & Risberg J (1990) Diagnostic criteria of Alzheimer's disease. In Maurer K, Riederer R & Beckman H (eds) *Alzheimer's Disease. Epidemiology, Neuropathology, Neurochemistry and Clinics*, pp 357–364. New York: Springer.

Gustafson L & Risberg J (1992) Deceptions and delusions in Alzheimer's disease and frontal lobe dementia. In Katona C & Levy R (eds) *Delusions and Hallucinations in Old Age*. London: Gaskell pp 218–229.

Hagberg B (1987) Behavior correlates to frontal lobe dysfunction. *Archives of Gerontology and Geriatrics* **6**: 311–321.

Heston LL (1978) The clinical genetics of Pick's disease. *Acta Psychiatrica Scandinavica* **57**: 202–206.

Jagust WJ, Reed BR, Seab JP, Kramer JH & Budinger TF (1989) Clinical-physiologic correlates of Alzheimer's disease and frontal lobe dementia. *American Journal of Physiologic Imaging* **4**: 89–96.

Johannesson G, Brun A, Gustafson L & Ingvar DH (1977) EEG in presenile dementia related to cerebral blood flow and autopsy findings. *Acta Neurologica Scandinavica* **56**: 89–103.

Johanson A & Hagberg B (1989) Psychometric characteristics in patients with frontal lobe degeneration of non-Alzheimer type. *Archives of Gerontology and Geriatrics* **8**: 129–137.

Johanson A, Gustafson L, Smith GJW et al (1990) Adaption in different types of dementia and in normal elderly subjects. *Dementia* **1**: 95–101.

Johanson A, Gustafson L, Brun A et al (1991) A longitudinal study of dementia of Alzheimer type in Down's syndrome. *Dementia* **2**: 159–168.

Kamo H, McGeer PL, Harrop R et al (1987) Positron emission tomography and histopathology in Pick's disease. *Neurology* **37**: 439–445.

Kanazawa I, Kwak S, Sasaki H et al (1988) Studies on neurotransmitter markers of the basal ganglia in Pick's disease, with special reference to dopamine reduction. *Journal of the Neurological Sciences* **83**: 63–74.

Kitamura S, Araki T, Sakamoto S, Iio M & Terashi A (1990) Cerebral blood flow and cerebral oxygen metabolism in patients with dementia of frontal lobe type. *Rinsho Shinkeigaku* **30**: 1171–1175.

Kim RC, Collins GH, Parisi JE, Wright AW & Chu YB (1981) Familial dementia of adult onset with pathological findings of a 'non-specific' nature. *Brain* **104**: 61–78.

Knopman DS, Christensen KJ, Schut LJ et al (1989) The spectrum of imaging and neuropsychological findings in Pick's disease. *Neurology* **39**: 362–368.

Knopman DS, Mastri AR, Frey WH et al (1990) Dementia lacking distinctive histologic features: a common non-Alzheimer degenerative dementia. *Neurology* **40**: 251–256.

Kuhl DE, Phelps ME, Markham CH et al (1982) Cerebral metabolism and atrophy in Huntington's disease determined by 18FDG and computed tomography. *Scan Annals of Neurology* **12**: 425–434.

Lhermitte F (1986) Human autonomy and the frontal lobes. Part II: Patient behavior in complex and social situations: the 'environmental dependency syndrome'. *Annals of Neurology* **19**: 335–343.

Lhermitte F, Pillon B & Serdaru M (1986) Human autonomy and the frontal lobes. Part I: Imitation and utilization behavior: a neuropsychological study of 75 patients. *Annals of Neurology* **19**: 326–334.

Lindvall O & Björklund A (1983) Dopamine- and norepinephrine containing neuron systems: their anatomy in the rat brain. In Emson PC (ed.) *Chemical Neuroanatomy*, pp 229–255. New York: Raven.

Luria AR (1973) *The Working Brain*. London: Penguin.

Mallison R (1947) Zur Klinik der Pickschen Atropic. *Nervenarzt* **6**: 247–356.

Masse G, Mikol J & Brion S (1981) Atypical presenile dementia. Report of an anatomo-clinical case and review of the literature. *Journal of the Neurological Sciences* **52**: 245–267.

Maurer K, Lowitzsch K & Stöhr M (1988) *Evozierte Potentiale. AEP-VEP-SEP.* Stuttgart: Enke.

Mazziotta JC (1989) Huntington's disease: studies with structural imaging techniques and positron emission tomography. *Seminars in Neurology* **9**: 360–369.

Mesulam MM (1982) Slowly progressive aphasia without generalized dementia. *Annals of Neurology* **11**: 592–598.

Miller BL, Lesser IM, Boone KB et al (1991a) Brain lesions and cognitive function in late-life psychosis. *British Journal of Psychiatry* **158**: 76–82.

Miller BL, Cummings JL, Villanueva-Meyer J et al (1991b) Frontal lobe degeneration: clinical, neuropsychological, and SPECT characteristics. *Neurology* **42**: 1374–1382.

Minthon L, Edvinsson L, Ekman R & Gustafson L (1990a) Cerebrospinal fluid neuropeptide Y-like immunoreactive levels in dementia of Alzheimer type and dementia with fronto-temporal degeneration of non-Alzheimer type. *Dementia* **1**: 262–266.

Minthon L, Edvinsson L, Ekman R & Gustafson L (1990b) Neuropeptide levels in Alzheimer's disease and dementia with frontotemporal degeneration. *Journal of Neural Transmission* **30**: 57–67.

Minthon L, Edvinsson L, Ekman R & Gustafson L (1991) Reduced lumbar cerebrospinal fluid somatostatin levels in Alzheimer's disease and dementia with frontotemporal degeneration. *Dementia* **2**: 273–277.

Mitsuyama Y, Kogoh H & Ata K (1985) Progressive dementia with motor neuron disease. *European Archives of Psychiatry and Neurological Sciences* **235**: 1–8.

Morita K, Kaiya H, Ikeda T & Namba M (1987) Presenile dementia combined with amyotrophy. A review of 34 Japanese cases. *Archives of Gerontology and Geriatrics* **6**: 263–277.

Neary D (1990) Dementia of frontal lobe type. *Journal of the American Geriatrics Society* **38**: 71–72.

Neary D, Snowden JS, Northen B & Gouldin P (1988) Dementia of frontal lobe type. *Journal of Neurology, Neurosurgery and Psychiatry* **51**: 353–361.

Neary D, Snowden JS, Mann DMA et al (1990) Frontal lobe dementia and motor neuron disease. *Journal of Neurology, Neurosurgery and Psychiatry* **53**: 23–32.

Nelson HE (1976) A modified card sorting test sensitive to frontal lobe deficits. *Cortex* **72**: 313–324.

Neumann MA (1949) Pick's disease. *Journal of Neuropathology and Experimental Neurology* **8**: 255–282.

Neumann MA & Cohn R (1967) Progressive subcortical gliosis—a rare form of presenile dementia. *Brain* **90**: 405–418.

Pilleri G (1966) The Klüver–Bucy syndrome in man. A clinico-anatomical contribution to the function of the medial temporal lobe structures. *Psychiatrie, Neurologie und Medizinische Psychologie* **152**: 65–103.

Risberg J (1987) Frontal lobe degeneration of non-Alzheimer type. III. Regional cerebral blood flow. *Archives of Gerontology and Geriatrics* **6**: 225–233.

Risberg J, Gustafson L & Brun A (1991) High resolution regional cerebral blood flow measurements in Alzheimer's disease and other dementia disorders. In Maurer K, Riederer P & Beckman H (eds) (1990) *Alzheimer's Disease. Epidemiology, Neuropathology, Neurochemistry, and Clinics*, pp 357–364. Wien: Springer.

Rosén J, Gustafson L & Risberg J (1992) Multichannel EEG Frequency Analysis and Somatosensory Evoked Potentials in Patients with Different Types of Organic Dementia. *Dementia* (in press).

Seibyl PJ, Krystal JH, Goodman WK & Lawrence HP (1989) Obsessive-compulsive symptoms in a patient with a right frontal lobe lesion—response to lithium augmentation of tranylcypromine. *Neuropsychiatry, Neuropsychology and Behavioral Neurology* **1**: 295–299.

Sjögren T, Sjögren H & Lindgren AGH (1952) *Morbus Alzheimer and Morbus Pick. A Genetic, Clinical and Patho-anatomical Study.* Copenhagen: Munksgaard.

Snowden JS, Goulding PJ & Neary D (1989) Semantic dementia: a form of circumscribed cerebral atrophy. *Behavioural Neurology* **2**: 167–182.

Snowden JS, Neary D, Mann MA, Goulding PJ & Testa HJ (1991) Progressive language disorder due to lobar atrophy. *Annals of Neurology* **31**: 174–183.

Stertz G (1926) Über die Picksche Atrophie. *Zeitschrift für Neurologie* **101:** 729–747.

Tonkonogy J & Barreira P (1989) Obsessive-compulsive disorder and caudate-frontal lesions. *Neuropsychiatry, Neuropsychology and Behavioral Neurology* **2:** 203–209.

Tyrrell PJ, Warrington EK, Frackowiak RSJ & Rossor MN (1990) Heterogeneity in progressive aphasia due to focal cortical atrophy. A clinical and PET study. *Brain* **113:** 1321–1336.

Van Mansvelt J (1954) *Pick's disease. A syndrome of lobar, cerebral atrophy; its clinicoanatomical and histopathological types.* Thesis, Enschede, Utrecht.

Verity MA & Wechsler AF (1987) Progressive subcortical gliosis of Neumann: a clinicopathologic study of two cases with review. *Archives of Gerontology and Geriatrics* **6:** 245–261.

Wallin A (ed.) (1990) Konsensus om demenssjukdomar. I: Klassifikation och utredning. *Läkartidningen* **87:** 3856–3865.

Wikström J, Paetau A, Palo J, Sulkava R & Haltia M (1982) Classic amyotrophic lateral sclerosis with dementia. *Archives of Neurology* **39:** 681–683.

6

Spectrum of primary progressive aphasia

M-MARSEL MESULAM
SANDRA WEINTRAUB

'Dementia' is a descriptive term. It can be used to designate any condition that leads to the gradual dissolution of cognition, comportment and daily living activities. Not all domains of mental function are equally affected. The relative degree of sparing and involvement across individual domains such as attention, memory, language and comportment has led to the identification of several different neuropsychological patterns in dementias caused by degenerative brain disease. We recently defined four neuropsychological profiles which we designated progressive amnestic dementia, progressive comportmental dysfunction, progressive visuospatial dysfunction and primary progressive aphasia (Weintraub and Mesulam, 1993). These profiles are non-overlapping but do not necessarily include all possible patterns that can be seen. Our purpose was to delineate those profiles that can be identified reliably and for which there is considerable clinical, anatomical and pathological information. The clinical classification of dementias according to these neuropsychological profiles has potential implications for predicting the underlying pathophysiology and for planning a management strategy based on the individual patient's strength and weaknesses.

The single most common symptom profile in adult onset dementia is one that involves a prominent deterioration of memory function. Included in this category of progressive amnestic dementia are patients who display the insidious appearance and progressive exacerbation of primary memory deficits within the first 2 years of putative onset. Deficits in other domains may coexist and may even be more salient at certain stages of the disease. When caused by degenerative brain diseases (that is when stroke, hydrocephalus, tumour, metabolic factors, nutritional deficiency, alcoholism, etc. are eliminated as aetiologies) this latter neuropsychological profile fulfils the McKhann et al (1984) criteria for probable Alzheimer's disease (PRAD). In a sample of 39 consecutive dementia cases from our clinic (the Beth Israel component of the Massachusetts Alzheimer's Disease Research Center (BI-ADRC)), that came to autopsy or brain biopsy, this profile was identified 21 times and was associated with the multifocal neurofibrillary tangles and neuritic plaques of Alzheimer's disease (AD) in 20 (95%) of the patients (Price et al, in press). Experience from other centres yields a concordance of 68–100% between the clinical syndrome of PRAD and the pathological diagnosis of AD (Morris et al, 1988; Risse et al, 1990). Other and less frequent pathological conditions associated with progressive amnestic dementia include non-specific degenerations, Pick's disease and Lewy body dementia (Risse et al, 1990).

Additional neuropsychological profiles of primary degenerative dementia include those of progressive comportmental dysfunction and progressive visuospatial disturbances. A patient is included in the group of Progressive Compartmental Dysfunction if gradual deficits of motivation, comportment and other executive functions emerge in relative isolation for at least the first 2 years of disease and if these deficits become the major factors that compromise daily living activities. In all six consecutive autopsies of patients with progressive comportmental dysfunction seen in the BI-ADRC clinical core sample, the neuropathological examination revealed neuronal loss, gliosis and atrophy, predominantly of the frontal lobes. Plaques, tangles and Pick bodies were not detected in any of those six cases. Results from other autopsy series are generally consistent with our observations but indicate that Pick's disease may also be seen in approximately 20% of patients with this neuropsychological profile (Brun, 1987) (see Chapter 5).

Patients in whom progressive deficits of complex visuospatial function (and related limitations of daily living activities) emerge without additional memory loss for at least the first 2 years of disease are included in the group of progressive visuospatial dysfunction. This profile is associated with a heterogeneous set of pathophysiological correlates that includes AD, Creutzfeldt–Jakob disease, adult onset glycogen storage disease and probably also non-specific gliosis and neuronal loss with an emphasis on the parieto-temporo-occipital regions of the brain (see Weintraub and Mesulam, 1993, for review).

This chapter deals with a fourth neuropsychological profile, one that we have identified as primary progressive aphasia (PPA). According to our current definition (Table 1), this diagnosis is made when a gradual dissolution of language (not just speech) is the only salient finding for at least 2 years and when this deficit becomes the only factor that compromises daily living activities. Attention, memory, visuospatial skills and comportment must be relatively intact during the first 2 years of disease. Other deficits of relatively lesser intensity are acceptable if they occur on tasks mediated by the left hemisphere language network (such as word fluency, verbal retrieval, digit span, calculations, ideomotor apraxia), if they are secondary to the language defect (due to an inability to process the linguistic or execute the praxic components of the task) and if they are reactive (such as depression and frustration caused by an awareness of the deficits). After the initial 2 years, deficits in other domains may emerge but the aphasia remains as the most salient feature.

The diagnosis of PPA should not be applied to patients who also develop memory or comportmental disturbances during the first 2 years of an otherwise progressive aphasia. The combination of a progressive aphasia and amnesia in the initial 2 years of disease leads to the diagnosis of progressive amnestic dementia and PRAD. PPA can thus be differentiated from PRAD on the basis of neuropsychological testing since a disturbance of memory

Table 1. Clinical criteria that differentiate PRAD from PPA.

PRAD[1]	PPA
Progressive worsening of memory and other cognitive functions	Progressive worsening of language (not just speech)
Deficits in two or more areas of cognition	Absence of deficits in other domains during the first 2 years or longer
No disturbance of consciousness	No disturbance of consciousness
Presence of 'dementia' syndrome	No additional signs of a more generalized 'dementia'[2] syndrome
Absence of systemic disorders or other brain disease that in and of themselves could account for the progressive deficits in memory and other cognitive functions	Absence of systemic disorders or other brain disease that in and of themselves could account for the progressive deficits in language

[1] According to the McKhann et al (1984)–NINCDS criteria.
[2] Depending on the definition that one chooses to use, the presence of the progressive aphasic disturbance itself would lead to the classification of these patients as having a dementing syndrome.

within 2 years of onset rules out PPA while it is a necessary criterion for the diagnosis of PRAD (Table 1).

Since the specificity of neuropsychological profiles tends to be blurred as the disease advances, our clinical experience has led us to base the definition of the four profiles described above on the cognitive and comportmental state within the first 2 years of disease. The choice of this 2 year interval is somewhat arbitrary, especially since specifying the exact date of disease onset can be particularly challenging. The 2 year period offers a heuristic guideline that may need to be changed when more reliable criteria become available.

CLINICAL AND NEURODIAGNOSTIC FEATURES OF PATIENTS WITH PPA: A REVIEW OF THE LITERATURE

The gradual dissolution of language in the context of degenerative disease has been appreciated for nearly 100 years. The reports of Pick (1892, 1904), Dejerine and Sérieux (1897), Franceschi (1908) and Rosenfeld (1909) provide examples of such patients. Among these cases, Dejerine and Sérieux's (1897) patient and Rosenfeld's (1909) first patient fit our definition of PPA. Dejerine and Sérieux describe a patient who developed pure word deafness at the age of 47 years. Gradual worsening of the language deficit occurred in the absence of other signs of dementia. Within 5 years, the patient's deficit progressed to a state of Wernicke's aphasia. She died 8 years after the emergence of the first symptoms. Autopsy revealed massive bitemporal atrophy with a loss of intracortical fibres and pyramidal cells. The first patient in Rosenfeld's report (as reviewed by Luzzatti and Poeck, 1991) sought medical advice at the age of 62 years with a history of progressive word finding difficulties. Other aspects of cognition and comportment remained relatively intact but some memory disturbances might have been detected at a time when he was examined 3 years after onset. At autopsy, atrophy and neuronal loss, especially marked in the left temporal lobe, were reported. There is insufficient clinical information to decide if patient 2 in Pick's 1904 report fits the definition of PPA. However, the patient reported by Pick in 1892, patients 1 and 3 in his 1904 paper, and the patient reported by Franceschi in 1908 do not fulfil the criteria for a diagnosis of PPA because they displayed additional and major abnormalities of memory and/or comportment at the very initial stages of gradually progressive aphasic disturbances.

One of the earliest contributions to the modern literature on progressive aphasia was Wechsler's 1977 report of a 60-year-old man with a progressive decline of language function who turned out to have Pick's disease at autopsy (Wechsler et al, 1982). As indicated in the 1977 paper, the patient had considerable comportmental disturbances in the early phases of the disease. One year after putative onset, for example, the patient started to shy away from people and became irritable and suspicious. He would catch flies, proceed to pull off their wings and set them afire with matches. Presumably such behaviour was not consistent with the patient's previous personality. In view of the early emergence of comportmental disturbances, Wechsler's patient does not fit our current definition of PPA and shares many features with the patients of Pick and Franceschi where progressive language deficits were associated early in the course of the disease with other comportmental and cognitive difficulties.

In 1982, we reported six patients with PPA (Mesulam, 1982). Many additional patients have been reported since then. Table 2 lists 63 reported cases that fit the definition of PPA outlined in Table 1. Omitted from this list were patients who had deficits other than aphasia in the first 2 years (such as those in reports by Snowden et al, 1989; Kobayashi et al, 1990) as well as reports that did not contain enough information to ascertain that the criteria in Table 1 had been fulfilled. In some of the papers reviewed, only some of the patients were included while others were excluded. Some patients have been reported in more than one publication but were entered only once in Table 2. None of the three patients who developed a progressive aphasia in association with Creutzfeldt–Jakob disease were included since the course was too rapid, leading to death within 2 years after onset (Shuttleworth et al, 1985; Yamanouchi et al, 1986; Mandell et al, 1989).

The cases listed in Table 2 demonstrate that the syndrome of PPA can emerge among speakers of Dutch, English, French, German, Italian, Japanese and Portuguese. Patient 4 in our 1982 report was a native speaker of Urdu, and we have correspondence indicating that PPA has been noted in speakers of Hebrew and Turkish. If one eliminates as an outlier patient 4 of our 1982 series, who developed progressive pure word deafness at the age of 17 years, the age of onset ranges from 40 to 75 years, with a mean of 60 ± 8 years. The age of onset was below 65 years in 46 patients and at 65 or above in 17 patients. The list in Table 2 contains 40 male and 23 female patients with a diagnosis of PPA.

Determining the type of language disturbance from published records offered a major challenge. In keeping with a common classification system, we designated the aphasias as fluent or non-fluent. Non-fluent aphasias are characterized by agrammatic spontaneous utterances with a reduced phrase length (under four words) and include Broca's aphasia and transcortical motor aphasia. The fluent aphasias include the anomic, conduction, Wernicke and transcortical sensory subtypes (Benson and Geschwind, 1985). If the clinical report of a given patient with PPA described a non-fluent aphasia and also deficits in language comprehension, we defined that patient as having a mixed (global) aphasia. Patients with speech disturbance (i.e. dysarthria) but without definitive proof for additional language difficulties were not included in Table 2. In some patients that we had reported in 1982, speech was fluent in the sense that phrase length was greater than four words and output was syntactically complete but there were also lengthy word finding pauses so that the overall rate of language production was decreased. We identified these patients as displaying a 'logopenic' but fluent aphasia to emphasize the preservation of grammar and phrase length. These patients are indicated in Table 2 with the designation of fluent($-$). In identifying a patient's aphasia, we relied most heavily (whenever such information was available) on the nature of the language deficit at a time when the disease was clearly established rather than at its very initial or terminal stages. According to these criteria, Table 2 contains 30 patients with fluent aphasias, 28 with non-fluent aphasias, and five patients with a mixed aphasia.

Time of onset was also difficult to pin-point and, in most reports, was based on unstructured interviews with the patient or family members. The time of onset for additional deficits in other domains of cognition and comportment was inferred by historical information and neuropsychological test results. Based on this type of information, we estimated the interval during which the patients with PPA had a 'pure' aphasia with no other significant cognitive or comportmental deficit (except for dyscalculia, apraxia and reactive dysthymia). Table 2 shows that the mean duration of this interval is 5.2 ± 2.8 years and that there are six patients who displayed a relatively isolated progressive aphasia for 10 years or longer. It is important to realize that these numbers underestimate the duration of the isolated aphasia since additional cognitive or comportmental deficits had not yet emerged at the time of the last examination of some patients and since some of the observed non-verbal deficits might have been secondary to the processing difficulties imposed by the severe aphasia.

Focal neurological signs such as right-sided weakness, right facial flattening, right-sided hyperreflexia, right body posturing, right upper extremity tremor or a right-sided Babinski sign were reported in 11 (17%) of the patients. Asymmetrical neurodiagnostic abnormalities over the left fronto-perisylvian region was reported in 41 (65%) of the patients. The most frequent findings were computerized tomographic (CT) or magnetic resonance imaging (MRI) scans with asymmetrically widened sylvian fissures and frontal horns on the left, electroencephalograms (EEG) demonstrating asymmetrical slowing on the left and reduced oxygen or glucose metabolisms and blood flow (as determined by positron emission tomography (PET) or

Table 2. Listing of patients with PPA who have been described in the literature between 1982 and early 1992[1].

No.	Authors	Patient no.	Gender/Age of onset[2] (years)	Aphasia only[3] (years)	Focal tests[4]	Focal signs[5]	Aphasia type[6]	Pathology
1	Mesulam (1982)	1	F69	5	+	+	Fluent(−)	
2		2	M57	11	+		Fluent(−)	FAtr-Bx[7]
3		3	F48	8	+		Non-fluent	
4		4	F17	10	+		Fluent	
5		5	M54	9	+		Fluent	
6		6	M61	6	+		Fluent (−)	
7	Heath et al (1983)		F69	4			Non-fluent	
8	Assal et al (1984)		F60	4			Mixed	
9	Pogacar and Williams (1984)		M56	2	+	+	Fluent	AD L>R[8]
10	Kirshner et al (1984)[9]	1	F64	4			Fluent	
11		2	M61	10	+		Mixed	FAtr-L>R
12		4	M58	4			Fluent	FAtr L>R
13	Holland et al (1985)		M66	11			Non-fluent	Pick L>R
14	Chawluck et al (1986)	1	F51	4			Fluent	
15	Case Records of the Massachusetts General Hospital (1986)		F68	5	+		Non-fluent	FAtr L>R[10]
16	Hamanaka and Yamagishi (1986)	1	F55	4	+		Fluent	
17		2	F60	4	+		Mixed	
18	Mehler et al (1987)	1	M54	3	+		Non-fluent	FAtr L>R
19	Mehler et al (1987)	2	M53	4	+		Non-fluent	
20	Basso et al (1988)		M68	6	+		Fluent	
21	Poeck and Luzzatti (1988)	1	F63	3	+		Fluent	
22		2	M53	4	+		Fluent	
23		3	M45	5	+		Fluent	
24	Goulding et al (1989)		M63	3	+	+	Non-fluent	
25	De Oliveira et al (1989)		M63	7	+		?Mixed	
26	Kushner (1989)		M71	4	+		Fluent	
27	Yamamoto et al (1989)	2	F67	6	+		Non-fluent	
28	Sapin et al (1989)	1	M66	3	+		Fluent	
29		2	M67	2	+		Fluent	
30	Graff-Radford et al (1990)		M56	5			Fluent	Pick
31	Berger and Porch (1990)		F57	5			Non-fluent	
32	Green et al (1990)	1	M60	5		+	Fluent	
33		2	M60	5			Fluent	
34		3	M75	2		+ +	Fluent	FAtr L>R
35		4	M57	3		+ +	Non-fluent	
36		5	F50	2		+	Fluent	

	Reference	Pt	Sex/Age	Years			Fluency	Diagnosis
39		8	F71	3	+		Non-fluent	AD L>R
40	Northen et al (1990)		M63	5	+	+	Non-fluent	AD L>R
41	Scheltens et al (1990)		M54	9			Fluent	
42	Weintraub et al (1990)	1	M47	9		+	Non-fluent	
43		2	M56	6		+	Non-fluent	
44		3	F40	8		+	Non-fluent	
45		4	M74	9			Non-fluent	
46	Kempler et al (1990)	3	M58	5	+	+	Fluent	AD
47	Tyrrell et al (1990)	1	M40	4		+	Fluent	
48		2	M59	4		+	Fluent	
49		5	M54	2		+	Fluent	
50		6	M60	2			Non-fluent	
51	DeLecluse et al (1990)		F66	3		+	Non-fluent	
52	Kartsounis et al (1991)		M58	8		+	Non-fluent	
53	Tyrrell et al (1991)	2	M59	6			Non-fluent	
54	Mendez and Zander (1991)	6	F55	14	+		Fluent	
55		9	M61	2		+	Non-fluent	
56		12	F59	4		+	Non-fluent	
57	Benson and Zaias (1991)		M58	7		+	Fluent	AD
58	McDaniel et al (1991)	1	F62	2		+	Non-fluent	
59		2	F73	2		+	Mixed	
60	Lippa et al (1991)		M66	3			Non-fluent	FAtr L>R[11]
61		1	F65	10			Non-fluent	
62	Snowden et al (1992)	4	M63	8	+	+	Non-fluent	FAtr L>R
63		5	M59	3			Non-fluent	

F, female; M, male; FAtr, focal atrophy; AD, Alzheimer's disease.

[1] This list includes articles published up to February 1992 that we have been able to identify and for which there were abstracts in English, French, German, Spanish or Italian.

[2] Age of onset was determined by history.

[3] Number of years during which the patient experienced a purely aphasic disorder without deficits in other domains.

[4] Neurodiagnostic tests such as EEG, CT, MRI, SPECT and PET were taken into consideration. A plus sign indicates that at least one of these tests showed a selective abnormality of the left hemisphere. A blank indicates that there were either no asymmetries noted or that the relevant tests were not reported.

[5] A positive sign indicates an abnormality of elementary neural function, such as hyperreflexia or facial flattening, on the right side of the body. A blank indicates either the absence of such a finding or the failure to report the elementary neurological examination.

[6] Patients with a logopenic anomic aphasia are indicated by the designation of fluent(−). If a patient initially displayed an anomic aphasia and subsequently a Broca's aphasia as the disease advanced, he or she was listed as having a non-fluent aphasia.

[7] The information on this patient is based on a biopsy from the left temporal lobe.

[8] The designation of L>R indicates that the pathological changes were described as being more severe in the left hemisphere.

[9] Patient numbers refer to those of Kirshner et al (1984) but the related pathological information is based on Kirshner et al (1987).

[10] The diagnosis of Pick's disease was raised in this case but no Pick bodies were detected.

[11] Neuronal achromasia was also reported in this case.

single photon emission computerized tomography (SPECT)) in the left frontal-perisylvian regions. In some patients, the reduced metabolic activity determined by PET was confined to the left hemisphere, while in others there were also lesser abnormalities in the right hemisphere (Chawluck et al, 1986; Tyrrell et al, 1990). The focality of the atrophy and the associated lucencies seen on CT scans occasionally raised the possibility of strokes. However, angiography or non-invasive diagnostic evaluation of the cerebral vasculature was invariably negative, patients rarely had risk factors for stroke, and CT and MRI scans provided evidence for a progressive atrophy over time (Figure 1). Table 3 summarizes some characteristics of the 63 patients that have been reported in the 10 year interval from 1982 to 1992.

CLINICAL AND NEUROPSYCHOLOGICAL PICTURE OF PATIENTS WITH PPA: OUR EXPERIENCE

On initial clinical encounter, the patient with PPA looks much more like a patient with focal stroke than one with dementia. The patient tends to be alert, attentive, cooperative, aware of the deficit, concerned with the predicament and remarkably adept at communicating despite the aphasia, by writing when nearly mute or by pantomime and gesture when necessary.

The patient is almost always the first to detect the presence of the language problem in the form of increased effort (or slowing) during word-finding and decreased efficiency in coming up with the most appropriate of several equally acceptable but perhaps not equally effective words. For several years, the patient may be the only one to notice the difficulty. One of our patients, who later became mute in the context of PPA, was sent to a psychiatrist in the early years of her condition in order to investigate the possibility of hypochondriasis.

Except for rare cases in which the difficulty may emerge in the form of word deafness (i.e. the patient of Dejerine and Sérieux and also patient 4 in our 1982 report), initial objective evidence for the language difficulty is almost always confined to tests of confrontation naming. The naming deficit usually leads to long word-finding pauses that give spontaneous speech a logopenic quality. The naming difficulty usually leads to phonemic rather than semantic paraphasias (Weintraub et al, 1990). In contrast, the naming difficulty associated with PRAD is frequently characterized by semantic paraphasias. The earliest difficulties in PPA may be detected in the naming of geometric forms and body parts, at the same time that other classes of objects are named correctly. In the initial stages, the patient is usually able to point to the correct object when the word is provided by the examiner despite being unable to name it spontaneously. This 'one-way' naming deficit indicates the preservation of word 'recognition' at a time when there is an impairment of word 'retrieval'.

Some patients remain at this stage of an anomic aphasia while others progress to develop more severe fluent or non-fluent aphasias. In the most advanced cases, mixed (global) aphasias can emerge. Writing and reading can show a relative sparing and the patient may come to the visit with a

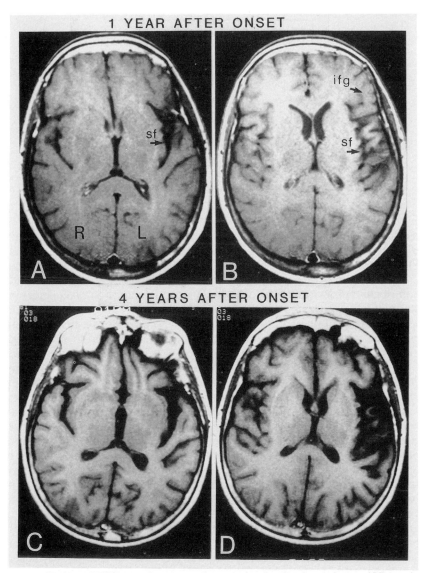

Figure 1. Horizontal MRI scan of a woman who started to develop the syndrome of PPA at the age of 61 years. Figures A and B on the top were obtained 1 year after putative onset and Figures C and D at the bottom 4 years after onset. There is a substantial increase in the size of the left sylvian fissure, indicating the increase of left perisylvian atrophy, during the 3 year interval between the two scans. ifg; inferior frontal gyrus; L, left hemisphere, R, right hemisphere; sf, sylvian fissure.

Table 3. Characteristics associated with the group of 63 patients with PPA that have been reported in the literature (1982–1992).

Total number of patients: 63
   Male: 40
   Female: 23

Presenile onset: 46 patients
Senile onset: 17 patients

Non-fluent aphasia: 28 patients
Fluent aphasia: 30 patients
Mixed aphasia: 5 patients

Duration of isolated aphasia: 5.2 ± 2.8 years

Frequency of focal signs: 17%

Frequency of focal neurodiagnostics: 65%

writing pad in an attempt to communicate with the examiner. The patients with the anomic and non-fluent aphasias are the easiest to diagnose as having PPA since the preserved comprehension enables them to give the clearest indication of intact performance in other domains. However, patients with non-fluent aphasias may also have severe ideomotor apraxia and may consequently say or signal 'no' when they mean 'yes', making conventional testing difficult to interpret. One patient would push the accelerator pedal when she meant to use the left foot for the clutch and had to stop driving because of the apraxia rather than because of other cognitive limitations.

In patients with the non-fluent aphasias (i.e. Broca's aphasia or transcortical motor aphasia), phrase length is diminished, naming is poor, there is almost always dysarthria and the output (spoken or written) tends to be terse but effective in communicating intent. Repetition is impaired in Broca's aphasia but is preserved in transcortical motor aphasia. Writing is never completely spared but is usually better than spoken language so that a patient may be able to write the name of an object that he or she is unable to utter. In some patients who may have extremely laboured and dysarthric spontaneous speech output, singing may improve speech intelligibility. The patients with the non-fluent aphasias also demonstrate a characteristic agrammatism. Their spoken and written language tends to show a paucity of grammatical relational words and morphological markers. While these patients may have excellent comprehension for most conversation, they start to show difficulties with syntactically difficult constructions such as those that include passive voice and embedded clauses. When asked to repeat, they have a greater difficulty with small grammatical words (prepositions, pronouns, etc.) than with semantically rich substantives. This discrepancy is also apparent when reading. For example, a patient may be much faster at detecting the written form of the word 'hippopotamus' than the word 'it' in a list of ten words. Buccofacial apraxia is common, especially for pharyngeal movements, constructions may show minor difficulties and calculations are impaired. These additional difficulties are also seen in patients who develop non-fluent aphasias on the basis of focal strokes in parts of the left hemisphere language network and therefore do not argue against the relative focality of the underlying pathological process.

Patients with the Wernicke and transcortical sensory subtypes of fluent aphasias are the most difficult to assess because of the associated comprehension difficulties. Transcortical sensory aphasia is differentiated from Wernicke's aphasia by the preservation of repetition. The comprehension impairment in some of these patients is at the level of sentences, whereas in others it is at the level of single words. For example, they can neither retrieve the appropriate word for an object they are shown nor match the word with the appropriate object, even at a time when they can accurately describe its use. This condition is defined as a 'two-way' naming deficit and reflects 'lexical lacunes'.

When comprehension is impaired, the patient may not understand verbal instructions so that attention, memory and visuospatial skills may be difficult to assess. Some of the patients with the fluent aphasias may also show agitation and lack of concern but it is important to remember that such comportmental disturbances are also seen in patients who develop Wernicke's aphasia in the context of focal strokes.

The assessment of cognitive and comportmental domains in patients with comprehension deficits is a challenging task that requires considerable improvisation. One patient with a fluent PPA was initially thought to be disorientated because he could not come up with accurate answers related to temporal orientation and topographic location. When given a calendar, however, the patient quickly pointed to the correct date and when provided with a map he was able to point to his location on a map even though he was being examined in a city far from his home.

The most critical factor in the differentiation of PPA from PRAD is the integrity of memory function. Some patients with PPA perform well in conventional tests of memory such as the Wechsler Memory Scale, the Rey–Osterreith Complex Figure, the Rey Auditory Verbal Learning List, and the Three Words Three Shapes Test (Weintraub et al, 1990). In other patients, however, there may be abnormalities in verbally mediated memory tasks. If scores in non-verbal memory tests are normal and if the daily living activities do not give evidence for abnormal forgetting, we assume that memory function is relatively spared and that the abnormal test scores reflect difficulties that are secondary to the aphasia.

In evaluating areas other than memory, we find the Visual Span subtest of the WMS-R (Wechsler Memory Scale-Revised) helpful for assessing attention, the Facial Recognition and Judgment of Line Orientation tests for assessing visuospatial abilities, and the Visual–Verbal Test or the Raven Progressive Matrices for assessing executive functions and conceptual abilities (Weintraub and Mesulam, 1985). Throughout the assessment, however, the clinician must be prepared to use intuition and inference and to improvise. Giving an aphasic patient a standard test battery (almost always based on verbal instructions if not on verbal responses) and then scoring it in standard form may lead to the erroneous conclusion that the patient has a more widespread (global) dementia.

The extent to which daily living activities can be preserved is the most characteristic feature of PPA. Many patients continue to drive, keep house, handle finances, and perform remarkably well and with exemplary creativity in virtually all tasks that can be done without intact language abilities. One patient helped his son build a log cabin while almost mute and could only explain his achievement by bringing a picture to the clinic and demonstrating the activities related to the construction with pantomime. Another patient extended her knowledge of organic gardening and would use gestures and diagrams to instruct us in the appropriate deployment of nasturtium and marigolds in fending off pests in the organic vegetable patch. One patient who was mute after 4 years of PPA carries on with her hobby of solving master-level jigsaw puzzles which adorn her bedroom walls. Two patients learned rudimentary sign language at a time when they were severely aphasic. These anecdotal examples provide clues to the maintenance of non-verbal cognitive skills, motivation and judgement.

There comes a time, however, when the patient loses all ability to communicate. At that time, it is virtually impossible to make any assessment of mental function except by interpreting gestures, facial expression and demeanor. One patient who is at that state after 9 years of PPA continues to attend church and other social functions, take care of her daily needs, including shopping and paying bills.

Two case descriptions (taken from Weintraub et al, 1990)

Case 1—patient 42 in Table 2

At the age of 47 years, a strongly right-handed industrial relations executive was aware of trouble pronouncing and finding words while giving public addresses. Over the next 5 years, his symptoms worsened and problems with oral reading and writing emerged. Detailed laboratory evaluation led to the diagnosis, by exclusion, of a degenerative brain disease. At the age of 52 years, he was referred to our clinic, 5 years after the onset of symptoms.

CT scans and an EEG were unremarkable. PET studies performed approximately 6 years after disease onset revealed reduced glucose metabolism in the left parietotemporal region but not in the right cerebral hemisphere. A SPECT study with iodoamphetamine yielded identical results (Figure 2).

In the initial examination (5 years after onset), the patient was meticulously groomed and fully orientated. Spontaneous speech was well articulated but marked by occasional hesitation, minor syntactical errors, and phonemic and semantic paraphasias. Repetition and oral reading were only mildly impaired. Confrontation naming contained phonemic paraphasic errors. Auditory and reading comprehension and writing were relatively intact, but the patient complained that he had difficulty composing letters. Buccofacial and limb apraxia were not noted. Performance on tests of memory, reasoning, calculations and visuospatial skills was within the normal range. Insight, judgement, comportment and effectiveness in most activities of daily living were unaffected.

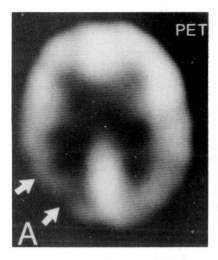 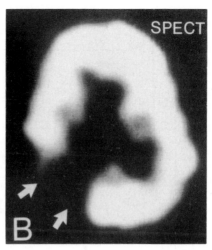

Figure 2. Regional cerebral metabolism and blood flow of patient 42 in Table 2, a right-handed man who started to experience symptoms of PPA at the age of 47 years. (A) PET scan with [^{18}F]2-deoxyglucose as the tracer. The scan indicates decreased glucose metabolism in the posterior perisylvian regions of the left hemisphere (arrows). This scan was obtained approximately 5 years after disease onset. See Chawluk et al (1986) for details of the PET studies. (B) SPECT of the same patient 6 years after disease onset. Iodoamphetamine was used as a marker of blood flow. Both scans were obtained at a time when the aphasia was predominantly anomic, albeit logopenic.

Over the next 5 years, language functions declined and evolved from an anomic aphasia to what appeared to represent Broca's aphasia. During the examination 9 years after onset, spontaneous speech was marked by frequent hesitation, paraphasias, less sophisticated syntax, and more grammatical errors. The dramatic change in the 4 year interval, from 5 to 9 years after onset, is apparent in the patient's oral description of the Cookie Theft picture (Figure 3). Narrative writing reflected a similar pattern of deterioration. Confrontation naming and repetition were more impaired as well, but auditory comprehension was impaired only for complex grammatical structures. Singing tended to improve the intelligibility of his verbal output.

With few exceptions and no consistent pattern, scores on tests of reasoning, non-verbal memory and visuospatial skills did not assume the course of deterioration over time seen in language (Figure 4). One strategy he devised to circumvent his increasing speech limitations consisted of displaying laminated index cards with written instructions that he had prepared for a number of commonly encountered situations, such as directing a cab driver. He travelled long-distance independently. Social graces were preserved. He remained concerned and appropriately saddened by his condition. He continued working in a reduced capacity and was forced to retire, 9 years after the onset of symptoms, because he was entirely unable to communicate with speech.

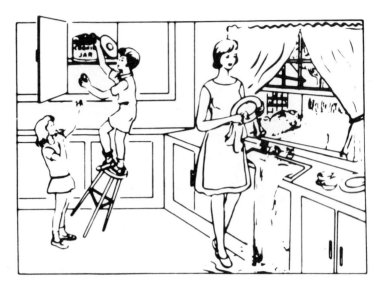

Figure 3. The descriptions of the Cookie Theft picture by patients 42 and 44 in Table 2. There is substantial deterioration over time in both patients.

Case 1
(5 years post onset): 'In the picture we have a boy ready to fall off the stool while he is getting cookies from the cookie jar, and the girl standing behind her on the floor is . . . is say "keep quite" so that the mother doesn't see whether the cookies are going. The mother's working at the kitchen looking out the window . . . wash . . . ah . . . driving plate. The water faucet is open—the water is going onto the floor.'

(9 years post onset): 'This is a picture of a woman . . . uh . . . who's . . . uh . . . lookin' out the . . . ah . . . win . . . uh . . . windshie . . . uh . . . windind and . . . uh . . . in the kitchen. And . . . uh . . . he's . . . uh (long pause) . . . she's . . . ah . . . he's dry, she is dryin' the . . . uh . . . plate while the water is comin' out from the sss . . . eh . . . (long pause). The water goin' on the floor . . . from the k-kitchen whatever it is. Behide her . . . There're boy is . . . it trying to goke up on the – the top of the . . . drawer for co-co-co . . . coke.eh . . . standing on a stool . . . Which wooks . . . looks it will falls . . . ss . . . This. The girl is there waking, waiting for the cookie, cookuk.'

Case 2
(6 years post onset): 'This is a crisis situation. Mother not watching the children. Boy goes up on the stool has a cookie in his hand and falling off the stool. Girl wants the cookie from his – her brother and the sink is overflowing.'

(9 years post onset): 'Uhm . . . co . . . co . . . uh . . . cookie . . . uhm . . . ss.um . . . ss . . . um s.sand . . . babuh, babuh [unintelligible] (patient pointed to the curtain). Sh . . . sh . . . sh . . . [unintelligible] (pointed to dishes) and call . . . uh . . . cup and . . . um . . . ca . . . ca . . . cu . . . cuya . . . uh window . . . um fall, fa . . . fa . . . falling (pointed to the boy falling). Uhm . . . apert (pointed to the apron). S.s . . . ssshow (pointed to the girl).' From Weintraub et al (1990).

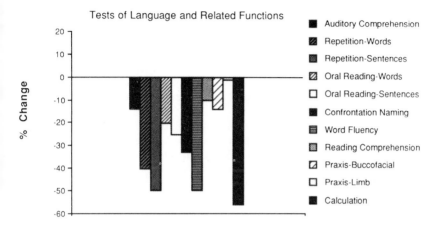

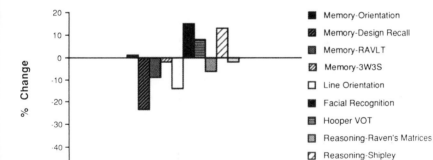

Figure 4. Performance in various neuropsychological tests by patient 42 in Table 2. The size of the bars indicates the change in test scores in a 4 year interval from 5 years after onset to 9 years after onset. There is a substantial deterioration in most language related tests whereas tasks of non-language functions are more stable and do not show consistent deterioration. From Weintraub et al (1990).

Case 2—patient 44 in Table 2

At the age of 40 years, a right-handed nursing professor and therapist experienced mild word-finding difficulties in the course of writing her doctoral dissertation. Four years later, in the wake of a series of tragic losses, these symptoms became very noticeable and gradually worsened. Her family did not report corresponding changes in personality and intellect. Her medical history was remarkable for rheumatoid arthritis, endometriosis, fibrocystic breast disease and treatment of breast cancer. Because of increasing difficulty delivering lectures, she took a medical leave of absence and sought neurological consultation 2 years later (6 years after the first sign of word-finding difficulty).

CT and MRI scans both showed bifrontal atrophy, probably greater on the left side. Auditory evoked responses showed some abnormalities in the cortical components, especially in the left temporal region.

She was well groomed, and orientation and comportment were normal. Her language deficit had many features of Broca's aphasia. Comprehension of spoken language, including grammatically complex constructions, was intact. Spontaneous speech was dysprosodic with occasional paraphasic errors, phonemic more than semantic. Grammatical form was simplified with numerous morphosyntactic errors. Dysarthria was not present. Repetition and oral reading was moderately impaired at the sentence level. Confrontation naming was relatively intact. Reading comprehension was good at the paragraph level. Praxis was normal with the exception of her inability to execute the command 'cough', in response to which she repeatedly uttered 'Cough, cough'. Narrative writing paralleled spontaneous speech, but sentences written to dictation contained only minor errors. Reasoning, memory and visuospatial test scores were in the superior range.

One year later (7 years after putative onset), evidence was present for a significant decline of speech and language functions, and the patient was forced to resign her teaching post. However, she remained very active as a member of several institutional boards and as a volunteer worker. The patient was motivated to learn functional sign language and, although it was not entirely normal, it allowed her to communicate effectively with deaf friends. Performance in other areas of testing remained unchanged, as were the results from the neurological examination.

Two years later, 9 years after onset, marked deterioration in the patient's ability to communicate was noted. With the exception of reading comprehension, the other language test scores decreased by at least 70%. Spontaneous speech was palilalic and, except for the rare occurrence of a clearly articulated word, unintelligible. Her oral description of the Cookie Theft picture 6 and 9 years after onset appears in Figure 3. She augmented speech with writing and was often able to communicate her ideas by writing words and short phrases. Narrative writing, however, was even more telegraphic than in the past. In the 3 year interval from 6 to 9 years after onset, deterioration was noted in repetition, oral reading, buccofacial praxis and confrontation naming. Neuropsychological test scores for memory,

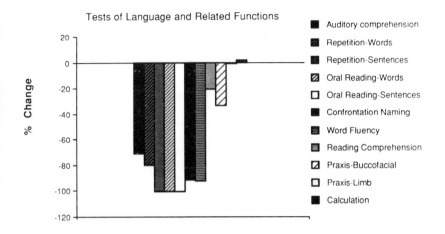

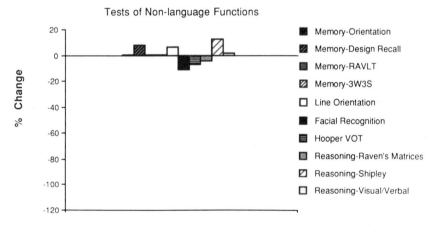

Figure 5. Performance in various neuropsychological tests by patient 44 in Table 2. The size of the bars indicates the change in test scores in a 3 year interval from 6 years after onset to 9 years after onset. There is a substantial deterioration in most language related tests whereas tasks of non-language functions are more stable and do not show consistent deterioration. From Weintraub et al (1990).

reasoning and visuospatial functions, with the exception of the Facial Recognition Test, remained stable (Figure 5). Insight, judgement and comportment also remained intact. She continued to be actively involved with her church and with the hearing-impaired community. Her signing was functional but further simplified. She purchased a teletype system so that she could maintain telephone contact with her sibling.

NATURE OF THE PATHOLOGICAL LESION

Of the 63 cases listed in Table 2, tissue information has been obtained on only 13, one by biopsy and 12 by autopsy. In four of these patients, a diagnosis of Alzheimer's disease (AD) was reached. In one of these four cases, the distribution of plaques and tangles was somewhat unusual since neurofibrillary tangles were distinctly rare in the nucleus basalis and in neocortical areas (Benson and Zaias, 1991). Furthermore, another patient who is included in Table 2 with a pathological diagnosis of AD, the patient of Pogacar and Williams (1984), appears to have displayed considerable deficits in domains other than language, probably within the initial 2 years, and therefore constitutes a borderline example of PPA. In two patients, Pick bodies were identified and a diagnosis of Pick's disease was established (Holland et al, 1985; Graff-Radford et al, 1990). In the remaining seven cases, non-specific neuronal loss with gliosis and some spongiform changes were reported. In one of these cases, the additional observation of neuronal achromasia was made (Lippa et al, 1991). In virtually all of the cases that came to autopsy, the frontoperisylvian regions of the left hemisphere were the most affected. In one case where biochemical analyses were undertaken, cortical somatostatin was decreased but cortical choline acetyltransferase was not (Mehler et al, 1987). The neuropathological experience in the group of patients with PPA is very limited and a considerably different picture may emerge as additional cases come to autopsy.

PPA COMPARED WITH CLINICALLY DIAGNOSED PRAD AND PATHOLOGICALLY PROVEN AD

PPA and PRAD represent two non-overlapping clinical syndromes. In Table 4, three groups of patients are compared: the 63 patients in Table 2 made up the PPA group; the first 63 consecutive cases of PRAD in the BI-ADRC core sample of 300 patients made up the PRAD group; and 20 consecutive patients with the pathological diagnosis of AD, where both the clinical and pathological examinations were done in our clinic, made up the AD group.

In the PPA group, disease onset was below the age of 65 years (presenile) in 73% of the patients and at the age of 65 years or older in 27%. The ratio was reversed for PRAD, where onset below the age of 65 years occurred in 32% of the patients and at, or above, the age of 65 years in 68%. In the AD group, the age of onset (70% at or above 65 years and 30% below the age of

Table 4. Comparison of patients with PPA, PRAD and pathologically-confirmed AD.

	PPA[1] (%)	PRAD[2] (%)	AD[3] (%)
Onset ≥65 years	27	68	70
Onset <65 years	73	32	30
Male	64	21	35
Female	36	79	65
Fluent	48[4]	100[5]	100[6]
Non-fluent	44	0	0
AD pathology	31[7]	68–100[8]	100
Non-AD pathology	69	32–0	0

[1] The numbers are based on the sample of 63 cases listed in Table 1.
[2] The numbers for age of onset and gender are based on a sample of the first consecutive 63 cases of PRAD entered into our clinical data base.
[3] The numbers are based on a sample of 20 consecutive cases of autopsy confirmed AD cases from our clinic.
[4] Logopenic aphasias are included in the fluent group. The four patients with mixed (global) aphasias were not included in any of the two groups.
[5] This information is based on the report of Appell et al (1982). Not all PRAD patients had aphasic disturbances. However, those that did had only fluent aphasia subtypes.
[6] Seventeen of the 20 AD cases had language deficits at initial examination. Only fluent aphasias were encountered. None of the patients developed a non-fluent aphasia (Broca or transcortical motor) at any point in the course of the disease.
[7] The total sample consists of the 13 cases from Table 2 for which there is tissue information.
[8] This range is derived from the reports of Morris et al (1988) and Risse et al (1990). In our sample 20 of 21 patients (95%) with clinically defined PRAD and who came to autopsy had AD.

65 years) was essentially identical to that of PRAD. Of the 63 patients with PPA, 64% were male and 36% female. This ratio was also reversed in the PRAD group where 21% of the patients were male and 79% were female. In the AD group, 35% of the patients were male and 65% were female, a ratio that was very similar to that of PRAD but very different from that of PPA. In order to eliminate the possibility that the gender difference was secondary to the difference in age of onset, we also looked at the subset of PRAD cases with onset under the age of 65 years. In that subset of 20 cases, 70% of the patients were female and 30% male, a distribution that remained distinctly different from that seen in the PPA sample. The prevalence of females in PRAD has been described in numerous epidemiological studies (Fratiglioni et al, 1991; Bachman et al, 1992). Since the total sample of PPA is relatively small, however, it is conceivable that there will be changes in the profile of gender and age of onset as additional patients are added to the list in Table 2.

Progressive aphasic disturbances are very common in PRAD and in pathologically confirmed cases of AD. In the BI-ADRC clinical core sample of 20 consecutive cases of AD, 17 had a disturbance of language at initial examination (Price et al, in press). In PRAD, the incidence of language difficulties varies from 36 to 100%, depending on disease severity (Faber-Langendoen et al, 1988). In both PRAD and AD, the associated language disturbances are almost exclusively of the fluent type and non-fluent aphasia such as Broca's aphasia or transcortical motor aphasia are never observed (Appell et al, 1982; Price et al, in press). In patients with PPA, however, 44% of the aphasias were non-fluent (Broca or transcortical motor) and even some of the aphasias that we classified as fluent were distinguished by a logopenic output.

These considerations suggest that PPA and PRAD are not only phenomenologically different but that they also represent two different (though perhaps partially overlapping) pools of susceptibilities, both with respect to individuals at risk and regions of the brain that are selectively affected (Table 5). It also appears that the characteristics of the PRAD group are nearly indistinguishable from those of pathologically-confirmed patients

Table 5. Differences between PRAD and PPA.

	PRAD	PPA
Populations at risk	F > M, senile > presenile onset	M > F, presenile > senile onset
Language function at risk	Fluency always preserved	Nearly 50% non-fluent
Brain regions at risk	Limbic cortex > others	Left fronto-perisylvian > others

with AD, whereas the characteristics of the PPA group are distinctly different from those of the AD group.

In the BI-ADRC sample of 39 consecutive autopsy cases of dementia, 21 patients had the clinical profile of PRAD and 20 of these, or 95%, were associated with the pathological features of AD. In contrast, at most, 31% of the PPA patients for whom there is pathological information have an underlying neuropathological process consistent with AD. It is interesting that three of the four PPA patients with AD pathology had a fluent aphasia. If only the PPA patients with non-fluent aphasias are considered ($n = 28$), only one of seven autopsied cases (14%) had the pathology of AD. These figures show that PPA has more than twice the likelihood of being associated with non-AD pathology than does PRAD (69% versus a maximum of 32%). It also appears that a progressive non-fluent aphasia is, by itself, a very strong predictor of non-AD pathology.

IS PPA A DISEASE, A SUBTYPE OF AD, A PRECURSOR TO DEMENTIA? HOW HETEROGENEOUS IS IT?

Is PPA a disease?

The literature on PPA contains several themes that have fuelled considerable discussion. In our initial report of 1982, and on several occasions since then, we stated that PPA is likely to represent a 'syndrome' rather than a 'disease' (Mesulam, 1982, 1987; Weintraub et al, 1990). A disease, such as AD, is based on at least one dimension of pathophysiological uniformity at the neuropathological or aetiological level. A syndrome, on the other hand, is uniform only at the semiological level and may be associated with one of several diseases that collectively constitute the list of differential diagnosis.

Both PPA and PRAD are syndromes but with substantially different implications for underlying pathophysiology. In PRAD, the incidence of multifocal plaques and tangles is extremely high, nearly 95–100% according to some authors, whereas in PPA this probability is approximately 31% and becomes even lower if one takes into account only those patients with a non-fluent aphasia.

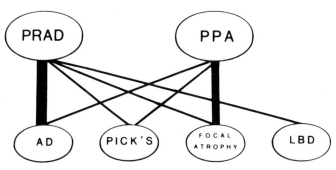

Figure 6. PRAD and PPA are clinical syndromes that can be caused by a variety of pathological processes. However, the frequency of association with a specific pathological process varies from one syndrome to the other. The thickness of the straight lines indicate the relative probability that links one of the clinical syndromes to specific underlying pathological processes. Focal atrophy, relatively focal neuronal loss with gliosis; LBD, Lewy body disease; Pick's, Pick's disease with Pick bodies.

PPA is neuropathologically heterogeneous in the sense that it can be associated with several entities including focal cortical degeneration, cortical achromasia, Pick's disease and AD. PRAD is also a heterogeneous syndrome in the sense that it can be associated not only with pathologically proven AD but also with Pick's disease, non-specific degeneration and Lewy body dementia. However, the probability of finding each of these neuro-pathological entities varies when PPA is compared with PRAD (Figure 6).

Is PPA heterogeneous?

The syndrome of PPA is clinically heterogeneous as well: some patients can have a fluent aphasia while others have a non-fluent aphasia; some can show an extremely indolent clinical progression while others show one with a brisker pace. A far greater degree of heterogeneity is introduced if the definition of PPA indicated in Table 1 is not followed, particularly if PPA becomes equated with all cases of progressive aphasia, including those that have early comportmental and memory deficits or those with a galloping course. This less restrictive definition leads to much greater heterogeneity by encompassing additional patients, many of whom would qualify for the diagnosis of PRAD.

Is PPA a subtype of AD?

There are some patients in whom the clinical picture of PPA has been associated with the pathological picture of AD. This probably represents an extremely small proportion of all AD cases, undoubtedly less than one in a 100. PPA could therefore join a list that now includes cortical blindness, Balint's syndrome, hemiparesis and right parietal lobe syndrome as one of several rare and idiosyncratic manifestations of AD-like pathology (see, for example, Jagust et al, 1990). It is quite likely that the incidence of AD pathology in PPA will tend to be inflated since some patients will come to autopsy many years after disease onset, in the advanced senium, when the probability of finding neuritic plaques and neurofibrillary tangles is very high even in cases when they may not have been causally related to the emergence of the PPA.

Is PPA a precursor to dementia?

Whether PPA is a precursor to dementia is very much dependent on one's definition of dementia. According to the criteria outlined here, PPA is a dementia confined for at least 2 years to the domain of language function. The anatomical substrate of language takes the form of a widely distributed network focused around the left perisylvian regions of the human brain (Mesulam, 1990). Individual components of this network also participate in other cognitive domains. It is therefore unlikely that a progressive degenerative disease, even one that is exclusively focused on the language network, could indefinitely leave other cognitive faculties unscathed. What is truly remarkable is that some patients with PPA experience a relatively isolated language deficit for more than 10 years. This clinical selectivity and the associated anatomical selectivity of the disease for the frontoperisylvian structures of the left hemisphere reveal a pattern that is very different from that of PRAD where the selectivity is focused on memory function and the limbic system.

SPECULATIONS ON THE SELECTIVE VULNERABILITY IN PPA

Patients with PPA show that a 'degenerative' process can selectively (though not necessarily exclusively) target an individual cognitive domain and its corresponding neural network. At least in some patients, the process in PPA may conceivably represent one subset of a larger family of 'focal degenerations' that afflict the brain in a regional fashion. When such focal atrophy affects the frontal lobes, the resulting syndrome is identified as progressive comportmental dysfunction (or frontal dementia); when it affects posterior cortices it leads to progressive Balint's syndrome or prosopagnosia in the context of progressive visuospatial dysfunction. In other patients, the focus of selective involvement may be the limbic system, giving rise to a syndrome of progressive amnestic dementia. When the focal atrophy tends to emphasize the left frontoperisylvian regions, the emergent syndrome is identified as PPA.

The factors that determine the distribution of the selective vulnerability are poorly understood. One of our patients, a retired businessman, had an abscess removed from the temporoparietal region of the left hemisphere when he was 11 years old. Recovery was complete with no residual language deficit. At the age of 70 he experienced the onset of a gradually progressive language deficit. When we examined him 6 years later, he had a logopenic fluent aphasia but a preservation of function in other domains, a pattern that was consistent with the diagnosis of PPA.

In the course of examining additional patients with suspected PPA, we were also struck by the number of patients reporting a history of early reading or spelling difficulties. We therefore undertook a preliminary study based on nine patients with a clinical diagnosis of PPA and compared them with two control groups, one consisting of 11 patients with a diagnosis of PRAD (but who also had anomic or aphasic impairments) and a third consisting of ten non-dementing age-matched control subjects. In a structured interview with subjects and family members, information was obtained about the incidence of developmental learning disabilities in the subjects themselves and in first-degree relatives.

We found that four of the nine patients with PPA reported an early history of reading and spelling difficulty and two reported difficulty with arithmetic. In contrast, none of the subjects in the other two groups reported early learning difficulties. With respect to relatives, Table 6 shows that a higher incidence of specific learning problems was reported by families of patients with PPA than by families of the other two groups. In one case, there was a family history of dyslexia in several generations. In another, all four siblings reported significant difficulties with writing and spelling and several nieces and nephews were diagnosed as having a learning disability. It is interesting to note that the incidence of PPA is distinctly higher in males, who are also more susceptible to dyslexia and allied learning disabilities. It will be useful to know if a similarly high familial incidence of learning disabilities will be

Table 6. Frequency of finding a history of learning disability in probands and first-degree relatives in PPA, PRAD and age-matched controls.

	Learning disability present	Learning disability absent	Probands + relatives
PPA $(n=9)$	18	56	$9+65$
PRAD $(n=10)$	3	88	$10+81$
Control $(n=11)$	2	88	$11+79$

χ^2 (d.f. 2) $= 32.41$, $P<0.0001$ (two-tail).
PPA versus PRAD Fisher Exact Test $P<0.0001$, PPA versus control $P<0.0001$.

found in patients with the Landau–Kleffner syndrome, a condition of acquired aphasia with convulsions seen in childhood (Paquier et al, 1992).

On the basis of our clinical observations and the preliminary results summarized in Table 6, we wonder if PPA reflects, at least in some patients, the tardive expression of a genetic or acquired vulnerability focused upon the left hemisphere language networks. In some patients, such a vulnerability may be the only determinant and may lead to non-specific abiotrophic changes. In others, this vulnerability can interact with other factors and may determine the site of least resistance for the emergence of pathological processes otherwise consistent with AD or Pick's disease.

There are at least three examples of temporally remote reactivations of previously acquired neurological impairments: (1) women who have recovered from Sydenham's chorea in childhood can experience chorea gravidarum during pregnancy in response to alterations in the hormonal milieu; (2) patients with a history of polymyelitis can develop, decades later, a progressive motor neurone disease (Cashman et al, 1987); (3) some individuals who have suffered brain injury early in life can develop, in midlife, a very slowly progressive hemiparkinsonism on the side opposite the early hemispheric lesion (Klawans, 1981). The mechanisms that mediate such delayed activations of early vulnerabilities remain very poorly understood. The syndrome of PPA, especially in patients with a family history of dyslexia, may provide an additional model for exploring these mechanisms.

CONCLUSIONS

We have identified a clinical syndrome, PPA, which is easily distinguishable from other clinical syndromes such as PRAD. The clinical syndrome of PPA is characterized by a relative preservation of memory and of language-independent daily living activities, despite a relentlessly progressive aphasia. The literature that we have been able to access contains reports of 63 patients that fit the criteria for PPA. When compared with patients with either PRAD or the pathological diagnosis of AD, the PPA group contains more males, a higher incidence of onset in the presenium and a greater incidence of non-fluent aphasias. The probability of finding AD-like pathology is 68–100% in PRAD but only 31% in the PPA sample represented in Table 2. PPA, like PRAD, is a syndrome, not a disease. Its unifying feature is not the underlying pathology but the anatomical distribution of the regions that are most severely affected by the disease process and the corresponding clinical picture.

PRAD and PPA are both clinical syndromes of progressive cognitive alterations but each has a different set of probabilities for being associated with specific types of neuropathological processes. Especially at a time when independent biological markers for the underlying disease processes in dementia are not available, the identification of such clinical syndromes is of considerable heuristic value for predicting the possible nature for the underlying pathophysiology and also for counselling patients and caregivers in matters related to course and management.

NOTE ADDED IN PROOF

At the stage of galleys we discovered that we had inadvertently overlooked a report by B. Croisile, B. Laurent, D. Michel, D. LeBras, L. Cinotti and F. Maugière (1991) (*Rev. Neurol.* (Paris), **147:** 192–199) in which three patients with PPA are described in extensive detail, including CT, MR and PET studies, bringing the current total of published PPA patients to 66.

Acknowledgements

We want to thank Leah Christie for expert secretarial assistance. Supported by NS-20285 and AG-05134.

This chapter is based on a report prepared for the IPSEN FOUNDATION COLLOQUIUM in Marseille on April 6, 1992.

REFERENCES

Appell J, Kertesz A & Fisman (1982) A study of language functioning in Alzheimer's patients. *Brain and Language* **17:** 73–91.

Assal G, Favre C & Regli F (1984) Aphasia as a first sign of dementia. *Senile Dementia: Outlook for the Future*, pp 279–282. New York: AR Liss.

Bachman DL, Wolf PA, Linn R et al (1992) Prevalence of dementia and probable senile dementia of the Alzheimer type in the Framingham study. *Neurology* **42:** 115–119.

Basso A, Capitani E & Laiacona M (1988) Progressive language impairment without dementia: a case with isolated category specific semantic defect. *Journal of Neurology, Neurosurgery and Psychiatry* **51:** 1201–1207.

Benson DF & Geschwind N (1985) Aphasia and related disorders: a clinical approach. In Mesulam M-M (ed.) *Principles of Behavioral Neurology*, pp 193–238. Contemporary Neurology Series. Philadelphia: FA Davis.

Benson DF & Zaias BW (1991) Progressive aphasia: a case with postmortem correlation. *Neuropsychiatry, Neuropsychology and Behavioral Neurology* **4:** 215–223.

Berger ML & Porch BE (1990) A longitudinal study of primary progressive aphasia. *Neurology* **40** (supplement 1): 198.

Brun A (1987) Frontal lobe degeneration of non-Alzheimer's type. I. Neuropathology. *Archives of Gerontology and Geriatrics* **6:** 193–208.

Case Records of the Massachusetts General Hospital (1986) *Weekly Clinicopathological Exercises* **314:** 111.

Cashman NR, Maselli R, Wollman RL, Roos R, Simon R & Antel JP (1987) Late denervation in patients with antecedent paralytic poliomyelitis. *New England Journal of Medicine* **317:** 7–12.

Chawluk JB, Mesulam M-M, Hurtig H et al (1986) Slowly progressive aphasia without generalized dementia: studies with positron emission tomography. *Annals of Neurology* **19:** 68–74.

Dejerine J & Sérieux P (1897) Un cas de surdité verbale pure terminée par aphasie sensorielle, suivi d'autopsie. *Comptes Rendus des Séances de la Société de Biologie (Paris)* **49:** 1074–1077.

DeLecluse F, Andersen AR, Waldemar G et al (1990) Cerebral blood flow in progressive aphasia without dementia. *Brain* **113:** 1395–1404.

De Oliveira SAV, DeO.Castro MJM & Bittencourt PRM (1989) Slowly progressive aphasia followed by Alzheimer's dementia, a case report. *Arquivos de Neuro-Psiquiatria* **47:** 72–75.

Faber-Langendoen K, Morris JC, Knesevich JW, LaBarge E, Miller JP & Berg L (1988) Aphasia in senile dementia of the Alzheimer type. *Annals of Neurology* **23:** 365–370.

Franceschi F (1908) Gliosi perivascolare in un caso di demenza afasica. *Annali di Neurologia* **26:** 281–290.

Fratiglioni L, Grut M, Forsell Y et al (1991) Prevalence of Alzheimer's disease and other dementias in an elderly urban population: relationship with age, sex and education. *Neurology* **41**: 1886–1892.

Goulding PJ, Northen B, Snowden JS, MacDermott N & Neary D (1989) Progressive aphasia with right-sided extrapyramidal signs: another manifestation of localised cerebral atrophy. *Journal of Neurology, Neurosurgery and Psychiatry* **52**: 128–130.

Graff-Radford NR, Damasio AR, Hyman BT et al (1990) Progressive aphasia in a patient with Pick's disease: a neuropsychological, radiologic and anatomic study. *Neurology* **40**: 620–626.

Green J, Morris JC, Sandson J, McKeel DW & Miller JW (1990) Progressive aphasia: a precursor of global dementia? *Neurology* **40**: 423–429.

Hamanaka T & Yamagishi H (1986) Slowly progressive aphasia in the praesenium with much later onset of generalized dementia: report of two cases. *Proceedings of the Joint Japan–China Stroke Conference*, Hirosaka and Tokyo, Japan, pp 33–40.

Heath PD, Kennedy P & Kapur N (1983) Slowly progressive aphasia without generalized dementia. *Annals of Neurology* **13**: 687–688.

Holland AL, McBurney DH, Moossy J & Reinmuth OM (1985) The dissolution of language in Pick's disease with neurofibrillary tangles: a case study. *Brain and Language* **24**: 36–58.

Jagust WJ, Davies P, Tiller-Borcich JK & Reed BR (1990) Focal Alzheimer's disease. *Neurology* **40**: 14–19.

Kartsounis LD, Crellin RF, Crewes H & Toone BK (1991) Primary progressive non-fluent aphasia: a case study. *Cortex* **27**: 121–129.

Kempler D, Metter EJ, Riege WH, Jackson CA, Benson DF & Hanson WR (1990) Slowly progressive aphasia: three cases with language, memory, CT and PET data. *Journal of Neurology, Neurosurgery and Psychiatry* **53**: 987–993.

Kirshner HS, Webb WG, Kelly MP & Wells CE (1984) Language disturbance: an initial symptom of cortical degeneration and dementia. *Archives of Neurology* **41**: 491–496.

Kirshner HS, Tanridag O, Thurman L & Whetsell WO (1987) Progressive aphasia without dementia: two cases with focal spongiform degeneration. *Annals of Neurology* **22**: 527–532.

Klawans HL (1984) Hemiparkinsonism as a late complication of hemiatrophy: a new syndrome. *Neurology* **31**: 625–628.

Kobayashi K, Kurachi M, Gyoubu T et al (1990) Progressive dysphasic dementia with localized cerebral atrophy: report of an autopsy. *Clinical Neuropathology* **9**: 254–261.

Kushner M (1989) MRI and ^{123}I-iodoamphetamine SPECT imaging of a patient with slowly progressing aphasia. *Advances in Functional Neuroimaging* (Winter) 17–20.

Lippa CF, Cohen R, Smith TW & Drachman DA (1991) Primary progressive aphasia with focal neuronal achromasia. *Neurology* **41**: 882–886.

Luzzatti C & Poeck K (1991) An early description of slowly progressive aphasia. *Archives of Neurology* **48**: 228–229.

McDaniel KD, Wagner MT & Greenspan BS (1991) The role of brain single photon emission computed tomography in the diagnosis of primary progressive aphasia. *Archives of Neurology* **48**: 1257–1260.

McKhann G, Drachman D, Folstein M et al (1984) Clinical diagnosis of Alzheimer's disease: report of the NINCDS–ADRDA Work Group under the auspices of the Department of Health and Human Services Task Force on Alzheimer's Disease. *Neurology* **34**: 939–944.

Mandell AM, Alexander MP & Carpenter S (1989) Creutzfeldt–Jakob disease presenting as isolated aphasia. *Neurology* **39**: 55–58.

Mehler MF, Horoupian DS, Davies P & Dickson DW (1987) Reduced somatostatin-like immunoreactivity in cerebral cortex in nonfamilial dysphasic dementia. *Neurology* **37**: 1448–1453.

Mendez MF & Zander BA (1991) Dementia presenting with aphasia: clinical characteristics. *Journal of Neurology, Neurosurgery and Psychiatry* **54**: 542–545.

Mesulam M-M (1982) Slowly progressive aphasia without generalized dementia. *Annals of Neurology* **11**: 592–598.

Mesulam M-M (1987) Primary progressive aphasia: differentiation from Alzheimer's disease. *Annals of Neurology* **22**: 533–534.

Mesulam M-M (1990) Large scale neurocognitive networks and distributed processing for attention, language and memory. *Annals of Neurology* **28**: 597–613.

Morris JC, McKeel DW, Fulling K, Torack RM & Berg L (1988) Validation of clinical diagnostic criteria for Alzheimer's disease. *Annals of Neurology* **24**: 17–22.

Northen B, Hopcutt B & Griffiths H (1990) Case study: progressive aphasia without generalized dementia. *Aphasiology* **4**: 55–65.

Paquier PF, VanDongen HR & Loonen CB (1992) The Landau–Kleffner syndrome or 'acquired aphasia with convulsive disorder'. *Archives of Neurology* **49**: 354–359.

Pick A (1892) Ueber die Beziehungen der senilen Hirnatrophie zur Aphasie. *Prager Medizinische Wochenschrift* **17**: 165–167.

Pick A (1904) Zur Symptomatologie der linksseitigen Schlafenlappenatrophie. *Monatsschrift für Psychiatrie und Neurologie* **16**: 378–388.

Poeck K & Luzzatti C (1988) Slowly progressive aphasia in three patients: the problem of accompanying neuropsychological deficit. *Brain* **111**: 151–168.

Pogacar S & Williams RS (1984) Alzheimer's disease presenting as slowly progressive aphasia. *Rhode Island Medical Journal* **67**: 181–185.

Price BH, Gurvit H, Weintraub S, Geula C, Leimkuhler E & Mesulam M-M (in press) Neuropsychological patterns and language deficits in autopsy-confirmed Alzheimer's disease. *Archives of Neurology*.

Risse SC, Raskind MA, Nochlin D et al (1990) Neuropathological findings in patients with clinical diagnoses of probable Alzheimer's disease. *American Journal of Psychiatry* **147**: 168–172.

Rosenfeld M (1909) Die partielle Grosshirnatrophie. *Journal of Psychology and Neurology* **14**: 115–130.

Sapin LR, Anderson FH & Pulaski PD (1989) Progressive aphasia without dementia: further documentation. *Annals of Neurology* **25**: 411–413.

Scheltens PH, Hazenberg GJ, Lindeboom J, Valk J & Wolters ECH (1990) A case of progressive aphasia without dementia: 'temporal' Pick's disease? *Journal of Neurology, Neurosurgery and Psychiatry* **53**: 79–80.

Shuttleworth EC, Yates AJ & Paltan-Ortiz JD (1985) Case report. Creutzfeldt–Jakob disease presenting as progressive aphasia. *Journal of the National Medical Association* **77**: 649–656.

Snowden JS, Goulding PJ & Neary D (1989) Semantic dementia: a form of circumscribed cerebral atrophy. *Behavioral Neurology* **2**: 167–182.

Snowden JS, Neary D, Mann DMA, Goulding PJ & Testa HJ (1992) Progressive language disorder due to lobar atrophy. *Annals of Neurology* **31**: 174–183.

Tyrrell PJ, Warrington EK, Frackowiak RSJ & Rossor MN (1990) Heterogeneity in progressive aphasia due to focal cortical atrophy. *Brain* **113**: 1321–1336.

Tyrrell PJ, Kartsounis LD, Frackowiak RSJ, Findley LJ & Rossor MN (1991) Progressive loss of speech output and orofacial dyspraxia associated with frontal lobe metabolism. *Journal of Neurology, Neurosurgery and Psychiatry* **54**: 351–357.

Wechsler AF (1977) Presenile dementia presenting as aphasia. *Journal of Neurology, Neurosurgery and Psychiatry* **40**: 303–305.

Wechsler AF, Verity A, Rosenschein S, Fried I & Scheibel AB (1982) Pick's Disease: a clinical, computed tomographic and histologic study with Golgi impregnation observations. *Archives of Neurology* **39**: 287–290.

Weintraub S & Mesulam M-M (1985) The examination of mental state. In Mesulam M-M (ed.) *Principles of Behavioral Neurology*, pp 71–123. Contemporary Neurology Series. Philadelphia: FA Davis.

Weintraub S & Mesulam M-M (1993) Four neuropsychological profiles in dementia. In Boller F & Spinnler H (eds) *Handbook of Neuropsychology*, vol. 8. Amsterdam: Elsevier (in press).

Weintraub S, Rubin NP & Mesulam M-M (1990) Primary progressive aphasia: longitudinal course, neuropsychological profile and language features. *Archives of Neurology* **47**: 1329–1335.

Yamamoto T, Fukuyama H & Yamadori A (1989) Two cases of slowly progressive aphasia without generalized dementia (Mesulam). A study with CT, MRI and [^{18}F] FDG–PET. *Neurological Medicine* **31**: 183–190.

Yamanouchi H, Budka H & Vass K (1986) Unilateral Creutzfeldt–Jakob disease. *Neurology* **36**: 1517–1520.

7

Dementia with motor neurone disease

JOHN KEW
NIGEL LEIGH

Dementia occurring with motor neurone disease (MND; amyotrophic lateral sclerosis; ALS) is rare, although the association has long been known and the last decade has witnessed increasing recognition of the disorder (Hudson, 1981; Wikstrom et al, 1982; Mitsuyama, 1984; Mitsuyama et al, 1985; Morita et al, 1987; Neary et al, 1990; Wightman et al, 1992). Dementia occurs with MND in approximately 2–3% of patients with the sporadic form but may be more common in familial cases (Hudson, 1981). As we shall see, the mental changes, which are often those of 'fronto-temporal' or 'anterior' dementia, are associated with characteristic changes in the brain and with a typical molecular pathology.

This chapter aims to provide a review of current knowledge and controversies concerning MND-dementia. Issues of particular importance include the relationships between typical MND (ALS) and MND-dementia, between prion disorders and MND with or without dementia, and between Pick's disease and other types of lobar atrophy and MND-dementia. As Hudson (1981) has pointed out, the tendency has been to dismiss the association between MND and dementia as coincidental, and to regard MND-dementia as unrelated to typical MND. In fact, MND-dementia may represent one end of a spectrum of cerebral involvement in a multi-system disorder that usually kills its victims by ventilatory failure before non-motor areas are significantly affected. On the other hand the notion that the intellect is preserved intact in MND holds true for most patients, although subtle changes of frontal or temporal lobe function, while leaving the intellectual abilities of the sufferer intact, may yet have significant consequences for the patient and the carers.

Although the cause of MND-dementia is unknown, there have been significant advances in the molecular genetics of familial MND (Siddique et al, 1991, 1992) and the identification of MND-dementia in families may provide a route to the identification of the molecular basis of this disorder and clues to the basis of phenotypic variation in MND.

Clinical features of MND-dementia

Although Charcot and Joffroy (1869) in their original description of amyotrophic lateral sclerosis did not link the disease with dementia, Westphal and

Baillière's Clinical Neurology—
Vol. 1, No. 3, November 1992
ISBN 0–7020–1631–4

Zacher (1886) (quoted by van Bogaert, 1925) described patients with MND and dementia paralytica. The complicating presence of syphilis makes these early reports difficult to interpret, and a report by Alzheimer (1891) is no exception. Alzheimer described a young man with progressive motor system degeneration and mental symptoms, although the patient had syphilis and carcinoma of the liver, and the 'psychosis' and the MND-like features may have been secondary to other factors. The patient was a 33-year-old man with a previous history of syphilis who developed wasting of the thenar muscles of the right hand 11 years before presenting with gastric pain and vomiting followed two months later by mental symptoms ('psychosis with prominent delirious confusion—*Verworrenheit*') and progressive wasting and weakness of the shoulder girdles and arms, fasciculations, and increased tendon reflexes. At autopsy, aside from carcinoma of the liver with lymph node and splenic involvement (perhaps lymphoma rather than carcinoma), there was atrophy of anterior roots and spinal motor neurones, degeneration of the nuclei of the floor of the fourth ventricle, widespread loss of cortical neurones, and involvement of the thalamus and striatum. Although there was no evidence of pachymeningitis or vascular disease of the cerebral hemispheres, the blood vessels at the base of the fourth ventricle were abnormal. Alzheimer concluded that the bulbar degeneration was probably not connected to the 'system disease' of the spinal cord, but could not connect the cortical pathology with the other features of the disease, or with other types of cortical pathology.

Oppenheim and Siemerling (1886) were probably the first to describe the syndrome of pseudobulbar emotional lability. Pierre Marie (1892) also provided an early account of the tendency for unprovoked laughing, weeping and generalized emotional lability in progressive bulbar palsy, and these symptoms were interpreted as reflecting 'feeble-mindedness' by Raymond and Cestan (1905), but these patients were probably not demented.

The first clear indications that MND might be complicated by a dementing illness were provided by Gerbert and Naville (1921), Büscher (1922), and especially by Van Bogaert (1925). In Van Bogaert's series of 31 ALS cases, 12 showed varying forms of mental change. Two exhibited emotional lability, while the remaining 10 showed both emotional and intellectual deficits. The latter were clearly organic and included defects of memory, attention, judgement and orientation. One patient was also aphasic. Bulbar symptoms were almost invariable, and in most cases the dementia was progressive.

Ziegler (1930) reviewed the clinical features of 101 ALS patients seen at the Mayo Clinic over a five year period. Nineteen patients had emotional lability associated with pseudobulbar palsy, but three patients developed dementia. Two of these patients, a man aged 51 years and a woman aged 59 years, presented with motor symptoms and subsequently developed features suggestive of fronto-temporal dementia. One patient, a woman aged 51 years, developed visual hallucinations, memory impairment, bizarre and inappropriate behaviour, and about 3 years later developed bulbar symptoms which evolved into typical ALS. Ziegler interpreted the mental abnormalities as due to a severe toxic psychosis, emphasizing the fluctuating symptoms and disorientation in time, place and sometimes person. No autopsies were performed of these patients.

Wechsler and Davison (1932) furnished a more detailed description of the clinical and pathological features of the syndrome of MND-dementia. Of three patients in their study who came to autopsy, one exhibited symptoms and signs which are now known to be characteristic of this disorder. The patient was a man aged 38 years who presented with impairment of memory. He later developed progressive loss of interest in his surroundings, became unkempt, and his social conduct deteriorated. Atrophy of the upper limb musculature became apparent six months after the onset of mental symptoms. On examination he was noted to have an expressionless, staring face, although when amused he would smile fatuously. His speech was dysarthric and monosyllabic and he showed perseveration of verbal response. He tended to wander about aimlessly, his behaviour was childish and inappropriate, and he showed emotional lability. There was asymmetrical facial weakness, atrophy and fasciculation of the tongue, fasciculations in the neck and shoulder musculature, and wasting and atrophy in the upper limbs. The patient's condition progressed to profound dementia with aphasia and he died from bronchopneumonia three years after the onset of symptoms. At autopsy the brain showed atrophy and neuronal loss in the frontal regions with fibrillary astrocytosis. The spinal cord showed demyelination of the pyramidal tracts and loss of anterior horn cells typical of MND (ALS).

A similar case of dementia complicated by the development of MND was reported by Friedlander and Kesert (1948) in a 50-year-old man. The initial manifestation of the disorder took the form of behavioural changes noticed by the patient's wife. These mental symptoms were rapidly followed by a severe progressive dysarthria, aphasia, and later distal amyotrophy of the limbs. The behavioural disorder was characterized by emotional lability and euphoria, at times interrupted by episodes of rage and violent behaviour. Inane grinning, restlessness and aimless wandering were other features. The patient died in a mute, bedridden state from terminal cachexia and respiratory failure 14 months after the onset of mental symptoms.

Familial occurrence of the disorder was reported by Robertson in 1953. The patient was a 69-year-old woman who presented with progressive bulbar palsy leading to death within 12 months of onset. Her father and cousin had both died from progressive bulbar palsy in their seventh decade. The inheritance pattern of the disorder suggested autosomal dominant transmission with incomplete penetrance. Other clinical features in the proband included progressive aphasia, memory impairment and behavioural changes. The latter took the form of general disinterest and lack of concern about her personal appearance, punctuated by episodes of restlessness, agitation and aimless wandering. Delusional ideation also suggested the coexistence of an organic psychosis. Autopsy disclosed generalized cerebral atrophy with fronto-temporal accentuation, loss of large pyramidal neurones from the motor cortex and neuronal loss with astrocytic proliferation in the frontal cortex. Although some argyrophilic plaques were present in the affected cortical areas, the author argued against the patient suffering from combined Alzheimer's disease and MND on clinical grounds and concluded that the intellectual deterioration was due to a cortical extension of the disease process causing the physical symptoms.

Major contributions to our understanding of the clinical and pathological features of MND-dementia have come from the extensive Japanese literature on the subject (Mitsuyama and Takamiya, 1979; Mitsuyama, 1984; Mitsuyama et al, 1985; Morita et al, 1987; Ohnishi et al, 1990). Many of the early papers are in Japanese, and both Mitsuyama et al (1985) and Morita et al (1987) provide detailed reviews of these sources, the latter authors identifying 34 cases including four of their own. Recent reports from North America (Salazar et al, 1983; Horoupian et al, 1984) and Europe (Bonduelle et al, 1968; Brion et al, 1980; Wikstrom et al, 1982; Neary et al, 1990; Ferrer et al, 1991; Wightman et al, 1992) have added to the literature, in which nearly 200 cases are now recorded, many with autopsy data. From these reports it is possible to build a fairly clear clinicopathological profile of this disorder.

Onset of the disease is usually in the sixth decade, with a mean age of about 55 years (Salazar et al, 1983). The duration from onset to death ranges from one to six years, with a mean of around 30 months (Wikstrom et al, 1982; Salazar et al, 1983; Mitsuyama, 1984; Morita et al, 1987). Men are more commonly affected than women, with a ratio of 2:1, as in typical MND. The onset of the disorder is insidious, the clinical picture being dominated at an early stage by signs of frontal lobe dysfunction including behavioural and personality changes, emotional disorder and memory loss. These changes tend to be noted by the patient's spouse or relatives, the patient remaining oblivious to his or her predicament. Patients frequently appear euphoric and childish, with a fatuous staring facial expression and a tendency to grin inanely. They may become rude, thoughtless, disinhibited and verbally aggressive. Restlessness and impulsivity are common, as is a tendency to wander about aimlessly or to collect objects at random (Morita et al, 1987). Obsessional traits, hyperphagia and hypersexuality may become apparent (Neary et al, 1990). Cases have been reported with elements of the Klüver–Bucy syndrome (Dickson et al, 1986), and with visual hallucinations and delusional ideation suggestive of an organic psychosis (Horoupian et al, 1984). Between periods of activity, patients may appear withdrawn and apathetic. Self-mutilation may occur as a late manifestation (Morita et al, 1987).

Neuropsychological evaluation is often difficult owing to lack of co-operation, poor attention and expressive dysphasia, but when possible shows abnormal performance on tests sensitive to frontal lobe function such as the Wisconsin card sorting test, the Weigl block task and verbal fluency tasks. In contrast, perceptual and spatial functions usually remain intact (Morita et al, 1987; Neary et al, 1990), and the discrepancy between verbal and performance intelligence quotient scores commonly found in patients with Alzheimer-type dementia is absent (Horoupian et al, 1984). Dyscalculia, on the other hand, is often present (Horoupian et al, 1984; Morita et al, 1987).

Progressive reduction in speech output due to motor aphasia commonly develops in parallel with the behavioural disorder, in time leading to stereotyped speech (*'stehende Redensarten'*), echolalia and eventually mutism (Mitsuyama, 1984; Neary et al, 1990). In spite of this, comprehension of the spoken word generally remains intact (Neary et al, 1990). Bulbar symptoms, particularly dysarthria, are common and may be present in up to 85% of cases (Wikstrom et al, 1982; Mitsuyama, 1984). Frontal release signs are frequently elicited (Neary et al, 1990).

Most commonly patients present with mental symptoms (Morita et al, 1987; Salazar, 1983; Horoupian et al, 1984; Neary et al, 1990). Signs of anterior horn cell involvement typically become apparent six to twelve months after the onset of the mental symptoms (Mitsuyama, 1984), although in some cases the two may evolve simultaneously, or muscular wasting and weakness may antedate the dementia (Morita et al, 1987). Unlike classical ALS, where the site of onset and pattern of disease progression are unpredictable, the distribution of the muscle atrophy in dementia with motor neurone disease tends to be relatively uniform. Wasting and fasciculation of the tongue, shoulder girdle, and proximal upper limb musculature is common and prominent, while atrophy in the hands is less severe, and the lower limbs tend largely to be spared (Wikstrom et al, 1982; Mitsuyama, 1984; Neary et al, 1990). Muscle weakness in the limbs may remain mild (Wikstrom et al, 1982; Neary et al, 1990). Thus patients often remain mobile until the late stages of the disease. Upper motor neurone features such as spasticity and extensor plantar responses may be less common in MND-dementia than in typical MND, although hyperreflexia is often present at some stage of the disorder. These findings concur with neuropathological studies showing degeneration of the anterior horns, but little involvement of the lateral corticospinal tracts. This pattern of bulbar and spinal involvement has led some authors to the conclusion that the disease may represent an atypical form of progressive spinal muscular atrophy, rather than a variant of ALS (Morita et al, 1987), but many patients with the classical combination of upper and lower motor neurone signs have been reported and there is no convincing evidence that MND-dementia should be separated from other forms of MND on the basis of the pattern of motor involvement alone.

Parkinsonism is quite commonly associated with MND and dementia, and probably represents a variant of the MND-dementia syndrome (Hudson, 1981).

Familial MND-dementia

Two to five per cent of MND patients with typical MND have a family history in a first-degree relative, and numerous kindreds have been described with multiple affected individuals (Siddique et al, 1989, 1991). The mode of inheritance in familial MND is usually of autosomal dominant type, and genetic linkage to chromosome 21q in the region of the amyloid precursor protein gene has been tentatively established in some families (Siddique et al, 1991, 1992). Reviewing 85 families in the literature, Hudson (1981) noted that 15% of all pedigrees contained one or more family members with a combination of dementia and MND, while 5% of pedigrees contained members with combined MND, dementia and extrapyramidal signs. The mean age of onset was slightly younger than in sporadic cases of dementia with MND, and mean disease duration was marginally longer. Another point of distinction from sporadic MND-dementia lay in the observation that although dementia could precede, accompany or follow the onset of MND in individual cases, mental changes most commonly developed after the features of anterior horn cell disease had become apparent. Otherwise, the clinical and pathological characteristics of the familial and sporadic forms of MND-dementia appear to be virtually indistinguishable. Memory loss, behavioural abnormalities, emotional lability and disordered social conduct are typical manifestations of the dementia (Finlayson et al, 1973). Bulbar involvement is usually prominent, and pathological lesions are similar in type and distribution to those of sporadic MND-dementia (Finlayson et al, 1973; Hudson, 1981), although hippocampal neurofibrillary tangle formation may also be present (Finlayson et al, 1973; Wightman et al, 1992).

A family recently described by Gunnarsson et al (1991) suggests that MND-dementia and non-Alzheimer's dementia with 'non-specific' pathological changes may represent variations of the same disorder. In this family, dementia of frontal lobe type (DFLT) occurred in three generations but in the fourth generation four members developed MND that was associated with minor cognitive abnormalities in three individuals and chronic psychosis in one. Pathological changes in the brain of one individual in the third generation showed 'non-specific' changes (see below) including vacuolar changes in neocortical layer 2, but no Alzheimer change. Aside from the appearance of MND in one generation, the clinical and pathological features are reminiscent of a kindred in which five of ten siblings in one generation developed dementia with frontal, temporal or parietal features and 'non-specific' pathological changes including vacuolar change in neocortical layers 2 and 3 (Kim et al, 1981). Although in this latter family the mode of inheritance is doubtful, in the family of Gunnarsson et al (1991) it is of autosomal dominant type, as is usually the case in MND-dementia.

Further evidence for a close relationship between non-Alzheimer dementia or dementia of frontal lobe type (DFLT) has been provided by Neary's description of a patient with MND and DFLT whose mother suffered for 14 years from a dementing illness with features of DFLT, but who never developed MND (Neary et al, 1990).

Pathology

Macroscopic changes in the brain consist of diffuse cerebral atrophy with fronto-temporal accentuation. Lobar atrophy may be very marked. Microscopically, the most characteristic finding is neuronal loss and spongy change with vacuolation of the neuropil in layers 2 and 3 of the frontal and temporal cortex (Hudson, 1981; Wikstrom et al, 1982; Salazar et al, 1983; Mitsuyama, 1984; Morita et al, 1987; Neary et al, 1990; Wightman et al, 1992). Golgi studies suggest that this appearance may be partly due to attenuation and reduction of the dendritic arbour of pyramidal neurones that expand in these cortical layers (Horoupian et al, 1984; Ferrer et al, 1991). In contrast to classical MND, there may be a normal complement of giant Betz cells in the motor cortex (Morita et al, 1987) although Betz cells may show shrinkage (Neary et al, 1990).

Ballooned neurones, Pick bodies, Alzheimer's neurofibrillary tangles and senile plaques are generally absent (Morita et al, 1987; Neary et al, 1990; Wightman et al, 1992). Immunocytochemical studies have clarified the relationship between MND-dementia and other types of dementia (Table 1). Thus antibodies against cytoskeletal proteins such as phosphorylated neurofilament (pNF) peptides or microtubule-associated protein tau identify Pick bodies (Murayama et al, 1990b) but not intra-neuronal inclusions in MND-dementia (Okamoto et al, 1991; Wightman et al, 1992). In contrast, antibodies against ubiquitin, a highly conserved protein implicated in the degradation of altered or short-lived proteins, identify inclusions in neurones of the frontal and temporal cortex and in the dentate granule cells of the hippocampus (Figure 1) in patients with MND-dementia (Okamoto et al, 1991; Wightman et al, 1992). These inclusions are difficult to identify with conventional stains, and unlike Pick bodies are not argyrophilic. They differ from cortical Lewy bodies in several ways (Table 1). They are thus similar in their staining and immunocytochemical properties to the characteristic ubiquitin-immunoreactive inclusions found in brainstem and spinal cord motor neurones in typical MND (Leigh et al, 1988, 1991; Lowe et al, 1988; Murayama et al, 1990a).

At a subcortical level, the disease is characterized by mild white matter gliosis (Mitsuyama, 1984). This may resemble, to some degree, the lesion of progressive subcortical gliosis (Neumann and Cohn, 1967), although the white matter changes are generally less severe. In addition, gliosis and neuronal loss may be prominent in the substantia nigra and basal ganglia in as many as half of all patients with MND dementia (Morita et al, 1987), whereas in progressive subcortical gliosis nigral pathology is absent (Neary et al, 1990). Despite the frequent presence of nigral degeneration in MND-dementia (Neary et al, 1990) clinical evidence of extrapyramidal disease remains rare (Mitsuyama et al, 1985), although cases with parkinsonism have been documented (Hudson, 1981; Horoupian et al, 1984). It is interesting, in view of the possibility that MND-dementia might represent a variant of familial MND/ALS, that nigral degeneration of the type seen in MND-dementia has been described in one member of a family with otherwise typical familial MND (Wolf et al, 1991).

In the brainstem, degeneration and gliosis are commonly present in the hypoglossal nucleus (Wikstrom et al, 1982). In the spinal cord there is loss of anterior horn cells. Remaining cells often show chromatolysis and neuronophagia, and some may contain large eosinophilic cytoplasmic inclusions and ubiquitin-immunoreactive inclusions as seen in typical MND (Wrightman et al, 1992; Wikstrom et al, 1982; Horoupian et al, 1984; Morita et al, 1987; Neary et al, 1990). However, as noted above, the spinal cord changes differ from those in classical MND in that demyelination of the corticospinal tracts is often mild or absent, in keeping with the clinical signs (Mitsuyama, 1984; Neary et al, 1990).

Table 1. Molecular pathology of MND-dementia.

	Distribution	UB	Ag	pNF	tau	CG-A	Anti-FAF	aBC	EM
Pick body	FT NC, DGCs, HC-PC	+	++	++	++	++	−	−	15–25 nm filaments
Cortical LBs	TP NC, PHG	++	+/−	+/−	−	?	+[1]	++[2]	10–15 nm filaments, granular material
MND	FT NC, DCGs	++	−	−	−	+/−	+[1]	++[2]	10–15 nm filaments, granular material

1. Courtesy of Professor Matti Hattia.
2. Courtesy of Dr James Lowe.

aBC = aB-crystallin; Ag = silver stains; CG-A = chromagranin A; DGCs = dentate granule cells; EM = electron microscope appearance; FAF = familial amyloid Finnish type; FT = fronto-temporal; HC-PC = hippocampal pyramidal cells; LB = Lewy bodies; NC = neocortex; PHG = parahippocampal gyrus; pNF = phosphorylated neurofilaments; TP = temporo-parietal.

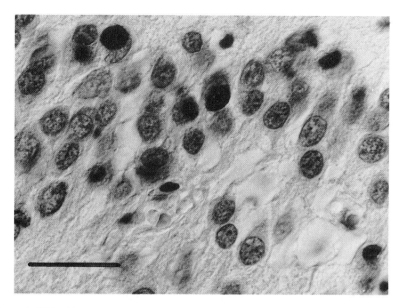

Figure 1. Ubiquitin cytochemistry on hippocampal dentate granule cells showing intra-neuronal inclusions in MND-dementia. Bar = 15 μm.

Investigations

Routine laboratory investigations and cerebrospinal fluid examination are generally normal. Electromyography and muscle biopsy confirm the presence of neurogenic atrophy (Mitsuyama et al, 1985). The electro-encephalogram (EEG) may show diffuse slowing of background activity, but high-voltage periodic spike discharges, as seen in Creutzfeldt–Jakob disease, are not present (Mitsuyama et al, 1985; Morita et al, 1987; Ohnishi et al, 1990). Computerized tomography of the brain typically shows fronto-temporal atrophy (Mitsuyama, 1984; Morita et al, 1987; Ohnishi et al, 1990). Recent functional brain imaging studies using single photon emission tomography (SPET) have demonstrated a pattern of reduced tracer uptake in the frontal (Neary et al, 1990), or fronto-temporal (Ohnishi et al, 1990) cortex with sparing of more posterior cortical areas; although striking, these abnormalities are non-specific and similar appearances may result from Pick's disease or progressive supranuclear palsy (Ohnishi et al, 1990).

MND-DEMENTIA AND OTHER NEURODEGENERATIVE DISORDERS

The precise nosological status of MND-dementia is unclear, and will remain so until the cause is known and specific molecular markers are identified. The neuropsychological and neuropathological correlates of cerebral involvement in MND-dementia are probably indistinguishable from those occurring in Pick's disease, using this term to indicate patients with fronto-temporal lobar atrophy with varying syndromes of 'anterior' dementia but lacking ballooned neurones and Pick bodies—types B and C Pick's disease of Constantinidis et al (1974). Other terms include 'frontal lobe degeneration of non-Alzheimer type' (FLD) (Brun, 1987) and 'dementia of frontal-lobe type' (DFLT) by Neary et al (1988, 1990). The difficulty in classification of the disorder is further illustrated by a number of cases in the literature where symptoms and signs of MND were manifestations of another pathologically-verified disease, and by recent reports of impaired frontal function in non-demented patients with classical MND.

Relationship to classical sporadic MND

Classical MND is not usually associated with impaired intellectual function. This view has been challenged, however, by a number of recent neuropsychological studies on patients with sporadic MND showing subtle but significant performance deficits on tests sensitive to frontal lobe function (Gallassi et al, 1985; David and Gillham, 1986; Gallassi et al, 1989; Ludolph et al, 1992). For example, David and Gilham (1986) found that 57% of their patients with MND failed the Wisconsin card sorting test compared to 11% of matched neurological controls, with 43% showing a complete inability to develop sorting strategies. Similarly, several studies have shown impaired verbal fluency in non-demented MND patients (Gallassi et al, 1985, 1989; Ludolph et al, 1992). The significance of these findings, and their neuro-anatomical basis, remain unclear. Functional brain imaging studies in typical MND using positron emission tomography (PET) have yielded conflicting results as to the site and extent of cortical involvement by the disease (Dalakas et al, 1987; Hoffman et al, 1987; Hatazawa et al, 1988; Ludolph et al, 1992). Two studies have reported reduced regional cerebral glucose metabolism at rest in the frontal cortex of ALS patients (Hoffman et al, 1987; Ludolph et al, 1992). The nature of frontal lobe involvement in classical MND clearly requires further investigation.

Relationship to frontal lobe degeneration (FLD)

As we have seen, MND-dementia shares features with FLD, a condition that may account for up to 10–20% of all cases of dementia (Brun, 1987). The cortical changes in FLD, consisting of fronto-temporal atrophy with neuronal loss, gliosis, and microvacuolation of layers 2 and 3, in the absence of ballooned neurones and Pick bodies, are indistinguishable from those in MND-dementia. In Brun's series of 16 cases, signs of MND were absent, although one case showed anterior horn cell changes.

It can therefore be seen that a close parallel exists, both in the nature of the dementia and in the pathological abnormalities, between DFLT and FLD and MND-dementia. FLD however often shows a protracted course, some patients surviving for more than 15 years from onset (Neary, 1990), whereas survival in patients with MND-dementia is typically only two to three years. It thus remains to be established whether the two disorders are separate clinico-pathological entities or whether they are different manifestations of the same disease.

Relationship to transmissible Creutzfeldt–Jakob disease (CJD)

In the so-called 'amyotrophic' form of Creutzfeldt–Jakob disease (CJD), typical spongiform change is absent and, with two possible exceptions, the disorder has not been transmitted to primates (Salazar et al, 1983; Connolly et al, 1988). In addition, myoclonus does not occur in the majority of patients, periodic sharp-wave discharges are not present in the electro-encephalogram and disease progression is considerably less rapid than in classical transmitted CJD. Furthermore, although status spongiosus of the superficial cortical layers is characteristic of dementia associated with MND, the classical spongiform change of CJD does not occur. The neuropathological lesion encountered in cases of rapidly progressive CJD is quite distinct from MND-dementia, being characterized by spongiform change that lacks a laminar distribution and by proliferation of hypertrophic astrocytes (Masters and Richardson, 1978; Salazar et al, 1983). It is therefore likely that many cases formerly classified as amyotrophic CJD are, in fact, cases of MND with frontal dementia (Hudson, 1981; Salazar et al, 1983).

Relationship to Pick's disease

As with transmissible CJD, cases of pathologically verified 'Pick body' Pick's disease have been described where the initial or predominant symptoms have been those of MND. One such patient presented with typical MND with some evidence of pseudobulbar palsy but without overt dementia (Sam et al, 1991). Neuropathologically atypical Pick bodies were present in the atrophic fronto-temporal cortex and the hippocampus. While the corticospinal tracts and hypoglossal nuclei were atrophic and gliotic, the anterior horn cells were relatively well preserved, and only a few axonal spheroids were encountered.

Relationship to western Pacific ALS-parkinsonism-dementia complex

This unique disease complex was first fully characterized by Hirano et al (1961) in the native Chamorro population of the western Pacific island of Guam at a time when the disease accounted for 10% of all adult deaths. The disorder is commoner in males, and a positive family history is obtained in about a third of cases, although it is not thought to be a genetic disorder. Presentation typically occurs in the fifth to seventh decade with progressive mental deterioration characterized by mental slowing, poor memory, lack of initiative, apathy and socially inappropriate behaviour, usually first noted by the patient's spouse or relatives. Features of parkinsonism almost always accompany the dementia. Typically patients show marked akinesia, mask-like expressionless faces, a stooped posture and a shuffling gait. In contrast to idiopathic Parkinson's disease, tremor is not prominent and, when present, occurs more commonly on action than at rest. Similarly, extra-pyramidal rigidity is present in less than half of all cases. Evidence of anterior horn cell degeneration is evident in about 25% of patients, but corticospinal tract involvement is more common, occurring in most patients (Rodgers-Johnson et al, 1986). In the later stages, progressive immobility and mutism occur, and the majority of patients die within four to five years of the onset of symptoms.

Another focus among the primitive Auyu and Jakai people of Western New Guinea bears close clinical resemblance to that on Guam, although age at onset is markedly lower and mean disease duration is longer (Gadjusek and Salazar, 1982).

Autopsy studies on Guam cases have shown atrophy of the frontal and temporal neocortex, loss of pigment in the substantia nigra and locus coeruleus, and atrophy of the globus pallidus. Histologically, severe Alzheimer's neurofibrillary degeneration is present in the pyramidal cell layer of the hippocampus, the substantia nigra and the amygdala, with similar but less prominent changes throughout the frontal and temporal cortices and brainstem (Hirano et al, 1961, 1966). These pathological features readily differentiate the disorder from MND-dementia, where Alzheimer-type changes are absent, or mild and commensurate with the patient's age.

Thus, although the ALS-parkinsonian dementia complex shares with MND-dementia the common clinical features of frontal lobe dementia and anterior horn cell disease, the consistent finding of extrapyramidal involve-ment in ALS-PD, and the markedly different neuropathological features suggest that the two conditions are, in fact, unrelated.

Alzheimer's disease and MND

Inevitably, considering how common Alzheimer's disease is in the elderly population, some patients with MND will have coexistent Alzheimer's change. There is no convincing evidence for a greater than chance associa-tion between the two conditions. However, a number of families have been reported in which MND and Alzheimer's disease have coexisted. Frecker et al (1990) reported a patient with pathologically proven MND (ALS) who had Alzheimer's disease changes in the temporal lobe, but who had not been clinically demented. This is reminiscent of one of our cases with MND and minor cognitive changes, a patient with familial MND of presumed autosomal-dominant inheritance (Wightman et al, 1992). They also reported two pedigrees in which Alzheimer's disease and MND (ALS) had coexisted. In their family too, a 65-year-old woman had pathologically proven Alzheimer's disease and MND, a brother with a clinical history suggestive of MND, but without dementia, and a father who died at the age of 69 years with a dementing illness thought to be Alzheimer's disease, but not pathologically proven. In another pedigree (family 3), Alzheimer's disease and MND were diagnosed in a mother and son respectively. In the mother's generation, four other siblings had a dementing illness thought to be Alzheimer's disease, but not confirmed by autopsy. Frecker et al found a probable or confirmed association between MND and Alzheimer's disease in three other published families. Unfortunately, in most cases, pathological confirmation is lacking.

Frecker et al (1990) also reported a patient, without any family history, who had pathologically proven MND and Alzheimer's disease change in the temporal lobe, although no evidence of dementia. They concluded that the association between MND and Alzheimer's disease in multi-generational families was more likely to be due to a genetic influence than to a chance association. This remains unproven, but in view of the fact that both disorders link to markers on chromosome 21, and recent linkage studies indicate an association between the chromosome 21 marker GT12 at the amyloid precursor protein (APP) locus, further examination of the association is warranted (Siddique et al, 1992).

Other associations

Finally, an intriguing association has been reported between MND (ALS) and the fragile X syndrome (Desai et al, 1990). The patient, a man of 41 years at the time of his death, had longstanding developmental delay associated with characteristic features of the phenotype, and the typical fragile site on 34% of his X chromosomes. He presented two years before death with bladder and bowel incontinence and progressive unsteadiness, and although these symptoms are clearly unlike typical MND, over the next two years he developed typical signs of anterior horn cell degeneration associated with upper motor neurone signs, and at autopsy a clinical diagnosis of MND was confirmed, including the presence of Bunina bodies in surviving spinal motor neurones, and selective degeneration of the corticospinal tracts in the spinal cord. There was marked atrophy of the pre-central gyri, with loss of pyramidal neurones from these regions, but no evidence of Alzheimer's disease, Pick's disease, or other specific cerebral pathology. This association may be coincidental, but could provide clues to the molecular basis of MND if further instances are identified.

CONCLUSIONS

Motor neurone disease with dementia emerges clinically as a condition leading to an initial disturbance of personality, behaviour and social conduct, often first noted by the patient's spouse or relatives, in conjunction with, or shortly followed by, symptoms of bulbar palsy. As the disease progresses, the mental changes evolve into a dementia of the frontal lobe type, and signs of amyotrophy become evident in the neck, shoulder and upper limb musculature. The picture is often complicated by aphasia and later mutism, and death usually occurs within two to three years of symptom onset. The aetiology is unknown, although heredofamilial occurrence in some examples of the disorder raises the possibility that the condition may be genetically determined. Characteristic but non-specific neuropatho-logical lesions are consistently found in the frontal and temporal cortex, but the pathogenesis of the condition remains obscure.

Acknowledgements

We are indebted to Dr Hans Forste for pointing out and translating Alzheimer's description of a patient with possible dementia and MND. John Kew was supported by the Medical Research Council.

REFERENCES

Alzheimer A (1891) On a case of spinal progressive muscle atrophy with accessory disease of bulbar nuclei and the cortex. *Archiv für Psychiatrie* 23: 459–485.

Bonduelle M, Bouygues P, Escourelle R & Lormeau G (1968) Evolution simultanée d'une sclerose latérale amyotrophique, d'un syndrome parkinsonien et d'une démence progressive: à propos de deux observations anatomo-cliniques essai d'interpretation. *Journal of the Neurological Sciences* 6: 315–332.

Brion S, Psimaras A, Chevalier F et al (1980) L'association maladie de Pick et sclérose latérale amyotrophique. Etude d'un cas anatomo-clinique et revue de la littérature. *L'Encéphale* VI: 259–286.

Brun A (1987) Frontal lobe degeneration of non-Alzheimer type. I. Neuropathology. *Archives of Gerontology and Geriatrics* 6: 193–208.

Büscher J (1922) Zur Symptomatologie der sogenannten amyotrophischen Lateralsklerose. *Archiv für Psychiatrie* 66: 61.

Charcot JM & Joffroy A (1869) Deux cas d'atrophie musculaire progressive avec les lésions de la substance grise et faisceaux antérolatéraux de la moelle épinière. *Archives de Physiologie Normale et Pathologique* 2: 354–367, 629–649, 744–760.

Connolly JH, Allen IV & Dermott E (1988) Transmissible agent in the amyotrophic form of Creutzfeldt–Jakob disease. *Journal of Neurology, Neurosurgery and Psychiatry* 51: 1459–1460.

Constantinidis J (1987) Syndrome familial: association de maladie de Pick et sclérose latérale amyotrophique. *Encéphale* 13: 285–293.

Constantinidis J, Richards J & Tissot R (1974) Pick's disease. *European Neurology* 11: 208–217.

Dalakas MC, Hatazawa J, Brooks RA & Di Chiro G (1987) Lowered cerebral glucose utilization in amyotrophic lateral sclerosis. *Annals of Neurology* 22: 580–586.

David AS & Gilham RA (1986) Neuropsychological study of motor neuron disease. *Psychosomatics* 27: 441–445.

Desai HB, Donat J, Shokeir MHK & Munoz DG (1990) Amyotrophic lateral sclerosis in a patient with fragile X syndrome. *Neurology* 40: 378–380.

Dickson DW, Horoupian DS, Thal LJ et al (1986) Kluver–Bucy syndrome and amyotrophic lateral sclerosis: a case report with biochemistry, morphometrics, and Golgi study. *Neurology* 36: 1323–1329.

Ferrer I, Roig C, Espino A et al (1991) Dementia of frontal lobe type and motor neuron disease. A Golgi study of the frontal cortex. *Journal of Neurology, Neurosurgery and Psychiatry* 54: 932–934.

Finlayson MH, Guberman A & Martin JB (1973) Cerebral lesions in familial amyotrophic lateral sclerosis and dementia. *Acta Neuropathologica* 26: 237–246.

Frecker MF, Fraser FC, Andermann E & Pryse-Phillips WEM (1990) Association between Alzheimer disease and amyotrophic lateral sclerosis? *Canadian Journal of Neurological Sciences* 17: 12–14.

Friedlander JW & Kesert BH (1948) The role of psychosis in amyotrophic lateral sclerosis. *Journal of Nervous and Mental Disease* 107: 243–250.

Gadjusek DC & Salazar AM (1982) Amyotrophic lateral sclerosis and parkinsonian syndromes in high incidence among the Auyu and Jakai people of West New Guinea. *Neurology* **32:** 107–126.

Gallassi R, Montagna P, Ciardulli C et al (1985) Cognitive impairment in motor neuron disease. *Acta Neurologica Scandinavica* **71:** 480–484.

Gallassi R, Montagna P, Morreale A et al (1989) Neuropsychological, electroencephalogram, and brain computed tomography findings in motor neurone disease. *European Neurology* **29:** 115–120.

Gerbert I & Naville F (1921) Contribution à l'étude histologique. *Encéphale* **1:** 113.

Gunnarsson L-G, Dahlbom K & Strandman E (1991) Motor neuron disease and dementia reported among 13 members of a single family. *Acta Neurologica Scandinavica* **84:** 429–433.

Gustafson L (1987) Frontal lobe degeneration of non-Alzheimer type. II. Clinical picture and differential diagnosis. *Archives of Gerontology and Geriatrics* **6:** 209–223.

Hatazawa J, Brooks RA, Dalakas MC et al (1988) Cortical motor-sensory hypometabolism in amyotrophic lateral sclerosis: a PET study. *Journal of Computer Assisted Tomography* **12:** 630–636.

Hirano A, Kurland LT, Krooth RS & Lessel S (1961) Parkinsonism-dementia complex, an endemic disease on the island of Guam. *Brain* **84:** 642–679.

Hirano A, Malamud N, Elizan TS & Kurland LT (1966) Amyotrophic lateral sclerosis and Parkinsonism-dementia complex on Guam. Further pathologic studies. *Archives of Neurology* **15:** 35–51.

Hoffman JM, Mazziota JC, Sumida R et al (1987) FDG PET studies in slowly progressive motor neurone disease. *Neurology* **37** (supplement): 163.

Horoupian DS, Thal L, Katzman R et al (1984) Dementia and motor neuron disease: morphometric, biochemical and Golgi studies. *Annals of Neurology* **16:** 305–313.

Hudson AJ (1981) Amyotrophic lateral sclerosis and its association with dementia, parkinsonism and other neurological disorders: A review. *Brain* **104:** 217–247.

Hughes JT (1982) Pathology of amyotrophic lateral sclerosis. In Rowland LP (ed.) *Human Motor Neuron Diseases*, pp 61–74. New York: Raven Press.

Kim RC, Collins GH, Parisi JE et al (1981) Familial dementia of adult onset with pathological findings of a 'non-specific' nature. *Brain* **104:** 61–78.

Lawyer T & Netsky MG (1953) Amyotrophic lateral sclerosis: a clinicoanatomic study of fifty-three cases. *Archives of Neurology and Psychiatry* **69:** 171–192.

Leigh PN, Anderton BH, Dodson A et al (1988) Ubiquitin deposits in anterior horn cells in motor neurone disease. *Neuroscience Letters* **93:** 197–203.

Leigh PN, Dodson A, Swash M et al (1989) Cytoskeletal abnormalities in motor neurone disease: an immunocytochemical study. *Brain* **112:** 521–535.

Leigh PN, Whitwell H, Garofalo O et al (1991) Ubiquitin-immunoreactive intraneuronal inclusions in amyotrophic lateral sclerosis: morphology, distribution, and specificity. *Brain* **114:** 775–788.

Lowe J, Lennox G, Jefferson D et al (1988) A filamentous inclusion body within anterior horn neurones in motor neurone disease defined by immunocytochemical localisation of ubiquitin. *Neuroscience Letters* **94:** 203–210.

Ludolph AC, Langen KJ, Regard M et al (1992) Frontal lobe function in amyotrophic lateral sclerosis: a neuropsychologic and positron emission tomography study. *Acta Neurologica Scandinavica* **85:** 81–89.

Marie P (1892) *Leçons sur les Maladies de la Moelle*, p 470. Paris: Masson & Cie.

Masters CL & Richardson EP (1978) Subacute spongiform encephalopathy (Creutzfeldt–Jakob disease). The nature and progression of spongiform change. *Brain* **101:** 333–344.

Mitsuyama Y & Takamiya S (1979) Presenile dementia with motor neurone disease in Japan. A new entity? *Archives of Neurology* **36:** 592–593.

Mitsuyama Y (1984) Presenile dementia with motor neuron disease in Japan: clinico-pathological review of 26 cases. *Journal of Neurology, Neurosurgery and Psychiatry* **47:** 953–959.

Mitsuyama Y, Kogoh H & Ata K (1985) Progressive dementia with motor neuron disease. An additional case report and neuropathological review of 20 cases in Japan. *Eur Arch Psychiatr Neurol Sci* **235:** 1–8.

Morita K, Kaiya H, Ikeda T & Namba M (1987) Presenile dementia combined with amyotrophy: a review of 34 Japanese cases. *Archives of Gerontology and Geriatrics* **6:** 263–277.

Murayama S, Mori H, Ihara Y et al (1990a) Immunocytochemical and ultrastructural studies of lower motor neurons in ALS. *Annals of Neurology* 27: 137–148.

Murayama S, Mori H, Ihara Y & Tomonaga M (1990b) Immunocytochemical and ultrastructural studies of Pick's disease. *Annals of Neurology* 27: 394–405.

Neary D, Snowden JS, Northen B & Goulding P (1988) Dementia of frontal lobe type. *Journal of Neurology, Neurosurgery and Psychiatry* 51: 353–361.

Neary D, Snowden JS, Mann DMA et al (1990) Frontal lobe dementia and motor neuron disease. *Journal of Neurology, Neurosurgery and Psychiatry* 53: 23–32.

Neary D (1990) Non Alzheimer's disease forms of cerebral atrophy. *Journal of Neurology, Neurosurgery and Psychiatry* 53: 929–931.

Neumann MA & Cohn R (1967) Progressive subcortical gliosis, a rare form of presenile dementia. *Brain* 40: 405–418.

Ohnishi T, Hoshi H, Jinnouchi S et al (1990) The utility of cerebral blood flow imaging in patients with the unique syndrome of progressive dementia with motor neuron disease. *Journal of Nuclear Medicine* 31: 688–691.

Okamoto K, Hirai S, Yamazaki T et al (1991) New ubiquitin-positive intraneuronal inclusions in the extra-motor cortices in patients with amyotrophic lateral sclerosis. *Neuroscience Letters* 129: 233–236.

Oppenheim H & Siemerling E (1886) Mitteilungen über pseudobulbär Paralyse und acute bulbär Paralyse. *Berl klin Wchnschr* 23: 791.

Raymond F & Cestan R (1905) Dix-huit cas de sclérose amyotrophique avec autopsie. *Revue Neurologique* 13: 504.

Robertson EE (1953) Progressive bulbar paralysis showing heredofamilial incidence and intellectual impairment. *Archives of Neurology and Psychiatry* 69: 197–207.

Rodgers-Johnson P, Garruto RM, Yanagihara R et al (1986) Amyotrophic lateral sclerosis and parkinsonism-dementia on Guam: a 30-year evaluation of clinical and neuropathologic trends. *Neurology* 36: 7–13.

Salazar AM, Masters CL, Gajdusek DC & Gibbs CJ (1983) Syndromes of amyotrophic lateral sclerosis and dementia: Relation to transmissible Creutzfeldt–Jakob disease. *Annals of Neurology* 14: 17–26.

Sam M, Gutmann L, Schochet SS & Doshi H (1991) Pick's disease: A case clinically resembling amyotrophic lateral sclerosis. *Neurology* 41: 1831–1833.

Siddique T, Pericak-Vance MA, Brooks BR et al (1989) Linkage analysis in familial amyotrophic lateral sclerosis. *Neurology* 39: 919–926.

Siddique T, Figlewicz DA, Pericak-Vance MA et al (1991) Linkage of a gene causing familial amyotrophic lateral sclerosis to chromosome 21 and evidence of genetic-locus heterogeneity. *New England Journal of Medicine* 324: 1381–1384.

Siddique T, Antonarakis S, Hu P et al (1992) Mapping a gene for familial amyotrophic lateral sclerosis (FALS) on chromosome 21. *Neurology* 42 (supplement): 201.

Smith MC (1960) Nerve fibre degeneration in the brain in amyotrophic lateral sclerosis. *Journal of Neurology, Neurosurgery and Psychiatry* 23: 269–282.

Van Bogaert L (1925) Les troubles mentaux dans la sclérose latérale amyotrophique. *Encéphale* 20: 315–321.

Wechsler IS & Davison C (1932) Amyotrophic lateral sclerosis with mental symptoms: a clinicopathologic study. *Archives of Neurology and Psychiatry* 27: 858–880.

Wightman G, Anderson VER, Martin J et al (1992) Hippocampal and neocortical ubiquitin-immunoreactive inclusions in amyotrophic lateral sclerosis with dementia. *Neuroscience Letters* 139: 269–274.

Wikstrom J, Paetau A, Palo J et al (1982) Classic amyotrophic lateral sclerosis with dementia. *Archives of Neurology* 39: 681–683.

Wolf HK, Crain BJ & Siddique T (1991) Degeneration of the substantia nigra in familial amyotrophic lateral sclerosis. *Clinical Neuropathology* 10(6): 291–296.

Zacher (1886) Ein Fall von progressiver Paralyse compliziert mit amyotrophischer Lateralsclerose. *Neurol. Centralbl.* 5: 551.

Ziegler LH (1930) Psychotic and emotional phenomena associated with amyotrophic lateral sclerosis. *Archives of Neurology and Psychiatry* 24: 930–936.

8

Human prion diseases

MARK S. PALMER
JOHN COLLINGE

SPONGIFORM ENCEPHALOPATHIES

The spongiform encephalopathies, Creutzfeldt–Jakob disease (CJD), Gerstmann–Sträussler–Sheinker syndrome (GSS) and kuru, are human neurodegenerative disorders that can be transmitted experimentally to animals. The original description by Creutzfeldt in 1920 (Creutzfeldt, 1920) of a progressive dementing illness in a 22-year-old woman was followed by reports a year later from Jakob of four older patients with a similar clinical presentation and course (Jakob, 1921a,b). Spielmeyer proposed the term Creutzfeldt–Jakob disease for these conditions (Spielmeyer, 1922) and CJD subsequently became the term for a range of similar neurodegenerative disorders. Clinical descriptions of CJD in the ensuing decades have typically portrayed a progressive dementia, characterized initially by loss of memory, diminished intellect and poor judgement. Today CJD is recognized clinically by the occurrence of a rapidly progressive dementia with myoclonus often accompanied by pyramidal signs, cerebellar ataxia or extrapyramidal features. The disease has a rapid clinical course and death usually follows within 12 months of onset. Diagnosis is not assisted by routine laboratory investigations and neuroimaging generally only reveals varying degrees of cerebral atrophy. The EEG may show characteristic pseudoperiodic sharp wave activity (Cathala and Baron, 1987). Neuropathological confirmation requires the demonstration of spongiosis affecting any part of the cerebral grey matter, neuronal loss and proliferation and hypertrophy of astrocytes (Beck and Daniel, 1987). These changes are sometimes accompanied by the accumulation of partially protease resistant amyloid plaques. Although these are often morphologically indistinguishable from those of Alzheimer's disease, immunocytochemistry has demonstrated that they are formed from an entirely different protein, as discussed below.

CJD has a remarkably uniform random world-wide distribution, with a peak incidence in late middle age of about 1 case per million people each year (Brown et al, 1987). In addition to the normal presentation of CJD as described above, about 10% of patients have an atypical presentation with a long duration of illness, usually over 2 years (Brown et al, 1984). About 15% of all cases are familial, while GSS is nearly always described in a familial context, both showing an autosomal dominant pattern of segregation. In

627

addition to the sporadic and familial forms of CJD a few cases world-wide have been recognized as being derived from iatrogenic causes.

In 1928 Gerstmann described a patient with a chronic cerebellar ataxia which progressed to dementia (Gerstmann, 1928). A more detailed report of this patient, and seven other affected cases from a single family, was written up by Gerstmann, Sträussler and Sheinker in 1936 as a 'peculiar heredo-familial disease of the central nervous system' (Gerstmann et al, 1936). This family showed an apparently autosomal dominant pattern of inheritance and a detailed clinical and pathological report of the family, covering six generations over 160 years, was presented by Seitelberger in 1962 (Seitelberger, 1962). The clinical features were similar to spinocerebellar degeneration and mild dementia. At autopsy the cerebellum and cerebral hemispheres were found to contain unusual multi-centric plaques. The definition of GSS has now expanded to include a range of neurodegenerative syndromes which include ataxic forms, telencephalic forms with dementia (Warter et al, 1982; Nochlin et al, 1989), parkinsonism and pyramidal features, as well as variants with neurofibrillary tangles (Farlow et al, 1989; Ghetti et al, 1989). Classically, patients present with a chronic cerebellar ataxia, and dementia occurs late in the clinical course, which is more protracted than in CJD. Clinical onset is usually in the third to fourth decade and the duration of illness is about 5 years, although there are recorded cases of up to 11 years duration. Amyloid plaques are a common feature of GSS pathology, but the multicentric forms, which are often described as the hallmark of GSS, are not a consistent finding and plaques are absent in many cases.

During the early 1950s an unusual epidemic was noted, predominantly amongst the Fore-speaking people of highland Papua New Guinea. Kuru, which means shivering or trembling in the Fore language, was characterized by a cerebellar ataxia and shivering-like tremor that progressed to complete motor incapacity with dysarthria, total loss of speech and death, usually within 3–9 months from onset (Zigas and Gajdusek, 1957; Gajdusek, 1990). Since the original investigations in 1956 at the height of the epidemic, over 2500 cases have been recorded, nearly all of which ended in death within 2 years of onset. The first, or ambulant, stage of kuru is a usually self-diagnosed instability of posture, truncal tremor and titubation and ataxia of gait. There is an early dysarthria, and speech progressively deteriorates. In the second, sedentary, stage the tremors and ataxia become more severe and are accompanied by widespread clonus. Despite the poor maintenance of muscle activity there is no fasciculation or real muscle weakness or atrophy. Patients show an emotional lability with inappropriate outbreaks of laughter and a resignation to the disease with a lack of concern that approaches euphoria. Although mental slowing is apparent there is no severe dementia. During the third, terminal, stage the patient cannot sit without support and the ataxia, tremor and dysarthria become progressively more severe and incapacitating. Urinary and faecal incontinence develop and dysphagia leads to thirst and starvation. The patient becomes mute and unresponsive as flaccidity, inanation and signs of bulbar involvement develop. Patients finally succumb to hypostatic pneumonia, usually with emaciation.

Throughout, the patient is afebrile (except for intercurrent or terminal infection) and there is no elevated CSF protein or pleocytosis; there is no renal or hepatic functional disturbance and endocrine functions remain normal.

Pathologically the kuru brain shows marked proliferation and hypertrophy of astrocytes, mild status spongiosis of the grey matter, diffuse neuronal degeneration, which is most severe in the cerebellum, and minimal demyelination (Klatzo et al, 1959). Spongiosis is the result of coalescing vacuolation within the pre- and postsynaptic processes of neurones, and to a lesser extent astrocytes and oligodendrocytes. All cases of kuru are cerebral amyloidoses, though only 75% show congophilic amyloid plaques, the rest show scrapie associated fibrils (SAFs) in density gradient preparations of brain suspensions seen by electron microscopy.

It is now well established that the spread of kuru throughout this population was due to contamination during its ritual cannibalistic consumption of dead relatives as a mark of respect and mourning. Cadaver dissection of the flesh and preparation for consumption was performed by the women and children. Liquefying brain tissue was scooped by hand into bamboo cylinders and would have been accompanied by scratching of ubiquitous itching scabies with impetiginous skin eruptions, insect bites and sores. As well as wiping their eyes and noses the women would have eaten with their bare hands without washing, so both oral and intradermal inoculations would have been common.

Since the cessation of such cannibalistic practices kuru has now essentially disappeared. Because of the detailed field work which accompanied this episode there is clear documentary evidence for inoculation periods of 30 years or more for the disease and the youngest known patients are now over 40 years of age. Although this disease is now an historical curiosity, studies on kuru have been central to the development of ideas that have led to our current thinking on the human spongiform encephalopathies, their animal counterparts and the bizarre phenomenon of being both genetic and transmissible diseases.

THE TRANSMISSIBLE AGENT

In 1959 the neuropathological similarities between kuru and CJD were noted by Klatzo et al (Klatzo et al, 1959) and the similarities between kuru and scrapie were noted by Hadlow (Hadlow, 1959). The pathological triad of astrocytosis, neuronal loss and spongiosis ('soap bubble vacuoles') together with the similarities in the course of the disease suggested that perhaps a similar aetiology underlay these disorders. Scrapie, an ovine spongiform encephalopathy, had been studied for many years and was known to be experimentally transmissible to both sheep and goats. Hadlow suggested that it would be profitable to examine the possibility that kuru might be experimentally induced in laboratory primates, and by 1968 both kuru and CJD had been transmitted to apes (Gajdusek et al, 1966; Gibbs et al, 1968; Beck et al, 1969). As a consequence the term transmissible spongiform encephalopathies was introduced to encompass scrapie, transmissible mink encephalopathy, kuru, CJD and GSS.

The nature of the transmissibility suggested that the spongiform encephalopathies were caused by a virus; the long incubation times implicated a slow virus such as the visna virus, a retrovirus which causes a progressive neurological disorder in sheep. Ultrafiltration experiments demonstrated that the agent could pass through filters with an average pore diameter of as low as 20–100 nm, a size range that is consistent with conventional viruses. However, unlike conventional viruses, the transmissible agent of scrapie was remarkably resistant to inactivation by ultraviolet ionizing radiation (Alper et al, 1966, 1967). All the radiobiological data suggested that the scrapie agent was fundamentally different from conventional viruses, and terms such as 'unconventional virus' and virino were introduced (Gajdusek, 1977; Dickinson and Outram, 1979). The original definition of virinos (by analogy with neutrinos) was 'small, immunologically neutral particles with high penetration properties but needing special criteria to detect their presence' (Dickinson & Outram, 1979). More recently the virinos have been described as 'host proteins sequestering the agent genome which may code for no product other than copies of itself' (Dickinson and Outram, 1988).

Transmissibility of the agent from brain preparations was established by inoculation of serial dilutions of material into mice or hamsters. The assay, despite its sensitivity, is extremely time consuming, though rodents were found to have shorter incubation times than the sheep that were originally used for transmission of scrapie. Through attempts to transmit scrapie to other species it was noted that primary agents isolated from the field took much longer to transmit: a number of years, compared with the 2–8 months for infectivity following passage in experimental mice. These properties gave rise to the concepts of a species barrier and host adapted strains for scrapie agents. It is now believed that the recent outbreak of bovine spongiform encephalopathy in the UK is due to the presence of scrapie affected material entering the meat and bone meal fed to cattle (Wilesmith et al, 1991).

The reduced incubation times for adapted strains, particularly in hamsters where the incubation times were as low as 90 days, increased the speed at which experiments could be performed and more chemicals and conditions evaluated for their capacity to inactivate the scrapie agent in order to cast light on its nature. The agent proved to be resistant to degradation by exposure to nucleases and to many other procedures that would modify or hydrolyse nucleic acids (Diener et al, 1982; Prusiner, 1982). The agent is also extremely resistant to proteinase-K, a broad-acting protease to which few proteins are resistant (Bolton et al, 1982).

Early attempts at purification of the transmissible scrapie agent involved the use of differential centrifugation and was improved by the use of density gradient centrifugation applied to brain homogenates solubilized in various detergents (Prusiner et al, 1980). During extraction of membranes, macromolecular fibrils (scrapie associated fibrils—SAFs), or rods were seen, morphologically and histochemically indistinguishable from many amyloids. The extraction procedure was improved by exploiting the agent's resistance to proteinase-K. However, the protein component which copurified with infectivity was not destroyed by this proteinase-K treatment (McKinley et al, 1983a). By the early 1980s all approaches at isolating the agent had resulted in the purification of a proteinaceous component that could not be dissociated from infectivity (Prusiner et al, 1982). All studies which attempted to demonstate the presence of nucleic acids failed, though it was argued that there may be a small amount of DNA present that was either too small or too intimately associated with the protein to be destroyed by the procedures used (McKinley et al, 1983b; Bellinger et al, 1987; Gabizon et al, 1987).

In 1982 the term 'prion' was coined for the transmissible agent of scrapie (Prusiner, 1982). The operational definition of 'a small proteinaceous infectious particle which is resistant to inactivation by procedures that modify nucleic acids' was careful to highlight the proteinaceous nature of the copurifying macromolecules but did not exclude the possibility that the isolated protein, prion protein, was associated with nucleic acid.

THE PRION PROTEIN

As purification of the infectious agent improved the nature of the prion protein could be assessed. Following proteinase-K treatment prion protein (PrP) was found to be a glycoprotein of relative molecular mass 27–30K, migrating in SDS-polyacrylamide gels as a broad band (McKinley et al, 1983a; Bolton et al, 1984). The microheterogeneity displayed by this product, PrP 27–30, is due to variation in its sialic acid content (Bolton et al, 1985; Endo et al, 1989). PrP 27–30 is derived from a larger protein of apparent M_r 33–35K, designated PrP^{Sc}, or the scrapie form of PrP (Oesch et al, 1985; Barry and Prusiner, 1986; Barry et al, 1986). The rod-shaped amyloid structures found in purified fractions are polymerized PrP 27–30 (Prusiner et al, 1983). A number of lines of evidence supported the view that the PrP was a component of the infectious particle. (1) PrP 27–30 and the scrapie agent copurify, PrP 27–30 being the most abundant macromolecule in purified preparations (Prusiner et al, 1982, 1983). (2) PrP 27–30 concentration is proportional to prion titre; PrP 27–30 and PrP^{Sc} are absent in normal uninfected animals (McKinley et al, 1983a). (3) Denaturation, hydrolysis or selective modification of PrP 27–30 diminishes the prion titre (McKinley et al, 1983b). (4) PrP 27–30 and scrapie infectivity partition together into different forms, membranes, rods, spheres, detergent–lipid–protein complexes and liposomes. These all contain PrP 27–30 and high prion titres (Prusiner et al, 1982, 1983, 1984). (5) Scrapie and CJD PrP have only been found in the tissues of those animals or humans with transmissible neurodegenerative diseases and not with other disorders such as systemic amyloidosis, human Alzheimer's disease, anoxic encephalopathy or non-neurological disorders (Bolton et al, 1984; Roberts et al, 1986). (6) Cultures of murine neuroblastoma cells have been infected with CJD and scrapie prion. Infected clones produce PrP^{Sc} while uninfected clones lack PrP^{Sc} (Butler et al, 1987). In addition, antisera against PrP 27–30 can neutralize infectivity in detergent–lipid–protein complexes, directly linking PrP 27–30 to the infective particle. To date, all attempts to separate PrP^{Sc} from infectivity have been unsuccessful (Gabizon et al, 1988).

Once PrP was sufficiently purified, partial amino acid sequence was obtained from the NH$_2$-terminal end (Prusiner et al, 1984), and isocoding oligonucleotides were used to probe a cDNA library from a scrapie infected hamster brain (Oesch et al, 1985). The cDNA isolated from this library was in turn used as a probe to screen Southern blots of normal and infected brain tissues. The results of these Southern blots showed that PrP was encoded by a cellular gene, present in a single copy, with the same restriction pattern in normal and infected animals, and that it was not the product of a viral genome. A single copy gene was soon also identified in mice and humans (Oesch et al, 1985; Kretzschmar et al, 1986b).

Careful screening of mRNA from infected and normal brain showed that there was no change in RNA expression associated with infection and that PrP transcripts were produced by a normal cellular gene in the absence of infection. Antisera to PrP 27–30 detect a protein of M$_r$ 33–35K in normal tissues. This protein (PrP^C) is the normal cellular product of the prion gene and, unlike the scrapie form, is completely digested by proteases (Oesch et al, 1985; Meyer et al, 1986). Both PrP^C and PrP^{Sc} are membrane proteins, but while PrP^C is solubilized on detergent extraction, PrP^{Sc} polymerizes into rods. The fibrils seen on detergent extraction are an artefact of the extraction procedure. The presence of normal PrP probably explains the lack of immune response during CJD as the host is tolerant to the abnormal isoform of PrP^{Sc}.

Complete sequencing of protein and cDNA clones revealed that both PrP^C and PrP^{Sc} are derived from the same transcriptional unit. The open reading frame is contained within a single exon, excluding the possibility of

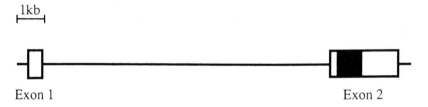

Figure 1. Genomic organization of the human PrP gene. Transcriptional unit is indicated by boxes with the open reading frame shaded black.

differential splicing generating different gene products (Figure 1). While this does not exclude the possibility of post-transcriptional editing of RNA, no differences have been found in the primary structure of the proteins by direct amino acid sequencing. So far, all attempts, including gas phased sequencing and mass spectroscopy, to identify a post-translational modification which may underlie the physical difference in susceptibility to degradation have failed to identify any such modification (Stahl and Prusiner, 1991). It is now clear that although both PrP^C and PrP^{Sc} are products of the same mRNA, PrP^{Sc} is derived from PrP^C and is not synthesized alone. Pulse chase experiments on [^{35}S]methionine-labelled cells infected with scrapie agent show that while PrP^C has a rapid turnover with a half-life of 5.5 h, PrP^{Sc} has a slow lag phase before appearance and steadily accumulates thereafter (Borchelt et al, 1990). The kinetics of turnover and appearance of this protein suggest that part of the pool of PrP^C is somehow converted into PrP^{Sc}, possibly after it has been on the cell surface and is internalized into the cell. There is now evidence to suggest that PrP^{Sc} accumulates within secondary lysosomes in infected cells (McKinley et al, 1991).

PrP is a protein of 253 amino acids in humans (254 in hamster and mouse). The amino terminus contains a 22 amino acid signal peptide which is cleaved during synthesis in the endoplasmic reticulum. The carboxy terminal also contains a signal sequence of 23 amino acids which is cleaved on addition of a glycoinositol phospholipid anchor to Ser231 (Stahl et al, 1987). This sialated phosphatidylinositol moiety anchors the protein on to the cell membrane (Stahl et al, 1990a,b). An internal disulphide bond forms a loop in the molecule, within which are attached two asparagine-linked oligosaccharides. Limited proteolysis of PrP^{Sc} removes 67 amino acids from the N-terminus of the mature PrP^{Sc} (generating PrP 27–30). This region contains an interesting set of repeated sequences. Two repeats of GG(S/N)RYP(Q/P)QG overlap with a longer set of five repeats, P(H/Q)GGG(−/T)WGQ. The significance of these repeats is unknown although they are highly conserved amongst all species sequenced so far (Figure 2). These repeats possess a high degree of β structure but are unnecessary for the amyloid properties of PrP polymers as they are absent from PrP 27–30. A short stretch between residues 96 and 112 contains a domain controlling the topology of PrP in artificial membranes, and is designated the stop transfer effector (Lopez et al, 1990; Yost et al, 1990).

HUMAN PrP GENETICS

The human PrP gene (*PRNP*) is located on the short arm of chromosome 20, in a region syntenic with the region of mouse chromosome 2 which encodes murine PrP (Liao et al, 1986; Robakis et al, 1986; Sparkes et al, 1986). It is constitutively expressed in the adult brain though it is regulated during development. PrP mRNA and choline acetyltransferase increase in parallel in the septum during development, whereas PrP expression occurs earlier in other brain regions (Mobley et al, 1988). The highest levels of PrP mRNA expression are found in neurones (Kretzschmar et al, 1986a).

Following the identification of the human PrP gene it was natural to ask whether in familial cases of CJD or GSS there was linkage of the disease to variants in the PrP gene, or indeed whether in these cases the gene contained pathogenic mutations. Hsiao et al demonstrated linkage between the PrP gene and GSS in two families (Hsiao et al, 1989). Affected members of these families contained a missense mutation in codon 102. A CpG to TpG substitution at codon 102, probably resulting from deamination of a methylated cytosine, altered the amino acid encoded at that position from a proline to a leucine. The change could be easily followed in these families

Positions 1–25

		1	2	3	4	5	6	7	8	9	10	11	12	13	14	15	16	17	18	19	20	21	22	23	24	25
HUMAN		M	A	N	L	G	C	W	M	L	V	L	F	V	A	T	W	S	D	L	G	L	C	K	K	R
MOUSE		M	A	N	L	G	Y	W	L	L	A	L	F	V	T	M	W	T	D	V	G	L	C	K	K	R
HAMSTER		M	A	N	L	S	Y	W	L	L	A	L	F	V	A	T	W	T	D	V	G	L	C	K	K	R
SHEEP	M V	K	S	H	I	G	S	W	I	L	V	L	F	V	A	M	W	S	D	V	G	L	C	K	K	R
COW	M V	K	S	H	I	G	S	W	I	L	V	L	F	V	A	M	W	S	D	V	G	L	C	K	K	R

Positions 26–51

	26	27	28	29	30	(ins)	31	32	33	34	35	36	37	38	39	40	41	42	43	44	45	46	47	48	49	50	51
HUMAN	P	K	P	G	G		W	N	T	G	G	S	R	Y	P	G	Q	G	S	P	G	G	N	R	Y	P	P
MOUSE	P	K	P	G	G		W	N	T	G	G	S	R	Y	P	G	Q	G	S	P	G	G	N	R	Y	P	P
HAMSTER	P	K	P	G	G		W	N	T	G	G	S	R	Y	P	G	Q	G	S	P	G	G	N	R	Y	P	P
SHEEP	P	K	P	G	G	G	W	N	T	G	G	S	R	Y	P	G	Q	G	S	P	G	G	N	R	Y	P	P
COW	P	K	P	G	G		W	N	T	G	G	S	R	Y	P	G	Q	G	S	P	G	G	N	R	Y	P	P

Positions 52–78

	52	53	54	55	56	57	58	59	60	61	62	63	64	65	66	67	68	69	70	71	72	73	74	75	76	77	78
HUMAN	Q	G	G	G	G	W	G	Q	P	H	G	G	G	W	G	Q	P	H	G	G	G	W	G	Q	P	H	G
MOUSE	Q	G	G		T	W	G	Q	P	H	G	G	G	W	G	Q	P	H	G	G	S	W	G	Q	P	H	G
HAMSTER	Q	G	G	G	T	W	G	Q	P	H	G	G	G	W	G	Q	P	H	G	G	G	W	G	Q	P	H	G
SHEEP	Q	G	G	G	G	W	G	Q	P	H	G	G	G	W	G	Q	P	H	G	G	G	W	G	Q	P	H	G
COW	Q	G	G	G	G	W	G	Q	P	H	G	G	G	W	G	Q	P	H	G	G	G	W	G	Q	P	H	G

Positions 79–96 (variable octarepeat region; insert shown where present)

	79	80	81	82	83	84	85	86	87	88	89	90	91	(insert)	92	93	94	95	96
HUMAN	G	G	W	G	Q	P	H	G	G	G	W	G	Q		G	G	G	T	H
MOUSE	G	S	W	G	Q	P	H	G	G	G	W	G	Q		G	G	G	T	H
HAMSTER	G	G	W	G	Q	P	H	G	G	G	W	G	Q		G	G	G	T	H
SHEEP	G	G	W	G	Q									P H G G G G W G Q	G	G	G	S	H
COW	G	G	W	G	Q	P	H	G	G	G	W	G	Q	P H G G G G W G Q	G	G	G	T	H

Positions 97–123

	97	98	99	100	101	102	103	104	105	106	107	108	109	110	111	112	113	114	115	116	117	118	119	120	121	122	123
HUMAN	S	Q	W	N	K	P	S	K	P	K	T	N	M	K	H	M	A	G	A	A	A	A	G	A	V	V	G
MOUSE	N	Q	W	N	K	P	S	K	P	K	T	N	F	K	H	V	A	G	A	A	A	A	G	A	V	V	G
HAMSTER	N	Q	W	N	K	P	S	K	P	K	T	N	F	K	H	V	A	G	A	A	A	A	G	A	V	V	G
SHEEP	S	Q	W	N	K	P	S	K	P	K	T	N	M	K	H	V	A	G	A	A	A	A	G	A	V	V	G
COW	G	Q	W	N	K	P	S	K	P	K	T	N	M	K	H	V	A	G	A	A	A	A	G	A	V	V	G

Positions 124–150

	124	125	126	127	128	129	130	131	132	133	134	135	136	137	138	139	140	141	142	143	144	145	146	147	148	149	150
HUMAN	G	L	G	G	Y	M	L	G	S	A	M	S	R	P	I	I	H	F	G	S	D	Y	E	D	R	Y	Y
MOUSE	G	L	G	G	Y	M	L	G	S	A	M	S	R	P	M	I	H	F	G	N	D	W	E	D	R	Y	Y
HAMSTER	G	L	G	G	Y	M	L	G	S	A	M	S	R	P	M	L	H	F	G	N	D	Y	E	D	R	Y	Y
SHEEP	G	L	G	G	Y	M	L	G	S	A	M	S	R	P	L	I	H	F	G	N	D	Y	E	D	R	Y	Y
COW	G	L	G	G	Y	M	L	G	S	A	M	S	R	P	L	I	H	F	G	S	D	Y	E	D	R	Y	Y

Positions 151–177

	151	152	153	154	155	156	157	158	159	160	161	162	163	164	165	166	167	168	169	170	171	172	173	174	175	176	177
HUMAN	R	E	N	M	H	R	Y	P	N	Q	V	Y	Y	R	P	M	D	E	Y	S	N	Q	N	N	F	V	H
MOUSE	R	E	N	M	Y	R	Y	P	N	Q	V	Y	Y	R	P	V	D	Q	Y	S	N	Q	N	N	F	V	H
HAMSTER	R	E	N	M	N	R	Y	P	N	Q	V	Y	Y	R	P	V	D	Q	Y	N	N	Q	N	N	F	V	H
SHEEP	R	E	N	M	Y	R	Y	P	N	Q	V	Y	Y	R	P	V	D	R/Q	Y	S	N	Q	N	N	F	V	H
COW	R	E	N	M	H	R	Y	P	N	Q	V	Y	Y	R	P	V	D	Q	Y	S	N	Q	N	N	F	V	H

Positions 178–204

	178	179	180	181	182	183	184	185	186	187	188	189	190	191	192	193	194	195	196	197	198	199	200	201	202	203	204
HUMAN	D	C	V	N	I	T	I	K	Q	H	T	V	T	T	T	T	K	G	E	N	F	T	E	T	D	V	K
MOUSE	D	C	V	N	I	T	I	K	Q	H	T	V	T	T	T	T	K	G	E	N	F	T	E	T	D	V	K
HAMSTER	D	C	V	N	I	T	I	K	Q	H	T	V	T	T	T	T	K	G	E	N	F	T	E	T	D	V	K
SHEEP	D	C	V	N	I	T	V	K	Q	H	T	V	T	T	T	T	K	G	E	N	F	T	E	T	D	I	K
COW	D	C	V	N	I	T	V	K	E	H	T	V	T	T	T	T	K	G	E	N	F	T	E	T	D	I	K

Positions 205–230

	205	206	207	208	209	210	211	212	213	214	215	216	217	218	219	220	221	222	223	224	225	226	(ins)	227	228	229	230
HUMAN	M	M	E	R	V	V	E	Q	M	C	I	T	Q	Y	E	R	E	S	Q	A	Y	Y		Q	R	G	S
MOUSE	M	M	E	R	V	V	E	Q	M	C	I	T	Q	Y	Q	K	E	S	Q	A	Y	Y	D	G	R	R	S
HAMSTER	M	M	E	R	V	V	E	Q	M	C	V	T	Q	Y	Q	K	E	S	Q	A	Y	Y	D	G	R	R	S
SHEEP	I	M	E	R	V	V	E	Q	M	C	I	T	Q	Y	Q	R	E	S	Q	A	Y	Y		Q	R	G	S
COW	M	M	E	R	V	V	E	Q	M	C	I	T	Q	Y	Q	R	E	S	Q	A	Y	Y		Q	R	G	A

Positions 231–253

	231	(ins)	232	233	234	235	236	237	238	239	240	241	242	243	244	245	246	247	248	249	250	251	252	253
HUMAN	S		M	V	L	F	S	S	P	P	V	I	L	L	I	S	F	L	I	F	L	I	V	G
MOUSE	S	S	T	V	L	F	S	S	P	P	V	I	L	L	I	S	F	L	I	F	L	I	V	G
HAMSTER	S		A	V	L	F	S	S	P	P	V	I	L	L	I	S	F	L	I	F	L	I	V	G
SHEEP			V	I	L	F	S	S	P	P	V	I	L	L	I	S	F	L	I	F	L	I	V	G
COW	S		V	I	L	F	S	S	P	P	V	I	L	L	I	S	F	L	I	F	L	I	V	G

since it creates a *Dde*I restriction site in the PrP open reading frame. This demonstration of linkage was the first formal proof that GSS was a genetic disease. However, linkage only establishes a significant probability that the target gene and the disease locus lie on the same chromosome. Although all other mammalian PrP open reading frames that have been sequenced encode proline at the equivalent position, it remained a possibility that proline-leucine substitution at codon 102 would be a benign, though uncommon, polymorphism that was in genetic linkage with the actual disease locus. The subsequent demonstration of this mutation cosegregating with disease in other GSS kindreds in Germany, the USA and Japan, and its absence from all control populations that have been looked at, strongly indicate that the mutation is indeed pathogenic. It has also been demonstrated in the original kindred reported by Gerstmann (Kretzschmar et al, 1991). To investigate further the pathogenicity of the leucine substitution at codon 102, Hsiao et al created transgenic mice in which mutant PrP genes were introduced containing a leucine encoding codon at the equivalent position in mouse PrP (Hsiao et al, 1990). These mice, expressing both normal mouse PrP and murine-PrP^{Leu}, spontaneously developed a neurological disease. Although only detected at low levels, PrP^{Sc} was present in the brains of the spontaneously sick mice and it has now proved possible to transmit the disease from these affected mice to unaffected ones (Hsiao et al, 1992). This experiment very clearly shows that not only is the Leu102 mutation pathogenic, but that the generation of abnormal PrP can follow from an alteration in the primary structure of PrP^{C} in the absence of exposure to infectious agents. It is a key observation in the argument that PrP^{Sc} alone is the infectious agent in these diseases.

Another mutation in the PrP open reading frame had been previously reported in the UK in a family with CJD (Collinge et al, 1989; Owen et al, 1989). This proved to be an insertion of 144 bp in the region encoding the octapeptide motif. Six extra octapeptide repeats were introduced by this insertion and seem to represent a complex recombination/mutational event as the nucleotide sequence inserted is not only larger than the naturally occurring repeat sequence, but presents repeat sequences in a unique order and includes additional non-coding third base pair variations (Figure 3). The insertion was subsequently found in five additional families in a screening of over 100 cases of neurodegenerative disease. In none of the five reference cases had the previous clinical diagnosis included CJD or GSS. Diagnoses included Alzheimer's disease, Huntington's disease, Pick's disease and familial presenile dementia. Genealogical work established that all of the families were in fact part of the same pedigree (Poulter et al, 1992). This pedigree, spanning eight generations, contains 47 affected family

---

Figure 2. Alignment of PrP amino acid sequence from five species. Single letter amino acid code is used and residues are numbered according to the human sequence. (The mouse sequence is from an I/LN strain mouse and the hamster sequence is from Chinese hamster.) Bovine alleles of PrP have five or six repeats in the octapeptide repeat region. The allele shown here for cow contains six repeats to illustrate that the sixth contains nine amino acids, as is found in the first repeat of all species except mouse and in the fifth repeat of sheep. Amino acids common to all five species are boxed.

members on whom information has been collected. This pedigree demonstrated considerable heterogeneity in both the clinical presentation and neuropathological features of individuals (Collinge et al, 1992), all of whom have the same mutations in the PrP gene. An individual who died in the 1940s had a rapid clinical course with a reported duration of 6 months, and

Wild Type Allele

CCT	CAg	GGC	GGT	GGT	GGC	TGG	GGG	CAG	R1
Pro	Gln	Gly	Gly	Gly	Gly	Trp	Gly	Gln	
CCT	CAT	—	GGT	GGT	GGC	TGG	GGG	CAG	R2
Pro	His	—	Gly	Gly	Gly	Trp	Gly	Gln	
CCT	CAT	—	GGT	GGT	GGC	TGG	GGG	CAG	R2
Pro	His	—	Gly	Gly	Gly	Trp	Gly	Gln	
CCc	CAT	—	GGT	GGT	GGC	TGG	GGa	CAG	R3
Pro	His	—	Gly	Gly	Gly	Trp	Gly	Gln	
CCT	CAT	—	GGT	GGT	GGC	TGG	GGt	CAa	R4
Pro	His	—	Gly	Gly	Gly	Trp	Gly	Gln	

Allele with Insertion

CCT	CAg	GGC	GGT	GGT	GGC	TGG	GGG	CAG	R1
Pro	Gln	Gly	Gly	Gly	Gly	Trp	Gly	Gln	
CCT	CAT	—	GGT	GGT	GGC	TGG	GGG	CAG	R2
Pro	His	—	Gly	Gly	Gly	Trp	Gly	Gln	
CCT	CAT	—	GGT	GGT	GGC	TGG	GGG	CAG	R2
Pro	His	—	Gly	Gly	Gly	Trp	Gly	Gln	
CCT	CAT	—	GGT	GGT	GGC	TGG	GGG	CAG	R2
Pro	His	—	Gly	Gly	Gly	Trp	Gly	Gln	
CCc	CAT	—	GGT	GGT	GGC	TGG	GGa	CAG	R3
Pro	His	—	Gly	Gly	Gly	Trp	Gly	Gln	
CCT	CAT	—	GGT	GGT	GGC	TGG	GGG	CAG	R2
Pro	His	—	Gly	Gly	Gly	Trp	Gly	Gln	
CCc	CAT	—	GGT	GGT	GGC	TGG	GGG	CAG	R3'
Pro	His	—	Gly	Gly	Gly	Trp	Gly	Gln	
CCT	CAT	—	GGT	GGT	GGC	TGG	GGG	CAG	R2
Pro	His	—	Gly	Gly	Gly	Trp	Gly	Gln	
CCT	CAT	—	GGT	GGT	GGC	TGG	GGG	CAG	R2
Pro	His	—	Gly	Gly	Gly	Trp	Gly	Gln	
CCc	CAT	—	GGT	GGT	GGC	TGG	GGa	CAG	R3
Pro	His	—	Gly	Gly	Gly	Trp	Gly	Gln	
CCT	CAT	—	GGT	GGT	GGC	TGG	GGt	CAa	R4
Pro	His	—	Gly	Gly	Gly	Trp	Gly	Gln	

Figure 3. Nucleotide and amino acid sequence of the octapeptide repeat region from individuals with the 144 bp insertion compared with the wild type allele. The individual repeat elements have been called R1–R4 on the basis of differences in the nucleotide sequence. Differences between repeats at the nucleotide level are indicated by lower case letters. Repeats R2, R3 and R4 have the same amino acid sequence. Because of the nature of the repeat region it is not possible to say exactly where the insertion event occurs. The repeat R3' differs from both R2 and R3 and is unique to the insertion.

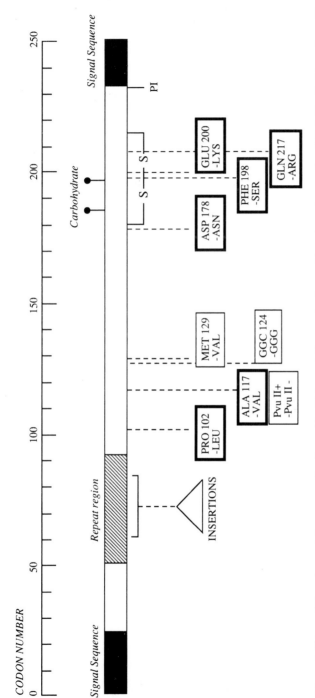

Figure 4. Figure of the prion protein open reading frame identifying mutations and polymorphisms by codon number (this is identical to amino acid residue number). Mutations are indicated in heavy boxes indicating change in the amino acid residue; polymorphisms are indicated in lighter boxes. The polymorphism at codon 117 is a silent change destroying a *Pvu*II restriction site. The polymorphism at codon 124 creates a third base change (GGC-GGG) in a glycine residue but is also silent and creates an *Eco*0 109I restriction site. An internal disulphide bond and the position of carbohydrate attachment are indicated. The signal sequences are cleaved during maturation of the protein and a phosphatidyl inositol anchor (PI) added at the new carboxy terminal.

was described as having Heidenhain's variant of CJD. Pathologically there was gross status spongiosis and astrocytosis affecting the entire cerebral cortex, and histology from this case was used to illustrate classic CJD pathology in Greenfield's Neuropathology textbook. By contrast, there are other family members with much longer duration of illness more typical of GSS (4–8 years) with only mild and subtle spongiform change, insufficient for a morphological diagnosis of CJD. Because of the difficulty in ascribing a diagnosis as CJD or GSS, even within the same family, it has been suggested that such diseases be renamed prion diseases, reflecting the central role of the prion protein in their aetiology (Collinge et al, 1990).

Screening of familial cases of CJD for mutations continues and a number of mutations have now been reported (Figure 4). The number continues to increase and for this reason no review can remain definitive for long. The recognition of mutations allows a subdivision of inherited prion diseases according to mutation, providing a nosology based on aetiological markers rather than descriptive terms. In the next section clinicopathological phenotypes are described in the context of the individual mutations.

INHERITED PRION DISEASE

In order to distinguish those prion diseases that are genetic in origin from the sporadic diseases it has been proposed that the term inherited prion diseases be used, followed by the name of the mutation in parentheses (Collinge and Prusiner, 1992). In this section we review those mutations that have been reported to date.

PrP insertions

Since the 144 bp insert a number of individuals have been reported with a range of inserts in the octapeptide repeat region, all of integer numbers of extra octapeptides. Four, five, six, seven, eight and nine extra repeats have now been reported.

PrP-96 bp insertion: (four extra repeats). This has so far only been reported in an individual without neurological disease and without any family history of a neurological disorder (Goldfarb et al, 1992).

PrP-120 bp insertion: (five extra repeats). The American patient with this mutation had a 15 year history of progressive dementia, abnormal behaviour, cerebellar signs, tremor rigidity and myoclonus. There was spongiform change on histological examination (Goldfarb et al, 1991a).

PrP-144 bp insertion: (six extra repeats). As mentioned above all individuals with this insertion have so far been found to belong to the same extended pedigree. Detailed clinical and pathological features have been described by Collinge et al (1992). The clinical phenotype in this family varies from cases with a rapidly progressing dementia, similar to classical CJD, to that of individuals with a course mimicking Alzheimer's disease with a long-standing history of antisocial personality disorder. The current and preceding generation have a picture of long-standing personality disorder, followed in early or mid-life by a slowly progressive multifocal dementia preceded by personality changes involving aggression and depression. This was accompanied by a varying combination of cerebellar ataxia and dysarthria, pyramidal signs, myoclonus and occasionally extrapyramidal signs, chorea or seizures.

The pathological variation ranges from the status spongiosis of classical CJD to cases showing no features of CJD despite extensive histological survey. Plaques with positive immunostaining for PrP were found in one patient who, interestingly, also had plaques that were immunostaining with antisera to βA4.

PrP-168 bp insertion: (seven extra repeats). This insert was found in an American family of English origin. Affected individuals had a prolonged disease with abnormal behaviour, clumsiness, cerebellar involvement, dementia and myoclonus. There is a heterogeneous neuropathological picture with severe spongiform change and gliosis in one woman but no spongiosis in her daughter (Goldfarb et al, 1991a).

PrP-192 bp insertion: (eight extra repeats). One patient in a PrP-192 bp insertion family had a brief 3 month illness with abnormal behaviour, mutism, cerebellar signs and myoclonus. Neuropathology was that of typical GSS. Eight other family members, including his mother, presented with similar symptoms but over a longer period (2–5 years) (Goldfarb et al, 1991a).

PrP-216 bp insertion: (nine extra repeats). This has been described in a patient with late onset dementia and myoclonus (Owen et al, 1991).

Point mutations

PrP-Leu102: Unrelated families from France, Germany, the UK, the USA and Japan have been found with this mutation, as well as the original family described by Gerstmann, which came from Austria. There is considerable variation in clinical and neuropathological presentation, and can include ataxia, amnesia and disorientation with spinocerebellar signs (Doh-ura et al, 1989; Hsiao et al, 1989).

PrP-Val117: Codon 117 is associated with two nucleotide changes. One is a non-coding third base change which is found in about 2.5% of the population (M. S. Palmer and J. Collinge, unpublished data) and is therefore a harmless polymorphism. It can be easily detected as it destroys a *Pvu*II restriction site in the open reading frame (Wu et al, 1987). The other change is a coding mutation changing an alanine to valine. This was first described in a French family (Doh-ura et al, 1989) and subsequently in an American family of German origin (Hsiao et al, 1991b). The American family was originally described as having familial Alzheimer's disease, but was reclassified to GSS upon finding PrP immunostaining amyloid plaques. The family had presenile dementia with extrapyramidal features. The French family had presenile dementia with pyramidal and pseudobulbar features, with cerebellar signs in some family members.

PrP-Asn178: This mutation, originally described in two Finnish families (Goldfarb et al, 1991b), has been demonstrated in seven additional CJD families in Hungary, The Netherlands, Canada, England, Finland and France (Nieto et al, 1991). Twenty-eight patients were neuropathologically confirmed to have CJD with widespread spongiosis. Patients with this mutation presented with an insidious memory loss, progressive presenile dementia with myoclonus, cerebellar and pyramidal features, but never showed the diphasic slow wave characteristic of other CJD patients. Duration of this disease was 1–2 years.

This mutation has also been found in two unrelated families described as having fatal familial insomnia (Manetto et al, 1992; Medori et al, 1992a,b). The first cases described had a rapidly progressive disease characterized clinically by untreatable insomnia, dysautonomia and motor signs, and neuropathologically by selective atrophy of the anterioventral and mediodorsal thalamic nuclei. Additional patients also had impairment of the autonomic, endocrine and motor systems. Only one patient showed a mild cerebral cortical spongiosis. Two individuals have been studied for their levels of PrP^{Sc} expression. The individual with spongiosis was one of the two. This individual, who had had a longer duration of illness, was found to have consistently higher levels of PrP^{Sc} than the other. Proteinase-K treatment of extracted PrP^{Sc} from these two subjects resulted in different bands on SDS-polyacrylamide gels than PrP^{Sc} from other sources, suggesting that there may be a number of different abnormal isoforms of PrP.

These families with fatal insomnia underline the point that there is probably a wider spectrum of prion disease than previously appreciated and that it is not always possible to correlate the basic genetic defect with the disease phenotype. Other genetic factors may well influence the consequences of having a specific mutation.

PrP-Ser198: This mutation has been recently described in a large American kindred (the Indiana kindred) with presenile dementia, ataxia and parkinsonism (Dlouhy et al, 1992). The duration of disease was more than 6 years. Of great interest was the observation in this family of neurofibrillary tangles, as seen in Alzheimer's disease. In addition there were PrP immunostaining plaques and mild spongiform changes.

PrP-Lys200: This subtype was originally described in a Polish sibling pair with CJD (Goldgaber et al, 1989). It accounts for ethnogeographic clustering of CJD in Slovakia, Libyan Jews in Israel, Sephardic Jews in Greece and familial CJD in Chile (Goldfarb et al, 1992). Two British families have also been identified: one had Libyan Jewish ancestry but the other appears to be a separate British focus (J. Collinge and M. S. Palmer, in press).

Patients with this subtype present with a rapidly progressive dementia, myoclonus and pyramidal, cerebellar or extrapyramidal signs. There is a characteristic pseudoperiodic picture on EEG. The average age at onset for this disease is 55 years. Histologically these patients are typical of CJD, plaques are absent but PrP^{Sc} can be demonstrated by immunoblotting. This is the only PrP mutation so far which has been described in the homozygous state. Homozygosity did not affect the phenotype, as would be predicted for a dominant disorder (Hsiao et al, 1991a). Also of interest is that a 78-year-old woman with this mutation has remained asymptomatic, suggesting that there is incomplete penetrance for the disease with this mutation.

PrP-Arg217. In addition to the Indiana kindred, neurofibrillary tangles have been found in two patients of a Swedish family with this mutation at codon 217. These patients had a history of symptoms of dementia 4 years before the development of gait ataxia, with dysphagia and confusion occurring in the months preceding death at the age of 67 and 71 years. The open reading frame of the PrP gene from one of these patients also revealed a new non-coding polymorphism at codon 124, in which there is a third base change in a glycine encoding codon (GGC-GGC) which can be detected by the creation of an *Eco*0 109I restriction site.

Presymptomatic testing and counselling

The identification of PrP mutations in families with inherited prion disease allows a direct gene test for subjects at risk as well as providing accurate diagnosis in affected individuals. Such tests have already been carried out following careful genetic counselling. For counselling purposes prion diseases are similar to Huntington's disease, for which protocols have been well established. Unlike Huntington's, however, for which there are many linked markers but no disease locus yet identified, the PrP gene test can be unambiguous as there is no possibility of recombination between the probe and the disease locus (Collinge et al, 1991b). However, the possibility of incomplete penetrance, as seen in PrP-Lys200 disease, needs also to be considered.

IATROGENIC PRION DISEASE

While transmissibility of the human diseases is mostly an experimental phenomenon, there are a small number of documented cases which show that CJD has been transmitted through contact with contaminated materials. These include the use of intracerebral electrodes which have not been sufficiently sterilized to remove the prion agent, dura mater grafting and corneal transplants. A particularly worrying finding was the appearance of CJD in a number of individuals who had been treated in childhood with growth hormone derived from cadaveric human pituitary glands (Buchanan et al, 1991). In the UK 1908 children were treated with human cadaveric pituitary derived growth hormone and by 1991 six individuals had developed

CJD. All presented with clinical features of a spongiform encephalopathy: rapidly progressing cerebellar dysfunction and ataxia followed by dementia and death within 12 months of onset. Neuropathological confirmation was established in each case examined. All the individuals appeared to develop the disease about 15 years after their first exposure to growth hormone. Each batch of hormone used was derived from a pool of up to 3000 pituitaries and there is no single batch that is common or unique to these six individuals. It is likely therefore that most of the children receiving growth hormone will have been treated with the same contaminated batches. Although there will have been differences in the dosage of prions to which individuals will have been exposed, it is also likely that genetic factors will to some extent determine susceptibility in these cases.

Analysis of the prion protein gene showed that none of the six cases, nor an additional individual who had died of CJD after pituitary derived gonadotrophin treatment, had any of the known mutations in their open reading frame (Collinge et al, 1991a). There was, however, a striking finding with respect to a coding polymorphism at codon 129. An amino acid change at codon 129 was originally described as a new mutation (Goldfarb et al, 1989). Screening of a control population in the UK demonstrated that this was actually a polymorphism (Owen et al, 1990), and further screening of larger numbers estimated the frequency of polymorphic alleles to be about 66% encoding methionine at codon 129, and 33% encoding valine. Valine homozygotes account for about one in nine of the population. Amongst the seven cases of iatrogenic CJD screened there were four valine homozygotes and two heterozygotes. This gave a frequency of 71% valine alleles. Although the numbers are small, statistical analysis confirms that this is significant. This finding implied that there is genetic susceptibility to iatogenic CJD. This may be a property of the valine-containing PrP molecule or linkage to another locus which confers susceptibility.

SPORADIC PRION DISEASE

Despite the extent of our knowledge of the inherited prion diseases we still know very little about the aetiology of sporadic cases of CJD, which account for about 85% of all cases. Although the epidemiological evidence suggests otherwise, it is a possibility that the sporadic cases are due to contamination with environmental prions. Since there is a uniform world-wide distribution of CJD which does not correlate with geographical distribution of endemic scrapie, it is difficult to know what the source of these environmental prions might be. Following from the observation of genetic susceptibility to iatrogenic CJD, the possibility that there is also a genetic predisposition towards sporadic CJD was investigated. When the genotype of a number of sporadic CJD cases were analysed it was found that, while there was not an increase in the number of valine alleles in that population, there was a striking increase in the number of homozygotes for either methionine or valine (Palmer et al, 1991). In a sample of 22 sporadic CJD cases meeting classical diagnostic criteria, only one was found to be heterozygous at amino acid residue 129. This dramatic increase in homozygosity associated with sporadic CJD has been confirmed in further studies. Of a further 45 individuals who were suspected to have sporadic CJD and who had been submitted to the UK's CJD surveillance survey, eight further heterozygous cases were found. Two of these individuals subsequently recovered and were clearly not affected with CJD. Of the other cases only one had the short duration of illness characteristic of typical CJD, although this case had an atypical EEG. All the others had an atypical presentation of disease with long duration times. We can therefore predict that in cases of suspected sporadic CJD, individuals who are heterozygous at codon 129 will generally fall into one of four categories: (1) individuals with an inherited disease that was not recognized as being familial; (2) individuals who will have been misdiagnosed and do not suffer from prion disease; (3) individuals who will have an atypical presentation and account for the differences between 'classical' and 'atypical' sporadic CJD; (4) a few individuals who appear to have classical CJD despite being heterozygous, perhaps reflecting quantitative differences in the number of disease foci.

This demonstration of genetic predisposition towards sporadic CJD does not explain the aetiology of this disorder; however, it has contributed enormously to our understanding of the likely mechanism underlying the biology of the prion diseases, which will be discussed in the final section of this chapter. The two most likely causes of sporadic prion disease are a somatic mutation in the PrP gene analogous to the inherited mutations or a spontaneous conversion of normal PrP^C into PrP^{Sc} in an individual with no genetic variation in PrP. Once PrP^{Sc} is present within an individual, whether by spontaneous conversion of normal PrP or because of a mutation which results in conversion, it will act like an exogenous source of infectious prions and lead to progression of the disease.

A PROTEIN MODEL FOR PRION DISEASES

While it has been seen as heretical by some to argue that a protein could be responsible for the transmission of the spongiform encephalopathies, in the absence of any nucleic acid, recent results from work on transgenic animals have suggested a possible mechanism that is consistent with conventional biological principles. The results on homozygosity in iatrogenic and sporadic human CJD seem, in part, to support this model, though there are many details remaining to be determined.

It is known that there is ordinarily a species barrier to transmission of scrapie (Pattison, 1965). Scrapie that has been passaged in mice is not easily transmitted to hamsters, while that passaged in hamsters is not transmissible to mice, although occasionally there is cross-species transmission after prolonged incubation times. To address the question of the role of the host PrP in determining transmissibility, mice were constructed that were transgenic for the hamster PrP gene so that they expressed both mouse and hamster PrP (Prusiner et al, 1990). The level of expression of hamster PrP depended upon the copy number of the transgene. These transgenic mice were as susceptible to mice prions as normal mice, but were also now susceptible to infection with hamster prions. The incubation time for infection with hamster prions depended upon the level of hamster PrP expression: the higher the levels of expression the shorter the incubation period. Transgenic mice that had been inoculated with hamster prions were also shown to generate hamster prions, since brain homogenates from these mice transmitted disease to normal hamsters but not to normal mice. Conversely, the inoculation of transgenic mice with mouse prions led to the generation of mice prions, as determined by the subsequent transmission to normal mice but not normal hamsters.

Since the only difference between normal and transgenic mice should be the expression of hamster PrP, it is difficult to argue that exogenous prions interact with a 'prion receptor' that is distinct from PrP, since this would not have changed between normal and transgenic animals (Prusiner et al, 1990). While there is almost certainly an involvement of other cellular components, the simplest interpretation of the transgenic transmission data is that there is a direct interaction between exogenous and endogenous PrP molecules required for initiation of the disease. Further, it can be argued that for this interaction to occur effectively the protein molecules must be homologous. Mouse–hamster PrP interaction would not normally be favourable for disease initiation.

The observation of homozygosity of PrP genotypes predisposing to sporadic CJD clearly supports the idea that interaction requires homologous PrP types. Whatever the cause of sporadic disease, if it is a truly stochastic event it should affect individuals with PrP genotypes in the same proportion as normal populations. The predominance of homozygotes suggests that heterozygosity is to some extent protective for the disease. If PrP interaction is required for progression of disease then clearly proteins homologous at residue 129 will facilitate that progression. This argues that residue 129 is at a site that is particularly important for the interaction of PrP molecules and that identity is required at this residue for efficient progression of disease.

Further evidence for the importance of residue 129 comes from observations on the large pedigree with a 144 bp insertion referred to above. Ages of onset of disease in a number of affected individuals have been correlated with codon 129 genotype. All individuals with an age of onset below 40 years were homozygous for methionine (the 144 bp insertion is on a methionine allele), while all those with onset above 40 years were heterozygous (Baker et al, 1991; Poulter et al, 1992). Again this implies that disease progression (which is inevitable because of the mutation) is facilitated by homologous protein types and takes longer when an individual is heterozygous.

How can the interaction of proteins lead to the progression of disease? Since disease is characterized by the accumulation of abnormal PrP (PrP^{Sc}), it is possible that the conversion of PrP^C to PrP^{Sc} is itself catalysed by the presence of PrP^{Sc}. In this autocatalytic cascade model PrP^{Sc} and PrP^C can be seen as coming together, perhaps to form dimers, and PrP^C adopting the conformation of the template PrP^{Sc} (Prusiner et al, 1990; Weissmann, 1991). As PrP^C is converted into PrP^{Sc} so PrP^{Sc} accumulates and provides a template for the conversion of more PrP^C (Figure 5). Alternatively, instead

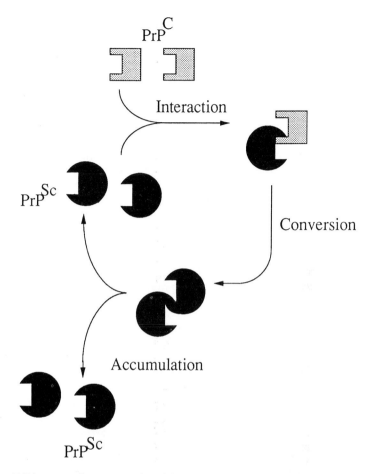

Figure 5. Diagrammatic representation of the protein model for prion replication. The normal and scrapie form of PrP are indicated by shaded motifs with different conformations. The model indicates that PrP^{Sc} and PrP^C might interact to form dimers. PrP^C is then converted into the PrP^{Sc} form and this leads to an accumulation of PrP^{Sc}. Since the nature of the difference between PrP^{Sc} and PrP^C is not known it is possible that there is no change in conformation of the molecule but that PrP^{Sc} is in a different aggregation state, for example, that acquires the property of protease resistance.

of a conversion of conformation, PrP^{Sc} may represent an aggregation of PrP^C, resulting in a form that is inaccessible to proteinase-K. Although this is a simplistic view of how PrP^{Sc} may accumulate, it is at least consistent with more conventional biological properties and provides an alternative view for considering how the disease is transmissible without requiring a self-replicating agent. There is considerable evidence from tissue culture models of infectivity that PrP^{Sc} is derived directly from PrP^C, supporting the central principle of this model. The excess of valine alleles associated with iatrogenic transmission is perhaps indicating that the valine variant is more susceptible to transformation into the disease related isoform during the initial stages of disease induction than the methionine variant.

CONCLUSIONS

Since the original reports of Creutzfeldt, Jakob, Gerstmann and Sträussler we have come to recognize a range of neurodegenerative disorders that can be categorized together as prion diseases, either on the basis of mutations in the PrP gene or by the demonstration of abnormal PrP in the brain. Both of these may be associated with transmissibility, though that is no longer the criterion by which these diseases need be classified. The diseases show a range of clinical presentations associated with dementia, though we are seeing families with mutations in the prion gene in which even dementia is a less obvious feature. Neuropathologically, prion diseases are proving to be quite heterogeneous, with the classical pathology of spongiform encephalopathies often absent, even after prolonged illness. The inherited prion diseases can now be classified on the basis of the PrP mutation associated with disease, and a broader classification of prion diseases encompassing all forms is shown in Table 1. The recognition of mutations in the PrP gene

Table 1. Classification of prion diseases.

Type	Syndrome	Aetiology
Inherited	CJD GSS Other*	Inherited mutation
Sporadic	CJD Typical Atypical Other†	Possibly somatic mutation: Codon 129 homozygotes Codon 129 heterozygotes
Acquired	Kuru Iatrogenic	Cannibalism Accidental inoculation

*For example fatal familial insomnia.
†For example possibly other sporadic neurodegenerative disorders will be prion diseases.

allows accurate diagnosis of prion disease in familial cases of dementia, and permits presymptomatic diagnosis in appropriate families. Many ethical questions are raised by the screening of individuals for PrP mutations. While counselling protocols for Huntington's disease can be followed where appropriate, the availability of a direct gene test has implications for many other family members and careful thought needs to be put into any diagnostic or research protocol that has the potential to diagnose a positive PrP mutation.

Research into prion diseases has now provided overwhelming evidence that the transmissible agent (the prion) is composed of a protease resistant isoform of a normal cellular gene product, the prion protein as its principal if not its sole constituent (Prusiner, 1991). The abnormal isoform, PrP^{Sc}, may function by catalysing the conversion of the normal protein PrP^C into the abnormal form. The nature of the difference between these two forms is still unknown and may reflect a conformational change or a change in aggregation state. Individuals with mutations in the PrP may spontaneously undergo the conformational conversion in the absence of exogenous PrP^{Sc} Once PrP^{Sc} is present it will drive the conversion of PrP^C, leading to accumulation of PrP^{Sc}. Disease will be initiated in iatrogenic cases by the inoculation with exogenous prions, though fortunately this is a rare cause of disease. In sporadic CJD the origin of PrP^{Sc} is not clear. It may follow from somatic mutation in the PrP gene which results in conversion as in familial cases, or alternatively sporadic cases may simply represent the rare natural background conversion of PrP^C into PrP^{Sc}.

Although there are many questions remaining to be answered in the prion field, we are now in a position to think clearly about non-viral models for transmissibility that may lead directly to therapeutic strategies. Ligands that interfere with the interaction of PrP^{Sc} and PrP^C may prove to be sufficient to prevent the progression of disease and lead to rational treatment for these neurodegenerative disorders.

REFERENCES

Alper T, Haig DA & Clarke MC (1966) The exceptionally small size of the scrapie agent. *Biochemical and Biophysical Research Communications* **22:** 278–284.

Alper T, Cramp WA, Haig DA & Clarke MC (1967) Does the agent of scrapie replicate without nucleic acid? *Nature* **214:** 764–766.

Baker HE, Poulter M, Crow TJ et al (1991) Aminoacid polymorphism in human prion protein and age at death in inherited prion disease. *Lancet* **337:** 1286.

Barry RA & Prusiner SB (1986) Monoclonal antibodies to the cellular and scrapie prion proteins. *Journal of Infectious Diseases* **154:** 518–521.

Barry RA, Kent SB, McKinley MP et al (1986) Scrapie and cellular prion proteins share polypeptide epitopes. *Journal of Infectious Diseases* **153:** 848–854.

Beck E & Daniel PM (1987) Neuropathology of transmissible spongiform encephalopathies. In Prusiner SB & McKinley MP (eds) *Prions: Novel Infectious Pathogens Causing Scrapie and Creutzfeldt–Jakob Disease*, pp 331–385. San Diego: Academic Press.

Beck E, Daniel PM, Alpers M, Gajdusek DC & Gibbs CJJ (1969) Neuropathological comparisons of experimental kuru in chimpanzees with human kuru. *International Archives of Allergy and Applied Immunology* **36:** 553–562.

Bellinger KC, Cleaver JE, Diener TO & Prusiner SB (1987) Purified scrapie prions resist inactivation by UV irradiation. *Journal of Virology* **61:** 159–166.

Bolton DC, McKinley MP & Prusiner SB (1982) Identification of a protein that purifies with the scrapie prion. *Science* **218:** 1309–1311.

Bolton DC, McKinley MP & Prusiner SB (1984) Molecular characteristics of the major scrapie prion protein. *Biochemistry* **23:** 5898–5906.

Bolton DC, Meyer RK & Prusiner SB (1985) Scrapie PrP 27–30 is a sialoglycoprotein. *Journal of Virology* **53:** 596–606.

Borchelt DR, Scott M, Taraboulos A, Stahl N & Prusiner SB (1990) Scrapie and cellular prion proteins differ in their kinetics of synthesis and topology in cultured cells. *Journal of Cell Biology* **110:** 743–752.

Brown P, Rodgers JP, Cathala F, Gibbs C & Gajdusek DC (1984) Creutzfeldt–Jakob disease of long duration: clinicopathological characteristics, transmissibility, and differential diagnosis. *Annals of Neurology* **16:** 295–304.

Brown P, Cathala F, Raubertas RF, Gajdusek DC & Castaigne P (1987) The epidemiology of Creutzfeldt–Jakob disease; conclusion of a 15-year investigation in France and review of the world literature. *Neurology* **37**: 895–904.

Buchanan CR, Preece MA & Milner RD (1991) Mortality, neoplasia, and Creutzfeldt–Jakob disease in patients treated with human pituitary growth hormone in the United Kingdom. *BMJ* **302**: 824–828.

Butler DA, Scott MRD, Kingsbury DT, Bockman JM & Prusiner SB (1987) Murine neuro-blastoma cell lines chronically infected with scrapie prions. *Neurology* **37** (supplement): 342 (abstract).

Cathala F & Baron H (1987) Clinical aspects of Creuzfeldt–Jakob disease. In Prusiner SB & McKinley MP (eds) *Prion: Novel Infectious Pathogens Causing Scrapie and Creutzfeldt–Jakob Disease*, pp 467–509. San Diego: Academic Press.

Collinge J & Prusiner SB (1992) Terminology of prion diseases. In Prusiner SB, Collinge J, Powell J & Anderson B (eds) *Prion Diseases of Humans and Animals*, 5–12 (in press). London: Ellis Horwood.

Collinge J, Harding AE, Owen F et al (1989) Diagnosis of Gerstmann–Sträussler syndrome in familial dementia with prion protein gene analysis. *Lancet* **ii**: 15–17.

Collinge J, Owen F, Poulter M et al (1990) Prion dementia without characteristic pathology. *Lancet* **336**: 7–9.

Collinge J, Palmer MS & Dryden AJ (1991a) Genetic predisposition to iatrogenic Creutzfeldt–Jakob disease. *Lancet* **337**: 1441–1442.

Collinge J, Poulter M, Davis MB et al (1991b) Presymptomatic detection or exclusion of prion protein gene defects in families with inherited prion diseases. *American Journal of Human Genetics* **49**: 1351–1354.

Collinge J, Brown J, Hardy J et al (1992) Inherited prion disease with 144 base pair gene insertion. 2: Clinical and pathological features. *Brain* **115**: 687–710.

Creutzfeldt HG (1920) Über eine eigenartige herdförmige Erkrankung des Zentralnerven-systems. *Zeitschrift für die Gesamte Neurologie und Psychiatrie* **57**: 1–18.

Dickinson AG & Outram GW (1979) The scrapie replication-site hypothesis and its impli-cations for pathogenesis. In Prusiner SB & Hadlow WJ (eds) *Slow Transmissible Diseases of the Central Nervous System*, pp 13–31. New York: Academic Press.

Dickinson AG & Outram GW (1988) Genetic aspects of unconventional virus infections: the basis of the virino hypothesis. *Ciba Foundation Symposium* **135**: 63–83.

Diener TO, McKinley MP & Prusiner SB (1982) Viroids and prions. *Proceedings of the National Academy of Sciences of the USA* **79**: 5220–5224.

Dlouhy SR, Hsiao K, Farlow MR et al (1992) Linkage of the Indiana kindred of Gerstmann–Sträussler–Scheinker disease to the prion protein gene. *Nature Genetics* **1**: 64–67.

Doh-ura K, Tateishi J, Sasaki H, Kitamoto T & Sakaki Y (1989) Pro-leu change at position 102 of prion protein is the most common but not the sole mutation related to Gerstmann–Sträussler syndrome. *Biochemical and Biophysical Research Communications* **163**: 974–979.

Endo T, Groth D, Prusiner SB & Kobata A (1989) Diversity of oligosaccharide structures linked to asparagines of the scrapie prion protein. *Biochemistry* **28**: 8380–8388.

Farlow MR, Yee RD, Dlouhy SR et al (1989) Gerstmann–Sträussler–Scheinker disease. I. Extending the clinical spectrum. *Neurology* **39**: 1446–1452.

Gabizon R, McKinley MP & Prusiner SB (1987) Purified prion proteins and scrapie infectivity copartition into liposomes. *Proceedings of the National Academy of Sciences of the USA* **84**: 4017–4021.

Gabizon R, McKinley MP, Groth D & Prusiner SB (1988) Immunoaffinity purification and neutralization of scrapie prion infectivity. (Published erratum appears in *Proc Natl Acad Sci USA* 1989 Feb; 86(4): 1223.) *Proceedings of the National Academy of Sciences of the USA* **85**: 6617–6621.

Gajdusek DC (1977) Unconventional viruses and the origin and disappearance of kuru. *Science* **197**: 943–960.

Gajdusek DC (1990) Subacute spongiform encephalopathies: transmissible cerebral amy-loidoses caused by unconventional viruses. In Fields BN & Knipe DM (eds) *Virology*, pp 2289–2324. New York: Raven.

Gajdusek DC, Gibbs CJ & Alpers M (1966) Experimental transmission of a kuru-like syndrome to chimpanzees. *Nature* **209**: 794–796.

Gerstmann J (1928) Über ein noch nicht beschriebenes Reflexphänomen bei einer Erkrankung des zerebellaren Systems. *Wiener Medizinische Wochenschrift* **78**: 906–908.

Gerstmann J, Sträussler E & Scheinker I (1936) Über eine eigenartige hereditär-familiäre Erkrankung des Zentralnervensystems. Zugleich ein Beitrag zur frage des vorzeitigen-lakalen Alterns. *Zeitschrift für Neurologie* **154**: 736–762.

Ghetti B, Tagliavini F, Masters CL et al (1989) Gerstmann–Sträussler–Scheinker disease. II. Neurofibrillary tangles and plaques with PrP-amyloid coexist in an affected family. *Neurology* **39**: 1453–1461.

Gibbs CJ, Gajdusek DC, Asher DM et al (1968) Creutzfeldt–Jakob disease (spongiform encephalopathy): transmission to the chimpanzee. *Science* **161**: 388–389.

Goldfarb LG, Brown P, Goldgaber D, Asher DM & Strass N (1989) Patients with Creutzfeldt–Jakob disease and kuru lack the mutation in the PRIP gene found in Gerstmann–Sträussler syndrome, but they show a different double allele mutation in the same gene. *American Journal of Human Genetics* **45**: A189.

Goldfarb LG, Brown P, McCombie WR et al (1991a) Transmissible familial Creutzfeldt–Jakob disease associated with five, seven, and eight extra octapeptide coding repeats in the PRNP gene. *Proceedings of the National Academy of Sciences of the USA* **88**: 10926–10930.

Goldfarb LG, Haltia M, Brown P et al (1991b) New mutation in scrapie amyloid precursor gene (at codon 178) in Finnish Creutzfeldt–Jakob kindred. *Lancet* **337**: 425.

Goldfarb LG, Brown P & Gajdusek DC (1992) The molecular genetics of human transmissible spongiform encephalopathy. In Prusiner SB, Collinge J, Powell J & Anderson B (eds) pp 139–152 (in press). London: Ellis Horwood.

Goldgaber D, Goldfarb LG, Brown P et al (1989) Mutations in familial Creutzfeldt-Jakob disease and Gerstmann–Sträussler–Scheinker's syndrome. *Experimental Neurology* **106**: 204–206.

Hadlow WJ (1959) Scrapie and kuru. *Lancet* **ii**: 289–290.

Hsiao KK, Baker HF, Crow TJ et al (1989) Linkage of a prion protein missense variant to Gerstmann–Sträussler syndrome. *Nature* **338**: 342–345.

Hsiao KK, Scott M, Foster D et al (1990) Spontaneous neurodegeneration in transgenic mice with mutant prion protein. *Science* **250**: 1587–1590.

Hsiao KK, Meiner Z, Kahana E et al (1991a) Mutation of the prion protein in Libyan Jews with Creutzfeldt–Jakob disease. *New England Journal of Medicine* **324**: 1091–1097.

Hsiao KK, Cass C, Schellenberg GD et al (1991b) A prion protein variant in a family with the telencephalic form of Gerstmann–Sträussler–Scheinker syndrome. *Neurology* **41**: 681–684.

Hsiao KK, Groth D, Scott M et al (1992) Genetic and transgenic studies in Gerstmann–Sträussler–Scheinker disease. In Prusiner SB, Collinge J, Powell J & Anderson B (eds) pp 120–128 (in press). London: Ellis Horwood.

Jakob A (1921a) Über eigenartige Erkrankungen des Zentralnervensystems mit bemerkenswertem anatomischen Befunde (spastische Pseudosclerose-Encephalomyelopathie mit disseminierten Degenerationsherden). Preliminary communication. *Deutsche Zeitschrift für Nervenheilkunde* **70**: 132–146.

Jakob A (1921b) Über eine der multiplen Sklerose klinisch nahestehende Erkrankung des Zentralnervensystems (spastische Pseudosklerose) mit bemerkenswertem anatomischen Befunde. Mitteilung eines vierten Falles. *Medizinische Klinik* **17**: 372–376.

Klatzo I, Gajdusek DC & Zigas V (1959) Pathology of kuru. *Laboratory Investigation* **8**: 799–847.

Kretzschmar HA, Prusiner SB, Stowring LE & DeArmond SJ (1986a) Scrapie prion proteins are synthesized in neurones. *American Journal of Pathology* **122**: 1–5.

Kretzschmar HA, Stowring LE, Westaway D et al (1986b) Molecular cloning of a human prion protein cDNA. *DNA* **5**: 315–324.

Kretzschmar HA, Honold G, Seitelberger F et al (1991) Prion protein mutation in family first reported by Gerstmann, Sträussler, and Scheinker. *Lancet* **337**: 1160.

Liao YC, Lebo RV, Clawson GA & Smuckler EA (1986) Human prion protein cDNA; molecular cloning, chromosomal mapping, and biological implications. *Science* **233**: 364–367.

Lopez CD, Yost CS, Prusiner SB, Myers RM & Lingappa VR (1990) Unusual topogenic sequence directs prion protein biogenesis. *Science* **248**: 226–229.

McKinley MP, Bolton DC & Prusiner SB (1983a) A protease-resistant protein is a structural component of the scrapie prion. *Cell* **35**: 57–62.

McKinley MP, Masiarz FR, Isaacs ST, Hearst JE & Prusiner SB (1983b) Resistance of the scrapie agent to inactivation by psoralens. *Photochemistry and Photobiology* **37:** 539–545.

McKinley MP, Taraboulos A, Kenaga L et al (1991) Ultrastructural localization of scrapie prion proteins in cytoplasmic vesicles of infected cultured cells. *Laboratory Investigation* **65:** 622–630.

Manetto V, Medori R, Cortelli P et al (1992) Fatal familial insomnia: clinical and pathologic study of five new cases. *Neurology* **42:** 312–319.

Medori R, Montagna P, Tritschler HJ et al (1992a) Fatal familial insomnia: a second kindred with mutation of prion protein gene at codon 178. *Neurology* **42:** 669–670.

Medori R, Tritschler HJ, LeBlanc A et al (1992b) Fatal familial insomnia, a prion disease with a mutation at codon 178 of the prion protein gene. *New England Journal of Medicine* **326:** 444–449.

Meyer RK, McKinley MP, Bowman KA et al (1986) Separation and properties of cellular and scrapie prion proteins. *Proceedings of the National Academy of Sciences of the USA* **83:** 2310–2314.

Mobley WC, Neve RL, Prusiner SB & McKinley MP (1988) Nerve growth factor increases mRNA levels for the prion protein and the beta-amyloid protein precursor in developing hamster brain. *Proceedings of the National Academy of Sciences of the USA* **85:** 9811–9815.

Nieto A, Goldfarb LG, Brown P et al (1991) Codon 178 mutation in ethnically diverse Creutzfeldt–Jakob disease families. *Lancet* **337:** 622–623.

Nochlin D, Sumi SM, Bird TD et al (1989) Familial dementia with PrP-positive amyloid plaques: a variant of Gerstmann–Sträussler syndrome. *Neurology* **39:** 910–918.

Oesch B, Westaway D, Walchli M et al (1985) A cellular gene encodes scrapie PrP 27–30 protein. *Cell* **40:** 735–746.

Owen F, Poulter M, Lofthouse R et al (1989) Insertion in prion protein gene in familial Creutzfeldt–Jakob disease *Lancet* **i:** 51–52.

Owen F, Poulter M, Collinge J & Crow TJ (1990) Codon 129 changes in the prion protein gene in Caucasians. *American Journal of Human Genetics* **46:** 1215–1216.

Owen F, Poulter M, Collinge J et al (1991) Insertions in the prion protein gene in atypical dementias. *Experimental Neurology* **112:** 240–242.

Palmer MS, Dryden AJ, Hughes JT & Collinge J (1991) Homozygous prion protein genotype predisposes to sporadic Creutzfeldt–Jakob disease. (Published erratum appears in *Nature* 1991 Aug 8; 352 (6335): 547.) *Nature* **353:** 340–342.

Pattison IH (1965) Experiments with scrapie and with special reference to the nature of the agent and the pathology of the disease. In Gajdusek DC, Gibbs CJ & Alpers MP (eds) *Slow, Latent and Temperate Virus Infections NINDB Monograph 2*, pp 249–257. Washington DC: US Government.

Poulter M, Baker HF, Frith CD et al (1992) Inherited prion disease with 144 base pair gene insertion. I: Genealogical and molecular studies. *Brain* (in press).

Prusiner SB (1982) Novel proteinaceous infectious particles cause scrapie. *Science* **216:** 136–144.

Prusiner SB (1991) Molecular biology of prion diseases. *Science* **252:** 1515–1522.

Prusiner SB, Groth DF, Cochran SP et al (1980) Molecular properties, partial purification, and assay by incubation period measurements of the hamster scrapie agent. *Biochemistry* **19:** 4883–4891.

Prusiner SB, Bolton DC, Groth DF et al (1982) Further purification and characterisation of scrapie prions. *Biochemistry* **21:** 6942–6950.

Prusiner SB, McKinley MP, Bowman KA et al (1983) Scrapie prions aggregate to form amyloid-like birefringent rods. *Cell* **35:** 349–358.

Prusiner SB, Groth DF, Bolton DC, Kent SB & Hood LE (1984) Purification and structural studies of a major scrapie prion protein. *Cell* **38:** 127–134.

Prusiner SB, Scott M, Foster D et al (1990) Trangenetic studies implicate interactions between homologous PrP isoforms in scrapie prion replication. *Cell* **63:** 673–686.

Robakis NK, Devine GE, Jenkins EC et al (1986) Localization of a human gene homologous to the PrP gene on the p arm of chromosome 20 and detection of PrP-related antigens in normal human brain. *Biochemical and Biophysical Research Communications* **140:** 758–765.

Roberts GW, Lofthouse R, Brown R et al (1986) Prion-protein immunoreactivity in human transmissible dementias. *New England Journal of Medicine* **315:** 1231–1233.

Seitelberger F (1962) Eigenartige familiäre-hereditare Krankheit des zentralen Nervensystems in einer niederösterreichischen Sippe. *Wiener Klinische Wochenschrift* **41/42:** 687–691.

Sparkes RS, Simon M, Cohn VH et al (1986) Assignment of the human and mouse prion protein genes to homologous chromosomes. *Proceedings of the National Academy of Sciences of the USA* **83:** 7358–7362.

Spielmeyer W (1922) Die histopathologische Forschung in der Psychiatrie. *Klinische Wochenschrift* **2:** 1817–1819.

Stahl N & Prusiner SB (1991) Prions and prion proteins. *FASEB J* **5:** 2799–2807.

Stahl N, Borchelt DR, Hsiao K & Prusiner SB (1987) Scrapie prion protein contains a phosphatidylinositol glycolipid. *Cell* **51:** 229–240.

Stahl N, Baldwin MA, Burlingame AL & Prusiner SB (1990a) Identification of glycoinositol phospholipid linked and truncated forms of the scrapie prion protein. *Biochemistry* **29:** 8879–8884.

Stahl N, Borchelt DR & Prusiner SB (1990b) Differential release of cellular and scrapie prion proteins from cellular membranes by phosphatidylinositol-specific phospholipase C. *Biochemistry* **29:** 5405–5412.

Warter JM, Steinmetz G, Heldt N et al (1982) Familial presenile dementia: Gerstmann–Sträussler–Scheinker syndrome. *Rev Neurol (Paris)* **138:** 107–121.

Weissmann C (1991) Spongiform encephalopathies. The prion's progress. *Nature* **349:** 569–571.

Wilesmith JW, Ryan JB & Atkinson MJ (1991) Bovine spongiform encephalopathy: epidemiological studies on the origin. *Veterinary Record* **128:** 199–203.

Wu Y, Brown WT, Robakis NK et al (1987) A *Pvu*II RFLP detected in the human prion protein (PrP) gene. *Nucleic Acids Research* **15:** 3191.

Yost CS, Lopez CD, Prusiner SB, Myers RM & Lingappa VR (1990) Non-hydrophobic extracytoplasmic determinant of stop transfer in the prion protein. *Nature* **343:** 669–672.

Zigas V & Gajdusek DC (1957) Kuru: clinical study of a new syndrome resembling paralysis agitans in natives of the Eastern Highlands of Australian New Guinea. *Medical Journal of Australia* **2:** 745–754.

9

Lewy body dementia

GRAHAM LENNOX

There are two reasons for wondering whether Lewy body dementia should appear in a volume entitled *Unusual Dementias*. The first is the continuing controversy over its status as a distinct entity. Is it a disease in its own right, or simply a variant of Alzheimer's disease? If you accept that it can be distinguished from other recognizable causes of dementia, the second reason is that it is almost certainly a common disease, unusual more for its belated recognition than for its prevalence.

These problems serve to emphasize that the concept of Lewy body dementia is an evolving one. First described in two American patients in 1961 (Okazaki et al, 1961), most of the early clinicopathological studies came from Japan (for review, see Kosaka, 1990). In the last 5 years an increasing number of centres have reported substantial series of cases, providing a broader and more coherent view of its clinical features. Despite this, the fundamental question of whether Lewy body dementia is a separate nosological entity remains open. The present evidence in favour of regarding it as a distinct pathological entity is discussed below (Neuropathology), but should not be regarded as complete; in particular, it seems likely that molecular genetic and cell biological studies will influence thinking on this issue within the next few years.

Of more immediate clinical interest is the emerging consensus that Lewy body dementia is associated with a parkinsonian dementia syndrome with potentially characteristic neuropsychiatric and neurological elements, posing particular problems of diagnosis and management; these are outlined later in this chapter. Ultimately, however, the best hope of effective treatment rests with the basic scientists and their search for an understanding of the molecular pathogenesis of Lewy body disease, which is outlined in the final section.

NEUROPATHOLOGY: THE CASE FOR A DISTINCT ENTITY

Lewy body dementia is defined by the presence of rounded eosinophilic inclusion bodies (Lewy bodies) within the cytoplasm of neurones, in certain brainstem, subcortical and cortical regions. These invariably include the locus coeruleus and substantia nigra (which provide the principal cortical noradrenergic and dopaminergic projections, respectively), which also show evidence of cell loss and gliosis. Other brainstem nuclei, such as the

Baillière's Clinical Neurology—
Vol. 1, No. 3, November 1992
ISBN 0–7020–1631–4

ventral tegmental area, the midbrain oculomotor structures and the dorsal vagal nucleus, are also often involved. In the diencephalon the nucleus basalis of Meynert (which provides the major cortical cholinergic projection) again invariably contains Lewy bodies with cell loss and gliosis. Within the cerebral cortex the most severe changes typically occur within limbic structures such as the mesial temporal lobe (largely sparing the hippocampus), insular cortex and anterior cingulate gyrus, with somewhat lower densities of Lewy bodies in neocortical parts of the frontal, temporal and parietal lobes. Areas of primary motor, sensory and visual cortex are spared. This pathology, which is reviewed in more detail in Chapter 2, closely resembles that of Parkinson's disease, with the important exception that there are much larger numbers of cortical Lewy bodies. Non-demented cases of Parkinson's disease generally have only small numbers of cortical Lewy bodies (Lennox et al, 1989a; Hughes et al, 1992). As in Parkinson's disease, Lewy bodies may also be found in the sympathetic ganglia.

Kosaka and colleagues (1980, 1984) and Yoshimura (1983) first drew attention to the possibility that Parkinson's disease and Lewy body dementia might represent different ends of a single disease spectrum. They called this Lewy body disease and classified it into three types: a brainstem type corresponding to Parkinson's disease; a diffuse type corresponding to Lewy body dementia; and an intermediate transitional type. The term 'diffuse Lewy body disease' is widely used by neuropathologists, but has been criticized on the grounds that it gives the impression that Lewy bodies are distributed uniformly throughout the nervous system instead of in the characteristic distribution outlined above.

Cortical Lewy bodies are difficult to identify using conventional staining, because (unlike Lewy bodies in the brainstem) they rarely have a halo separating the eosinophilic inclusion body from the surrounding eosinophilic cytoplasm. Immunohistochemical techniques such as antiubiquitin immunohistochemistry are more sensitive, provided that care is taken to distinguish Lewy bodies from other spherical inclusions such as Pick bodies and small spherical neurofibrillary tangles (Lennox, 1989b). Cortical Lewy bodies are not an entirely specific marker for Lewy body dementia. They have been reported in a few cases of rare diseases such as Hallervorden–Spatz disease and neuroaxonal dystrophy (Dooling et al, 1974; Hayashi et al, 1992), subacute sclerosing panencephalitis and ataxia-telangectasia (Gibb, 1986; Gibb et al, 1990); similar inclusions are seen in the motor cortex in motor neurone disease (Lowe et al, 1989). They are also a very occasional finding in normal old age where they may represent a presymptomatic stage of Lewy body dementia (Perry et al, 1990a).

In young onset cases of Lewy body dementia there is rarely any other associated pathology (for review, see Kosaka, 1990). Most older cases also have cortical senile plaques in substantial numbers, proportional to the number of cortical Lewy bodies (Lennox et al, 1989a). Senile plaques are most familiar to neuropathologists as a feature of Alzheimer's disease, although they also occur in a wide range of other neurodegenerative diseases and in normal old age. In Lewy body dementia (as in old age) the plaques tend to be of a diffuse type and lack the classical amyloid cores and neuritic

Table 1. Histopathological differences between Lewy body dementia and Alzheimer's disease.

Area	Lewy body dementia	Alzheimer's disease
Brainstem pigmented nuclei	Classical Lewy bodies Severe neurone loss	Neurofibrillary tangles Variable neurone loss
Nucleus basalis of Meynert	Classical Lewy bodies Loss of large neurones	Neurofibrillary tangles Loss of large neurones
Hippocampus	Usually few or no tangles; dystrophic neurites in CA2–3	Many tangles, with granulo-vacuolar degeneration and Hirano bodies
Limbic cortex	Many cortical Lewy bodies Variable numbers of diffuse plaques; usually few or no tangles Occasional spongiform change	No cortical Lewy bodies Many tangles, and senile plaques of diffuse and classical type Occasional spongiform change
Neocortex	Moderate numbers of cortical Lewy bodies and diffuse plaques Relatively few or no tangles	No Lewy bodies Many tangles and senile plaques of all types, with dystrophic neurites/threads

elements that are seen in most cases of Alzheimer's disease. Where they do contain dystrophic neurites these are unusually rounded and granular and do not generally contain the paired helical filaments (PHF) characteristic of Alzheimer's disease, nor are they immunoreactive for tau (Dickson et al, 1989). PHF-negative abnormal neurites are found in the CA2–3 region of the hippocampus but are rare in the neocortical neuropil (Dickson et al, 1991); the converse is true of Alzheimer's disease which spares the CA2–3 region and where PHF-positive neocortical neuropil threads are invariably present.

A smaller proportion (approximately one-third) of cases of Lewy body dementia also have neurofibrillary tangles (Dickson et al, 1989; Lennox et al, 1989a). Interestingly, a larger proportion of these patients are female than one would expect from chance. Even in these cases there are significantly fewer tangles than in Alzheimer's disease (Hansen et al, 1991) and many are morphologically unimpressive, consisting of little more than a wisp of fibrillary material.

The interpretation of these findings remains a matter of debate. Hansen and colleagues (1990) have suggested that Lewy body dementia should be regarded as a variant of Alzheimer's disease. Most other groups have resisted this view (Kosaka et al, 1984; Lennox et al, 1989a; Dickson, 1990; Fearnley et al, 1990), citing the differences in pathology described above as well as clinical differences (see below, Clinical Features). Molecular studies may eventually settle the issue. Goate and colleagues (1991) have recently reported a family with autosomal dominant Alzheimer's disease associated with a missense mutation at codon 717 of the amyloid precursor protein gene (see Chapter 3); neuropathological examination of one affected member revealed cortical plaques, tangles and Lewy bodies, suggesting that all three forms of pathology can arise from a defect in a single gene (Lantos et al, 1992). Lewy body pathology has not, however, been reported in other families with mutations at this site (Hardy et al, 1991; Mann et al, 1992), nor have such mutations been reported in sporadic cases of either Alzheimer's disease or Lewy body dementia. Furthermore, differences in the molecular composition of Lewy bodies and neurofibrillary tangles (particularly with regard to components of the cell stress system) suggest that they represent fundamentally different strategies of neurones attempting to cope with disease (Lowe et al, 1990; and see below, Towards Effective Treatment).

One final aspect of the neuropathology of Lewy body dementia is worth mentioning, again in relation to advances in molecular genetics, and this is the presence of spongiform vacuolation in the temporal lobes in some cases (Burkhardt et al, 1988; Hansen et al, 1989). Spongiform change is characteristic of the transmissible prion encephalopathies such as Creutzfeldt–Jakob disease. Lewy body dementia does not appear to be transmissible, but the spongiform change raises the possibility that its pathogenesis may share molecular mechanisms with the prion diseases.

In this chapter the term Lewy body dementia will refer to cases with disordered higher mental function and numerous brainstem and cortical Lewy bodies, regardless of the presence or absence of associated features. The precise definition of 'numerous' remains difficult; quantitative criteria have been proposed (Lennox et al, 1989a) but are difficult to standardize between laboratories and have not been prospectively validated. For the purposes of this review, this broad definition excludes non-demented Parkinson's disease patients with a few cortical Lewy bodies but encompasses cases reported under other rubrics such as diffuse (cortical) Lewy body disease, the Lewy body variant of Alzheimer's disease and senile dementia of Lewy body type. The last of these terms is worthy of note in that it draws attention to the observation that the pathology of Lewy body dementia may vary somewhat with age, older patients showing similar clinical features to their younger counterparts but in general having larger numbers of senile plaques and smaller numbers of cortical Lewy bodies (Perry et al, 1990b). At our present stage of knowledge, however, a 'lumping' approach has the advantages of simplicity and numerical power, despite running the risk of being overinclusive and upsetting enthusiastic 'splitters.' The term Lewy body dementia is at any rate less cumbersome, more descriptive and can be regarded as nosologically neutral.

EPIDEMIOLOGY AND AETIOLOGY

Several pathological studies have provided information about the epidemiology of Lewy body dementia (as defined above). Such studies are inevitably subject to bias, partly because of the tendency to seek post-mortem neuropathological examination preferentially in unusual or difficult cases, and partly because of preselection of the population under study. Two groups have reduced the latter bias by systematically looking at a large number of unselected consecutive autopsies. Forno and Langston (1988) examined 260 brains from consecutive autopsies at a Veterans Administration hospital in California; they do not state how many of the patients were demented. Thirteen brains contained brainstem and cortical Lewy bodies, and 12 of these cases had suffered from dementia. Lewy body dementia therefore occurred in 5% of the series as a whole, but it is not possible to calculate how frequently it formed the pathological basis of dementia from their abstract. Interestingly, they also identified three cases with Lewy bodies confined exclusively to the periamygdaloid cortex but do not give details about the clinical features of these cases. The Nottingham group examined all 216 brains referred (for a wide variety of reasons) from within a single health district during a single year; 55 were from patients who had suffered from dementia. They found 15 cases of Lewy body dementia, representing 7% of the entire series and 27% of the cases of dementia (Byrne et al, 1989; Lennox et al, 1989a); Lewy body dementia was the second most common cause of dementia after Alzheimer's disease in this series.

Other groups have studied preselected groups of patients with dementia. Joachim et al (1988) examined 150 brains from patients with a clinical diagnosis of Alzheimer's disease. The brains were referred from a wide range of sources with no formal clinical diagnostic criteria. Twenty-six brains (17%) were found to have brainstem and cortical Lewy bodies, although the authors comment that the numbers of the latter varied greatly from case to case, and remain neutral about their nosological status. Dickson et al (1989) examined 216 consecutive brains referred for evaluation of degenerative brain disease over a 3 year period. They identified 27 brains (13%) with numerous brainstem and cortical Lewy bodies; as in Nottingham, Lewy body dementia was the second most common cause of dementia after Alzheimer's disease. The Newcastle group examined 93 brains of elderly patients (>70 years) with dementia referred from local psychogeriatric units over a 5 year period (Perry et al, 1990b): 20 brains (22%) (from patients with atypical dementia syndromes) contained numerous brainstem and cortical Lewy bodies; a further five brains (5%) (from patients with Parkinson's disease complicated by dementia) contained numerous brainstem and smaller numbers of cortical Lewy bodies, the latter being confined to limbic cortex in two cases. Hansen et al (1990) in San Diego examined the brains of 36 patients with dementia who fulfilled clinical diagnostic criteria for Alzheimer's disease which exclude patients presenting with parkinsonism: 13 (36%) had numerous brainstem and cortical Lewy bodies.

Combining the studies that looked specifically at patients with dementia, 106 of 550 cases (19%) fulfil the present diagnosis of Lewy body dementia. The same proportion (75 of 400; 19%) is obtained if one excludes the series of Joachim and colleagues because of their doubts about the numerical significance of the cortical Lewy bodies, and the seven Parkinson's disease patients from the Newcastle series who had what they regarded as small numbers of cortical Lewy bodies.

Lewy body dementia should therefore be regarded as relatively common. It is probably slightly more common than vascular dementia, and definitely more common than Pick's disease or Creutzfeldt–Jakob disease. Its aetiology remains unknown. On the assumption that it forms part of the same spectrum of Lewy body disease as Parkinson's disease, both environmental and genetic causes seem possible. At the moment the pendulum of evidence is swinging towards a substantial genetic component. Familial cases of Lewy body dementia have been described (Muenter et al, 1986; Golbe et al, 1990); it is possible that in some families Lewy body disease is transmitted as an autosomal dominant trait with different individuals manifesting the disorder as Parkinson's disease (or 'oligosymptomatic' fragments thereof), dementia or both. Perhaps environmental factors influence the phenotypic expression of a fundamentally genetic disorder.

CLINICAL FEATURES

The initial reports of Lewy body dementia described a wide range of clinical features, perhaps reflecting the bias of single case reports towards the unusual and the bizarre. As larger groups of patients have come to be described a more coherent picture has emerged, of a disorder predominantly causing dementia with parkinsonism.

Neuropsychological and neuropsychiatric features

The central feature is progressive deterioration in higher mental function. This occurs in all cases eventually and comes to dominate the clinical picture, creating the greatest management problems. Memory loss, inattention and difficulty in sustaining a line of thought are often the earliest manifestations and are gradually followed by irritability, personality change and symptoms of temporoparietal cortical dysfunction such as aphasia, acalculia, apraxia, agnosia and spatial disorientation (Gibb et al, 1987, 1989; Gibb et al, 1989a; Byrne et al, 1989). Common complaints are difficulty with naming everyday objects, handling money, solving problems, recognizing acquaintances and finding one's way around strange places. These familiar symptoms (similar in many ways to those of early Alzheimer's disease) are often accompanied by a puzzling and more distinctive fluctuation in cognitive performance which is usually attributed to a confusional state. Carers comment that the patient has very obvious good and bad days, and often the latter lead to acute hospital admissions in a fruitless attempt to identify some intercurrent illness that might be exacerbating the cognitive impairment. These exacerbations appear to be partly related to decreased attention and lead to a global deterioration on simple bedside tests of mental function. They are not, however, invariably associated with drowsiness or frank delerium; they cannot be attributed to identifiable toxic, metabolic or iatrogenic processes and are not associated with any specific changes in electroencephalographic activity. At present their cause remains obscure. They are much more common in Lewy body dementia than Alzheimer's disease, and were observed in approximately 80% of patients in both the Nottingham and Newcastle series (Byrne et al, 1989; Perry et al, 1990b). In both centres they frequently led to an erroneous diagnosis of multi-infarct dementia (even in the absence of vascular risk factors or focal neurological signs); the presence of striking cognitive fluctuations in a patient with dementia should in fact raise the possibility of Lewy body dementia unless a more plausible alternative explanation can be found.

As time goes by, and the dementia becomes more profound, the fluctuations diminish and disappear. Visuospatial problems become more obvious, with an increasing tendency to disorientation. Language disturbance becomes troublesome, with paraphasic errors and echolalia and later a progressive reduction in spontaneous speech which sometimes leaves the patient mute. Apraxia becomes more severe and assistance with even simple everyday activities gradually becomes necessary. Emotional lability and aggression give way to apathy, and the patient eventually enters into a vegetative state of total dependency, with incontinence of urine and faeces. Death commonly intervenes through bronchopneumonia, pulmonary embolism or intestinal volvulus. On average the duration of survival from the onset of dementia is approximately 6 years, although cases with much more rapid decline (occasionally over months; Armstrong et al, 1991) or much longer survival have been recorded.

Hansen and colleagues (1990) have prospectively performed detailed neuropsychological testing in their series of patients who were thought in life to have early Alzheimer's disease but were later found to have the pathology of Lewy body dementia. They compared nine of these cases to a group with pathologically confirmed Alzheimer's disease, which was matched for overall dementia severity on the Blessed scale as well as age and educational status. The groups were similarly poor at tests of naming (a shortened version of the Boston Naming Test) and memory (the Buschke Selective Reminding Test and the Visual Reproduction Test). The Lewy body dementia patients made significantly more mistakes than the Alzheimer disease patients on tests of visuospatial and constructional ability (the Block Design subtest from the revised Wechsler Intelligence Scale for Children, and a simple drawing copying task). This was thought to reflect a greater degree of parietal lobe dysfunction, although the two groups scored similarly on Luria's motor sequencing task. The Lewy body patients also had slightly shorter digit spans and performed more poorly on certain verbal fluency tests (although the authors did not comment on whether this defect of attention and frontal lobe function correlated with fluctuating episodes of confusion). These findings confirm the bedside impression of major temporoparietal and attentional difficulties with less marked impairment on tests thought to be sensitive to frontal lobe dysfunction.

Returning to the symptoms at presentation, psychotic features are sometimes prominent, with visual, auditory or occasionally olfactory hallucinations and paranoid delusions. These may be worse during episodes of confusion but characteristically also occur during periods of clear consciousness and optimal cognitive function. The visual hallucinations are usually formed and complex, and the patient can often describe them in detail. After a while some patients come to recognize them as unreal and accept, for example, the sight of the local football team practising in their garden as an unthreatening or even welcome distraction from the mundane. The auditory hallucinations are usually more unpleasant, frequently consisting of a critical commentary, and are often accompanied by paranoid ideation. The form and severity of this varies greatly from case to case, from unusual overvalued ideas (such as a man whose first symptom was the constant conviction that his testicles had been damaged by analgesic drugs) to frank paranoid psychosis (such as a woman who heard strangers in her flat plotting to poison her and in consequence subsisted on tinned dog food for several weeks). These symptoms may occasionally precede other manifestations of Lewy body dementia by months or even years (Kosaka and Mehraein, 1979) and in some cases may be the only manifestation of Lewy body disease (Perry et al, 1990a), again giving rise to diagnostic difficulty. Other psychiatric symptoms may feature early on, including anxiety and depression. These too may precede other manifestations of Lewy body dementia (Gibb et al, 1987) and appear to be part of the disease process rather than a reaction to it.

Psychiatric manifestations of this sort were the presenting symptom in five (14%) of the 37 Japanese cases reviewed by Kosaka (1990). They occur at some stage in the illness in about half of all cases (Burkhardt et al, 1988; Byrne et al, 1989; Perry et al, 1990b) and should be regarded as a possible pointer to the diagnosis of Lewy body dementia. Although similar symptoms occur in Alzheimer's disease, they are less common and generally occur later in the course of the disease, at a time when dementia is at least moderately severe.

A wide range of behavioural manifestations of dementia occur, including wandering, disruption of the sleep–wake cycle and eating disorders (including excessive food consumption with apparent loss of satiety, attempts to eat inedible objects, which may be due to an agnosia or the Kluver–Bucy syndrome, and reduced food consumption with apparent loss of appetite despite substantial weight loss).

Neurological features

Parkinsonism (i.e. the movement disorder syndrome characteristic of Parkinson's disease) forms part of the picture of Lewy body dementia to a variable degree, ranging from a minor feature, of interest only as a diagnostic aid, to a major cause of disability. In patients presenting with early dementia or neuropsychiatric disturbance parkinsonism may be subtle, with, for example, a slow, shuffling or unsteady gait, a flexed posture or limb rigidity. In this group of patients a broader range of parkinsonian features tends to become apparent, and each feature more severe, as time passes. Parkinsonian features are significantly more common in these patients than in those who subsequently prove to have Alzheimer's disease (Hansen et al, 1990; Perry et al, 1990b).

Other patients present with parkinsonism, and only later develop dementia. In the unselected Nottingham series such patients are as common as those presenting with pure cognitive impairment (Byrne et al, 1989). Usually this group of patients to all intents and purposes has typical late onset Parkinson's disease, with a slowly progressive, asymmetrical, levodopa-responsive akinetic–rigid syndrome, often accompanied by classical rest tremor. Dementia follows months or years after the onset of parkinsonism, in the manner described above. Again, visual hallucinations are frequently the first indication of impending trouble; these often settle for a while if levodopa and anticholinergic drugs are withdrawn, only to reappear later, together with cognitive impairment, even if the patient remains off antiparkinsonian therapy.

This presentation of Lewy body dementia has been under-recognized (Lennox et al, 1989a). Dementia frequently complicates late onset Parkinson's disease (Brown and Marsden, 1984; Godwin-Austen and Lowe, 1987; Mayeux et al, 1990) and in most cases Lewy body dementia is the underlying cause (Yoshimura, 1988).

There is, therefore, a spectrum of clinical manifestations in Lewy body disease, which presumably reflects the development of pathology in different brain regions at different times. When the disease begins in the brainstem and spreads to the cerebral cortex the patient will manifest Parkinson's disease followed by dementia; when the reverse pathological process occurs the earliest symptoms will be those of dementia followed by parkinsonism. Both disease courses eventually culminate in the syndrome of Lewy body dementia.

It is not surprising that all of the motor features of Parkinson's disease have been described in patients with Lewy body dementia (Table 2). Reviewing 75 case reports published between 1961 and 1991 (which vary considerably in the amount of clinical detail provided), 58 cases (77%) were noted to have increased limb tone; this was generally extrapyramidal rigidity, although in some reports it is difficult to make the distinction between rigidity, spasticity and *gegenhalten* (the fascinating phenomenon found in some normal people and many demented patients in which they resist with increasing force the examiner's attempts to move their limbs, despite all encouragement to relax). Axial rigidity was less frequently noted, but is not uncommon. Thirty-seven cases (49%) had limb tremor. Again this took various forms, from the classical parkinsonian pill-rolling tremor at rest to postural and action tremors more akin to those of familial essential tremor. A jerky postural tremor involving proximal muscles seems to be particularly common when actively sought; it is sometimes difficult to distinguish from myoclonus (see below). A reduction or slowing of spontaneous movements was noted in 30 cases (40%) and was often accompanied by a reduction in facial expression. Gait disturbance was recorded in 36 cases (48%); this was sometimes thought to be typically parkinsonian, with start hesitancy, festination, reduced armswing, freezing and unsteadiness on turning, although many reports describe less specific abnormalities of gait, like slowness, staggering and instability. In elderly patients with Parkinson's disease a tendency for the gait to become more chaotic (or 'dyspraxic') with frequent falls often goes hand in hand with the onset of cognitive impairment, suggesting that the classical parkinsonian gait disorder may be mediated through brainstem pathology, whilst the recognizable but less specific later disintegration of gait and stability may reflect the development of cortical pathology. Abnormalities of resting posture were noted in 21 cases (28%), most frequently taking the form of increasing cervical and thoracic flexion. This can become very severe, doubling the patients over and making it difficult for them to look forwards, communicate or eat.

Minor parkinsonian features such as blepharospasm, sialorrhoea and seborrhoeic dermatitis have all been described.

Overall, in only eight of these 75 cases (11%) were none of the cardinal parkinsonian features (tremor, akinesia, rigidity, gait disturbance and abnormal posture) noted. Fifteen cases (20%) were reported to have only one of these parkinsonian features, which was almost always limb rigidity; 16 cases (21%) showed only two parkinsonian features, which again almost always included rigidity. The remaining 36 cases (48%) showed three (19 cases; 25%), four (seven cases; 9%) or all five features (ten cases; 13%).

Table 2. The clinical features of Lewy body dementia.

Feature	Frequency* (%)	Notes
Dementia	100	Present by definition†
Fluctuations or episodic confusion	10++‡	Noted in 80% of the patients in Byrne et al (1989) and Perry et al (1990)
Psychosis	33	Mainly visual hallucinations and/or paranoid delusions
Depression	15	
Parkinsonism	90	May be the presenting feature
Rigidity	80+	Both limb and axial rigidity
Tremor	50+	Not always classical: see text
Bradykinesia	40+	
Gait disorder	50+	Often early in the disease
Flexed posture	30+	
1 or 2 of these	40−	
3 or more of these	50+	
Myoclonus	10	Probably much more common (unpublished observations)
Other movement disorder	10	Includes dystonia, chorea and drug-induced dyskinesia
Pyramidal signs	25	Usually late in disease
Other brainstem features	10	Includes dysphagia and supranuclear gaze palsies
Autonomic failure	10	i.e. symptomatic orthostatic hypotension

* Approximate frequency derived from a review of published case reports giving individual clinical details, i.e. Okazaki et al (1961), Kosaka et al (1973, 1976, 1984), Kono (1976), Forno et al (1978), Ikeda et al (1978, 1980), Kosaka (1978), Kuroda et al (1978), Ogasawara et al (1978), Kosaka and Mehrein (1979), Kayano et al (1980), Minagawa et al (1980), Monma et al (1981), Yagishita et al (1980), Yoshimura et al (1980), Itoh et al (1982), Yoshimura (1983), Clark et al (1986), Eggertson and Sima (1986), Philpot et al (1986), Sima et al (1986), Delisle et al (1987), Dickson et al (1987), Gibb et al (1987, 1989), Kuyama et al (1987), Popovitch et al (1987), Burkhardt et al (1988), Yamamoto and Imai (1988), Byrne et al (1989), Commons et al (1989), Crystal et al (1990), Lewis and Gawel (1990), Armstrong et al (1991) and Fearnley et al (1991). Some cases have been described in more than one report, including some reports not cited here; for summaries of many of the individual cases and additional references see Burkhardt et al (1988) and Kosaka (1990).

† Ikeda et al (1977) described a man with young onset Parkinson's disease and diffuse Lewy body pathology who died suddenly aged 38 years without dementia. Non-demented patients with Parkinson's disease may have a few cortical Lewy bodies. None of these cases has Lewy body dementia as defined here.

‡ + or ++, Denotes an increased or much increased prevalence of a particular feature in recent reports of large unselected series; − denotes the opposite.

However, two trends can be discerned from analysis of this literature. First, the later case reports, and particularly the recent papers describing larger series of cases, have described more parkinsonian features than the early ones, suggesting that there may be an element of under-reporting of parkinsonism in the early literature. The exception to this trend is the study of Hansen et al (1990), which excluded patients presenting with parkinsonism. Secondly, the cases with few parkinsonian features tend to be those (perhaps unsurprisingly) who presented with neuropsychiatric symptoms; this may be because death from the complications of dementia intervenes before parkinsonism becomes apparent or because of the difficulties of performing a neurological examination on an uncooperative patient.

Other neurological features are less common. Generalized seizures are rare. Myoclonus is more often observed, particularly when dementia is severe. It usually takes the form of mild, spontaneous, multifocal jerks, predominantly affecting the upper limbs (i.e. the pattern seen in a wide range of cerebral cortical degenerations), but it is occasionally a very prominent feature, leading to confusion with Creutzfeldt–Jakob disease (Burkhardt et al, 1988). Other spontaneous movement disorders are much less common, although dyskinetic neck movements (Kosaka et al, 1976), chorea (Yoshimura, 1983) and dystonia affecting axial and limb muscles have all been observed. Dyskinesia due to the drugs used to treat parkinsonism is uncommon, although it is seen in younger patients.

Primitive reflexes (such as grasp, pout and palmomental reflexes) can be elicited with a frequency that probably reflects the enthusiasm of the examiner; it is increasingly recognized that they are of little diagnostic or localizing value. More reliable signs of frontal lobe dysfunction, such as forced grasping and utilization behaviour, are unusual except in severely demented patients. Similarly, pyramidal signs such as spasticity and extensor plantar responses occur in the later stages of the disease in approximately 25% of patients (Burkhardt et al, 1988) but early or prominent involvement of the corticospinal pathways appears to be rare. More distal involvement of the motor pathways is even more unusual. Delisle et al (1987) and Gibb et al (1989a) have described individual patients with lower motor neurone signs of wasting, fasciculation and areflexia due to destruction of anterior horn cells (accompanied by Lewy body formation). The author has seen a single patient with Lewy body dementia and a hereditary demyelinating sensory and motor neuropathy (G. Lennox & A. E. Harding, unpublished observation).

Dysarthria is common, particularly in patients with parkinsonism. A few patients become completely mute, but it is often difficult to establish whether this is due to cortical or brainstem disease. Severe bulbar involvement causing dysphagia occurs in a substantial minority of patients and is easy to overlook. Recently two patients have been reported with striking supranuclear disorders of vertical and horizontal gaze resembling those seen in Steele–Richardson–Olszewski syndrome (Lewis and Gawel, 1990; Fearnley et al, 1991.)

Autonomic involvement has been reported in several cases, with symptomatic orthostatic hypotension occasionally constituting the presenting problem (Kono et al, 1976.) There has been no systematic or detailed study of autonomic function in patients with Lewy body dementia, no doubt because many of the tests rely upon reasonable patient cooperation and become difficult to interpret in older subjects. On pathological grounds (see above, Neuropathology) one might predict that autonomic failure would be more common in Lewy body dementia than other forms of dementia, and if suitable tests could be devised they might provide diagnostic information.

DIFFERENTIAL DIAGNOSIS AND ANCILLARY INVESTIGATIONS

At present Lewy body dementia can only be diagnosed with certainty by neuropathological examination. Diagnosis in life remains based upon that balancing of probabilities tempered by prejudice, known as clinical judgement. A set of clinical diagnostic criteria has been proposed, but has not yet been validated (Byrne et al, 1991). These suggest that the diagnosis of Lewy body dementia can probably be made when the patient has the core syndrome of gradually progressive dementia with prominent attentional

Table 3. Some diseases causing parkinsonism and cognitive impairment.

Disease	Notes
Lewy body dementia	Most common cause of parkinsonian dementia (see text)
Alzheimer's disease	Most common cause of non-parkinsonian dementia; can cause parkinsonism in its own right (Daniel and Lees, 1991)
Alzheimer's disease plus Parkinson's disease	Probably the chance association of two common pathologies of old age, i.e. cortical tangles and brainstem Lewy bodies
Cerebrovascular disease	Rarely closely mimics Parkinson's disease; more commonly produces a syndrome of gait disorder with focal neurological signs including patchy cognitive deficits. History of strokes and risk factors common. Pathology includes Binswanger's disease, amyloid angiopathy, cerebral vasculitis, etc
Cerebral anoxia (or carbon monoxide poisoning)	Akinetic–rigid syndrome with pyramidal signs, memory loss and variable additional cognitive impairment following a defined anoxic-ischaemic insult; sometimes action myoclonus develops later
Hydrocephalus	Like cerebrovascular disease, usually only superficially resembles parkinsonism with a dyspraxic gait disorder, together with incontinence and cognitive impairment
Steele–Richardson– Olszewski syndrome	Usually mainly axial dystonia/rigidity with gait disturbance and instability, supranuclear gaze palsy, pseudobulbar palsy and bradykinesia; impaired frontolimbic function without temporoparietal features; rest tremor and levodopa response rare (Lees, 1987)
Multiple system atrophy	Combinations of parkinsonism, cerebellar ataxia, autonomic failure, pyramidal deficit and peripheral neuropathy; cognitive deficit mild and of frontal lobe type (Quinn, 1989)
Pick's disease and its variants	Classically progressive impairment of frontal lobe function, language and memory; extrapyramidal pathology is common and occasionally clinically manifest (Constantinidis et al, 1974)

deficits or episodic confusional states, accompanied by a substantial constellation of parkinsonian features (at least three out of tremor, rigidity, bradykinesia, flexed posture and gait disturbance), in the absence of a history or signs suggestive of cerebrovascular disease and following attempts to exclude other identifiable causes of parkinsonian dementia. They also allow the *possible* diagnosis of Lewy body dementia in cases where the dementia is more rapid in onset and associated with psychiatric symptoms, and only one or two parkinsonian features are present.

Burkhardt et al (1988) and Crystal et al (1990) have emphasized the diagnostic importance of assessing the evolution of the clinical features over time. For example, they suggest that early gait disturbance, occurring when dementia is only mild or moderate, may be more suggestive of Lewy body dementia than later gait deterioration when dementia is severe. Again, such observations have not been tested prospectively.

Clinical criteria such as these are an important first step in establishing ways of making an accurate diagnosis during life, which in turn is vital for studies of therapeutic intervention. There are, however, many other causes of a parkinsonian dementia syndrome (Table 3); the greatest problem arises in distinguishing Lewy body dementia from Alzheimer's disease. Recent

Table 3. (*continued*)

Creutzfeldt–Jakob disease	Rapidly progressive dementia with ataxia and myoclonus; occasionally parkinsonism
Corticobasal degeneration	Usually presents with a rigid, dyspraxic, jerky limb; later becomes generalized with parietal sensory and cognitive deficits and supranuclear gaze palsy. Global dementia not described (Gibb et al, 1989b)
Huntington's disease	Classically presents with chorea followed by frontolimbic dementia; rigidity is seen in juvenile cases and late in the adult disease (Quarrell and Harper, 1991)
Neuroacanthocytosis	Similar to Huntington's disease with additional features of orolingual dystonia, neuropathy and abnormal red cells (Hardie et al, 1991)
Wilson's disease	Early adult onset of autosomal recessive mixed movement disorder (often parkinsonism, dystonia and tremor) with Kayser–Fleischer rings; important because of potential cure with copper chelation therapy
Hallervorden–Spatz disease	Usually presents before the age of 20 years with dystonia, rigidity and dementia and ataxia and pyramidal signs; MRI may show 'eye of the tiger' sign in globus pallidus; occasional adult-onset cases (Jankovic et al, 1985)
Dementia pugilistica	Dementia, parkinsonism and often ataxia, following repetitive head trauma
Encephalitis lethargica	A few survivors of the epidemics still show static parkinsonism, dystonia and cognitive impairment; rare sporadic cases occur following an encephalitic illness (Howard and Lees, 1987)
Parkinsonism–dementia complex of Guam	A geographically clustered syndrome often accompanied by motor neurone disease; possible environmental toxin
Rare familial syndromes	e.g. forms of familial motor neurone disease (Hudson, 1981); hereditary dysphasic dementia (Morris et al, 1984); familial parkinsonism and dementia with granulovacuolar degeneration (unpublished observations), etc

clinicopathological studies have shown that Alzheimer-type pathology affecting the striatum and substantia nigra can mimic closely the clinical features of Parkinson's disease (Morris et al, 1989; Daniel and Lees, 1991; Hughes et al, 1992). Similarly it is inevitable that some patients will develop both Parkinson's disease and Alzheimer's disease, if only through the chance association of two of the common diseases of later life (Quinn et al, 1986). These cases could not be distinguished from Lewy body dementia on the basis of their parkinsonian features; the unusual neuropsychiatric features of Lewy body dementia discussed above (prominent fluctuations in cognitive performance, apparent acute confusional states, visual hallucinations and delusions) might provide guidance but their pathological basis is not known. It is possible that they may also occur in other disorders causing damage to the brainstem monoaminergic nuclei (see below, Neurochemistry), in which case their specificity and discriminating power would be low. Large prospective studies are required to clarify these issues.

Crystal and colleagues (1990) have also commented upon the value of electroencephalography (EEG) in distinguishing between Lewy body dementia and Alzheimer's disease. They found that four out of six patients with Lewy body dementia had abnormal EEGs with background slowing and bursts of frontal 2–4 Hz activity at a time when they were only mildly demented, and comment that EEG abnormalities in early Alzheimer's disease are generally less severe. Again these observations have not been validated in a larger series, although similar non-specific EEG abnormalities have been reported by others (e.g. Gibb et al, 1987, 1989a). A few patients show striking periodic complexes reminiscent of Creutzfeldt–Jakob disease (Yamamoto and Imai, 1988; Byrne et al, 1989); usually continued observation makes the distinction between these two conditions clear, with Lewy body dementia patients surviving longer (sometimes with a plateau of stable functioning after an initial rapid decline), failing to develop cerebellar ataxia and showing less striking myoclonus and startle reflexes than are characteristically seen in Creutzfeldt–Jakob disease.

Neuroimaging has not yet been shown to be of any value in discriminating between Lewy body dementia and Alzheimer's disease. Pathological studies have in general shown greater cerebral atrophy (and brain weight reduction) in Alzheimer's disease but generalized atrophy is notoriously difficult to quantify (and to distinguish from the effects of ageing) with conventional structural neuroimaging. Anecdotally one occasionally sees patients who show clinical features suggestive of severe Lewy body dementia and have relatively normal computerized tomography (CT) and magnetic resonance imaging (MRI) brain scans. This clinicoradiological disparity is not unique to Lewy body dementia (also occurring, for example, in Creutzfeldt–Jakob disease) but should at any rate raise the possibility of diagnoses other than Alzheimer's disease. More detailed radiological studies may have greater specificity; it is the author's impression that atrophy may be more marked in selected areas (such as the anterior cingulate gyrus) in Lewy body dementia and in others (such as the hippocampus) in Alzheimer's disease. This might form the basis of a diagnostic test but would require the use of special scanning orientations.

Functional neuroimaging has been studied in patients with parkinsonian dementia, but without subsequent confirmation of the underlying pathological process. Both positron emission tomography (PET) and single photon emission computerized tomography (SPECT) scanning can detect striatal dopaminergic deficiency in parkinsonian patients using special ligands; PET scanning is capable of picking this up before clinical features of parkinsonism become apparent. It remains to be seen whether this is useful in assessing individual patients with dementia. Both techniques show a similar bitemporoparietal deficit in cortical blood flow and metabolism in patients with parkinsonian and non-parkinsonian dementia, presumably reflecting the damage to association areas which is common to both Lewy body dementia and Alzheimer's disease (Spampinato et al, 1991); at present the main value of these techniques seems to be in differentiating temporoparietal forms of primary degenerative dementia from ones causing a mainly frontal deficit (see Chapter 5) and multi-infarct dementia.

Multi-infarct dementia can, however, usually be diagnosed without recourse to specialized imaging. A background of cerebrovascular risk factors and in particular hypertension, a history of stroke-like events and stepwise deterioration, focal motor and sensory signs, early urinary disturbance and patchy cognitive defects all raise the possibility of vascular pathology. Most cases (with striatal infarction) show what has been termed pseudoparkinsonism, with an unsteady and disorganized ('dyspraxic') gait and predominantly lower limb rigidity rather than bradykinesia and rest tremor; much less frequently infarction in the substantia nigra causes a syndrome indistinguishable from Parkinson's disease. CT scans usually show multiple lacunar infarcts involving the striatum, or diffuse low attenuation within ischaemic areas of subcortical white matter; MRI is even more sensitive to these changes. SPECT and PET show patchy defects of cerebral blood flow and metabolism.

Two other disorders present particular diagnostic difficulties: Steele–Richardson–Olszewski syndrome and Pick's disease. Steele–Richardson–Olszewski syndrome usually presents with an unsteady gait, frequent falls and visual problems. The patient usually goes on to develop dysarthria, dysphagia, severe axial rigidity (often without distal limb rigidity), emotional lability and cognitive impairment. Almost always a supranuclear disorder of gaze evolves, starting with impairment of saccades and progressing to complete loss of voluntary upward, and then downward and horizontal eye movements; reflex eye movements (particularly the vestibulo-ocular reflex) are spared. This disorder is so striking that when present it always leads to consideration of Steele–Richardson–Olszewski syndrome, but it also occurs in other degenerative diseases affecting the mesencephalic eye movement centres (Lees, 1987), including Lewy body dementia (Lewis and Gawel, 1990; Fearnley et al, 1991). The pattern of cognitive impairment is different in Steele–Richardson–Olszewski syndrome, affecting mainly memory and frontal lobe function, with poor abstract reasoning and set shifting ability. However, in some cases profound slowness in response to questions and prominent distractibility can give the impression of a more global dementia. Manual function deteriorates (often with the development of grasp reflexes and utilization behaviour) and speech often becomes incomprehensible because of pseudobulbar and bulbar problems, making detailed cognitive testing impossible. At this stage Steele–Richardson–Olszewski syndrome may be very difficult to distinguish from severe Lewy body dementia, unless rest tremor or levodopa-responsiveness suggestive of the latter are present. Functional neuroimaging might be of assistance, showing a frontal distribution of cerebral hypometabolism in clinically diagnosed cases of Steele–Richardson–Olszewski syndrome (D'Antona et al, 1985).

Pick's disease can present problems for similar reasons. Its pattern of cognitive abnormalities (see Chapter 4) is characteristic but again may sometimes be difficult to elicit. Behavioural abnormalities, such as social or sexual disinhibition suggestive of frontal lobe dysfunction and excessive eating thought to be attributable to amygdala pathology, may be observed early in the illness, but also occur in some cases of Lewy body dementia. Parkinsonian features such as rigidity and gait disturbance are also reported in Pick's disease, particularly where a broad pathological definition of the disorder is used (Constantinidis et al, 1974). Laboratory investigations may help to make the distinction between Pick's disease and Lewy body dementia. The EEG remains relatively normal even in advanced Pick's disease, and functional neuroimaging may show frontal cerebral hypometabolism extending into the caudate nuclei (Kamo et al, 1987).

Most of the other causes of parkinsonian dementia are more readily differentiated from Lewy body dementia (Table 3). For example, the history will usually identify cases with postanoxic or postencephalitic damage to the basal ganglia and cerebral cortex, cases with dementia pugilistica due to repetitive head trauma and cases with the combination of parkinsonism and dementia from the island of Guam. The family history may be useful in patients with, for example, juvenile Huntington's disease (usually transmitted from the father) and the clinically similar but genetically less clear-cut neuroacanthocytosis. Additional neurological signs characterize multiple system atrophy and corticobasal degeneration (see Chapter 10), in which localized defects of cognitive function are found, rather than severe global dementia. General examination should not be omitted and is occasionally diagnostic, as when the Kayser–Fleischer corneal rings of Wilson's disease are present (although their exclusion requires slit lamp examination by an experienced ophthalmologist). Wilson's disease is also an example of a disorder where special tests are helpful, low serum copper and caeruloplasmin levels confirming the diagnosis; other examples are neuroacanthocytosis where abnormal red cell morphology is found (albeit sometimes intermittently) (Hardie et al, 1991) and Hallervorden–Spatz disease where striking 'eye-of-the-tiger' appearances are seen in the basal ganglia with MRI (Schaffert et al, 1989), although the specificity of these abnormalities is not absolute (Higgins et al, 1992). The techniques of molecular biology may become increasingly valuable in forthcoming years, and already have a place in Huntington's disease (for counselling rather than diagnosis) and in familial cases of Alzheimer's disease and prion dementia (see Chapters 3 and 8).

NEUROCHEMISTRY

A number of studies have demonstrated interesting correlations between post-mortem neurochemical abnormalities and clinical and pathological features. Clark and colleagues (1986) described an 80% reduction in the activity of the cholinergic marker enzyme choline acetyltransferase (ChAT) in the neocortex of two cases of Lewy body dementia. Dickson and colleagues (1987) confirmed this severe ChAT reduction in several neo-cortical regions in six cases, and made the additional observation that the hippocampus was much less severely affected. These biochemical findings parallel the pathological changes, with severe cell loss in the basal forebrain cholinergic nuclei and much more subtle abnormalities in the hippocampus (Lennox et al, 1989a; Dickson et al, 1991; see above, Neuropathology). The severity of ChAT reduction was similar to cases of Alzheimer's disease, except that hippocampal ChAT is not spared in the latter condition. Dickson et al (1987) also showed a severe reduction in neocortical somatostatin-like immunoreactivity, which again resembled the reduction found in Alzheimer's disease except that the hippocampus was relatively spared.

These observations have been extended by the Newcastle group, who found a reduction in caudate dopamine levels in a series of elderly cases of Lewy body dementia (Perry et al, 1990c); again this parallels the substantia nigra pathology. They confirmed the reduction in temporal cortex ChAT activity which, together with cortical nicotinic acetylcholine receptor binding levels, was particularly low in patients who had experienced halluci-nations (falling to 20% of normal levels in this subgroup). Conversely, they found that monoaminergic markers (including the serotonin and dopamine metabolites 5-hydroxyindoleacetic acid and homovanillic acid, and sero-tonin receptor subtype S2 binding) were only significantly reduced in patients who had not experienced hallucinations (Perry et al, 1990d). This dissociation could not be explained on the basis of prior drug treatment. They suggest that hallucinations in Lewy body dementia are due to an imbalance between the cholinergic and monoaminergic systems in the temporal lobe, and that hallucinating patients with very severe but relatively selective cholinergic deficits might be particularly suitable for attempts at cholinergic replacement therapy.

This attempt to subdivide patients into potential treatment groups is made all the more important by the finding that other neurotransmitter systems are also impaired in Lewy body dementia. The Newcastle group has, for example, reported that corticotrophin releasing hormone levels are reduced in temporal cortex in Lewy body dementia (but not in non-demented Parkinson's disease), although arginine vasopressin levels were unchanged (Leake et al, 1991).

MANAGEMENT

There is at present no specific curative treatment for Lewy body dementia, and this makes a pragmatic approach aimed at maximizing residual abilities and supporting carers as important here as it is in other forms of irreversible dementia (Arie, 1986). Some aspects of the palliative drug treatment are, however, worthy of specific comment, because of the particular problems and dilemmas that they pose.

When patients initially present with Parkinson's disease and then develop dementia, the first step is to consider reducing their anti-parkinsonian therapy in an attempt to reduce unwanted effects on cognitive function. Anticholinergic drugs are particularly liable to exacerbate confusion, memory loss and hallucinations and should almost always be withdrawn. It sometimes takes several weeks for their deleterious effects to wear off; the patient's parkinsonism usually deteriorates more rapidly and it may require considerable persuasion that the trade-off between reduced mobility and increased lucidity is likely to be worthwhile. Unfortunately, as already outlined, the subsequent improvement is often only a temporary reprieve, with symptoms returning after a few months or a year as the pathological process progresses. Amantadine again seems to cause more problems than benefit in the dementing patient (despite its potentially neuroprotective NMDA antagonist properties), and should probably also be withdrawn; this must be done gradually because rapid cessation sometimes precipitates severe rebound parkinsonism. Dopaminergic drugs, including levodopa and all the direct dopamine receptor agonists such as bromocriptine and lysuride, have a particular tendency to provoke hallucinations but can also exacerbate behavioural manifestations of dementia such as wandering and irritability. Because these drugs usually represent the mainstay of antiparkinsonian therapy, the author's policy is to try to simplify the regimen to a single drug such as levodopa (with a peripheral decarboxylase inhibitor), and then titrate the dose down until the best compromise between immobility and confusion is achieved. This tends to lean towards immobility, most patients and their carers finding this more acceptable and certainly safer. Slow release levodopa preparations are sometimes helpful in achieving an appropriate dose reduction without completely disabling the patient. Increasingly, patients with established Parkinson's disease find themselves taking the monoamine oxidase B (MAOB) inhibitor selegiline in the hope that it will slow the progression of their disease; whether it reduces the incidence or subsequent progression of dementia is not known (see below). Selegiline has arousing effects due to amphetamine-like metabolites and this can exacerbate agitation and precipitate psychosis. When these symptoms occur, selegiline should be discontinued. There is no rationale for continuing its use in any patient once dementia has become severe.

In patients who present with dementia and subsequently develop parkinsonism, the use of antiparkinsonian drugs is even more difficult. All of the same arguments with regard to deleterious side-effects apply, and in this setting the risks of transforming an immobile demented patient into one capable of wandering out of the house or falling down the stairs become obvious to all concerned. Some groups have found that parkinsonism in Lewy body dementia is unresponsive to levodopa therapy, although this has not been the experience in Nottingham. The author's practice is to restrict levodopa therapy to patients with relatively mild cognitive impairment and specific parkinsonian disabilities (such as intolerable akathisia) and to severely demented and well-supervised patients where a modest reduction in parkinsonism makes nursing easier. Even in these groups, levodopa should be introduced very cautiously and withdrawn if on balance it makes matters worse. There are theoretical reasons for supposing that selegiline might slow the progression of Lewy body dementia, and pilot studies to test this hypothesis are in progress. The author's anecdotal experience has been disappointing, with no discernible benefit and a high incidence of side-effects.

The relatively recent recognition of Lewy body dementia as a clinical entity has delayed studies of neurotransmitter replacement therapy. Cholinergic therapy (such as tacrine) has been tried with limited success in patients with a clinical diagnosis of Alzheimer's disease; no such study has been performed in patients thought to have Lewy body dementia. There are some grounds for cautious optimism, including the relative sparing of the hippocampus and the relatively selective neurochemical deficit in some patients with Lewy body dementia, but it remains to be seen whether this will be borne out by clinical trials. Once again the reciprocal balance between the motor and cognitive aspects of the disease may prove troublesome.

Similar considerations hamper management of hallucinations and delusions, where conventional treatment with neuroleptics exacerbates parkinsonism. As always, non-pharmacological approaches should be tried where appropriate. Visual hallucinations are probably best left untreated when they are not distressing or precipitating dangerous activity. Restlessness and wandering sometimes respond to small doses of levodopa or conventional doses of β-adrenoreceptor blockers, and excessive eating to fluoxetine. Night-time confusion and hallucination can often be managed with non-specific sedatives such as benzodiazepines or chlormethiazole. Where neuroleptics have to be employed it is the author's practice to start with small doses of thioridazine or sulpiride, moving on to drugs with more parkinsonian side-effects like haloperidol as a last resort. Such drugs often render the patient totally immobile; the physical risks of this are considerable. Clozapine is a neuroleptic without parkinsonian side-effects; unfortunately it has a tendency to cause agranulocytosis and the need for regular monitoring of blood counts makes it difficult to use in practice.

Depression is an exception to this litany of therapeutic difficulties. It usually responds well to conventional tricyclic antidepressant therapy, and improvement in mood is often accompanied by improvement in cognitive performance. For this reason the author has a low threshold for trying antidepressants if there is any hint of affective disorder. In severely depressed and mildly demented patients electroconvulsive therapy can be useful, any transient worsening of memory being offset by the rapid improvement in mood and often by a transient improvement in parkinsonism as well.

TOWARDS EFFECTIVE TREATMENT

Effective treatment to prevent, halt or reverse the disease remains elusive. There are several possible ways forward. Molecular genetic studies may confirm that there is indeed a genetic component to the Lewy body diseases. In addition to the work on the amyloid precursor protein gene described above (Neuropathology), research is in progress into the role of genes responsible for mitochondrial function and xenobiotic metabolism (for example, Armstrong et al, 1992). Work of this kind may eventually enable the identification of individuals who may be at risk of developing Lewy body dementia later in life, and lead to an improved understanding of the disease mechanisms. Genetic treatment, however, remains a distant prospect. Attempts to understand the way in which Lewy bodies are formed may represent a more rapid route to therapeutic intervention. Lewy bodies contain ubiquitin, a highly-conserved molecule which is rapidly expressed in cells in response to stress and which conjugates with abnormal proteins to 'tag' them for degradation. Ubiquitin is also a component of many of the other inclusion bodies seen in neurodegenerative disease such as neuro-fibrillary tangles (for review, see Lowe and Mayer, 1991), but unlike tangles, Lewy bodies also contain an enzyme that frees ubiquitin from its target proteins to allow further conjugation (Lowe et al, 1990). Lewy bodies also differ from tangles in containing $\alpha\beta$-crystallin, a small protein which again appears to be related to the cell stress system (Lowe et al, 1992). These latter two components suggest that Lewy body formation may represent an active and 'cytoprotective' (i.e. helpful) response of the neurone to stress, and it may be possible to harness and enhance this response in the treatment of Lewy body disease. Alternative strategies would be to identify the key target proteins and alter their metabolism. Even if research of this kind does not result in direct therapeutic intervention, it is likely to generate specific biological markers of Lewy body dementia which will improve clinical diagnosis and allow attempts at pharmacological palliation to be prescribed on a rational basis.

The concept of Lewy body dementia has come a long way in the 30 years since its first description, with an exceptionally swift transition from patho-logical curiosity to widely-recognized dementia syndrome. We must hope that the coming years see equally rapid progress towards effective treatment.

SUMMARY

Lewy body dementia is common. It presents either with cognitive impair-ment and neuropsychiatric disturbance followed by parkinsonism or as dementia complicating established Parkinson's disease. It is unusual both in its pathological features and in its clinical manifestations. Although both overlap to some extent with those of Alzheimer's disease, Lewy body dementia is at least potentially recognizable during life. Some of its manifestations can be ameliorated by established methods, and it has pathological and neurochemical features which offer some hope for the development of useful palliative therapy. Major progress towards effective treatment is, however, likely to depend upon an improved understanding of the molecular mechanisms underlying its aetiology.

Acknowledgements

I am grateful to my colleagues in Nottingham who have collaborated in studies of Lewy body dementia, including Jim Lowe, Jane Byrne, Mike Landon, John Mayer and Richard Godwin-Austen, and especially to Jim Lowe for his helpful comments on this manuscript.

REFERENCES

Arie T (1986) Management of dementia: a review. *British Medical Bulletin* **42:** 91–96.

Armstrong M, Daly AK, Cholerton S, Bateman DN & Idle JR (1992) Mutant debrisoquine hydroxylation genes in Parkinson's disease. *Lancet* **339:** 1017–1018.

Armstrong TP, Hansen LA, Salmon DP et al (1991) Rapidly progressive dementia in a patient with the Lewy body variant of Alzheimer's disease. *Neurology* **41:** 1178–1180.

Brown RG & Marsden CD (1984) How common is dementia in Parkinson's disease? *Lancet* **ii:** 1262–1265.

Burkhardt CR, Filley CM, Kleinschmidt-DeMasters BK et al (1988) Diffuse Lewy body disease and progressive dementia. *Neurology* **38:** 1520–1528.

Byrne EJ, Lennox G, Lowe J & Godwin-Austen RB (1989) Diffuse Lewy body disease: clinical features in 15 cases. *Journal of Neurology, Neurosurgery and Psychiatry* **52:** 709–717.

Clark AW, White CL, Manz HJ et al (1986) Primary degenerative dementia without Alzheimer pathology. *Canadian Journal of Neurological Sciences* **13:** 462–470.

Commons S, Dancea S & Montpeit VJA (1989) Ultrastructural study of an unusual case of diffuse Lewy body disease (LBD) without senile changes. *Journal of Neuropathology and Experimental Neurology* **48:** 341.

Constantinidis J, Richard J & Tissot R (1974) Pick's disease. Histological and clinical correlations. *European Neurology* **11:** 208–217.

Crystal HA, Dickson DW, Lizardi JE, Davies P & Wolfson LI (1990) Antemortem diagnosis of diffuse Lewy body disease. *Neurology* **40:** 1523–1528.

Daniel SE & Lees AJ (1991) Neuropathological features of Alzheimer's disease in non-demented parkinsonian patients. *Journal of Neurology, Neurosurgery and Psychiatry* **54:** 972–975.

D'Antona R, Baron JC, Samson Y et al (1985) Subcortical dementia: frontal cortex hypo-metabolism detected by positron emission tomography in patients with progressive supra-nuclear palsy. *Brain* **108:** 785–799.

Delisle MB, Gorce P, Hirsch E et al (1987) Motor neuron disease, parkinsonism and dementia: report of a case with diffuse Lewy body-like intracytoplasmic inclusions. *Acta Neuropathologica* **75:** 104–108.

Dickson DW (1990) Lewy body variant. *Neurology* **40:** 1147–1148 (letter).

Dickson DW, Davies P, Mayeux R et al (1987) Diffuse Lewy body disease. Neuropathological and biochemical studies of six patients. *Acta Neuropathologica* **75:** 8–15.

Dickson DW, Crystal H, Mattiace LA et al (1989) Diffuse Lewy body disease: light and electron microscopic immunocytochemistry of senile plaques. *Acta Neuropathologica* **78:** 572–584.

Dickson DW, Ruan D, Crystal H et al (1991) Hippocampal degeneration differentiates diffuse Lewy body disease (DLBD) from Alzheimer's disease: light and electron microscopic immunocytochemistry of CA 2–3 neurites specific to DLBD. *Neurology* **41:** 1402–1409.

Dooling EC, Schoene WC & Richardson EP (1974) Hallervorden–Spatz syndrome. *Archives of Neurology* **30:** 70–83.

Eggertson DE & Sima AAF (1986) Dementia with cerebral Lewy bodies: a mesocortical dopaminergic defect? *Archives of Neurology* **43:** 524–527.

Fearnley J, Daniel SE & Lees A (1990) Lewy body variant. *Neurology:* 1149 (letter).

Fearnley JM, Revesz T, Brooks DJ, Frackowiak RS & Lees AJ (1991) Diffuse Lewy body disease presenting with a supranuclear gaze palsy. *Journal of Neurology, Neurosurgery and Psychiatry* **54:** 159–161.

Forno LS & Langston JW (1988) The amygdala-parahippocampal region: a predilection site for Lewy bodies. *Journal of Neuropathology and Experimental Neurology* **47:** 354 (abstract).

Forno LS, Barbour PJ & Norville RL (1978) Presenile dementia with Lewy bodies and neurofibrillary tangles. *Archives of Neurology* **35**: 818–822.

Gibb WRG (1986) Idiopathic Parkinson's disease and the Lewy body disorders. *Neuropathology and Applied Neurobiology* **12**: 223–234.

Gibb WRG, Esiri MM & Lees AJ (1987) Clinical and pathological features of diffuse cortical Lewy body disease (Lewy body dementia). *Brain* **110**: 1131–1153.

Gibb WRG, Luthert PJ & Lantos PL (1989a) Cortical Lewy body dementia: clinical features and classification. *Journal of Neurology, Neurosurgery and Psychiatry* **52**: 185–192.

Gibb WRG, Luthert PJ & Marsden CD (1989b) Corticobasal degeneration. *Brain* **112**: 1171–1192.

Gibb WRG, Scaravilli F & Michaud J (1990) Lewy bodies of subacute sclerosing panencephalitis. *Journal of Neurology, Neurosurgery and Psychiatry* **53**: 710–711.

Goate A, Chartier-Harlin MC, Mullan M et al (1991) Segregation of a missense mutation in the amyloid precursor protein gene with familial Alzheimer's disease. *Nature* **349**: 704–706.

Godwin-Austen RB & Lowe JS (1987) The two types of Parkinson's disease. In Rose FC (ed.) *Current Problems in Neurology (Volume 6). Parkinson's disease—clinical and experimental advances*, pp 79–82. London: Libbey.

Golbe LI, Di Iorio G, Bonavita V, Miller DC & Duvoisin RC (1990) A large kindred with autosomal dominant Parkinson's disease. *Annals of Neurology* **27**: 276–282.

Hansen LA, Masliah E, Terry RD & Mirra SS (1989) A neuropathological subset of Alzheimer's disease with concomitant Lewy body disease and spongiform change. *Acta Neuropathologica* **78**: 194–201.

Hansen L, Salmon D, Galasko D et al (1990) The Lewy body variant of Alzheimer's disease: a clinical and pathologic entity. *Neurology* **40**: 1–8.

Hansen LA, Masliah E, Quijada-Fawcett S & Rexin D (1991) Entorhinal neurofibrillary tangles in Alzheimer disease with Lewy bodies. *Neuroscience Letters* **129**: 269–272.

Hardie RJ, Pullon HWH, Harding AE et al (1991) Neuroacanthocytosis: a clinical, haematological and pathological study of 19 cases. *Brain* **114**: 13–50.

Hardy J, Mullan M, Chartier-Harlin et al (for the Alzheimer's Disease Research Group) (1991) Molecular classification of Alzheimer's disease. *Lancet* **337**: 1342–1343.

Hayashi S, Akasaki Y, Morimura Y et al (1992) An autopsy case of late infantile and juvenile neuroaxonal dystrophy with diffuse Lewy bodies and neurofibrillary tangles. *Clinical Neuropathology* **11**: 1–5.

Higgins JJ, Patterson MC, Papadopoulos NM et al (1992) Hypoprebetalipoproteinemia, acanthocytosis, retinitis pigmentosa, and pallidal degeneration (HARP syndrome). *Neurology* **42**: 194–198.

Howard RS & Lees AJ (1987) Encephalitis lethargica: a report of four recent cases. *Brain* **110**: 19–33.

Hudson AJ (1981) Amyotrophic lateral sclerosis and its association with dementia, parkinsonism and other neurological disorders. *Brain* **104**: 217–247.

Hughes AJ, Daniel SE, Kilford L & Lees AJ (1992) Accuracy of clinical diagnosis of idiopathic Parkinson's disease: a clinico-pathological study of 100 cases. *Journal of Neurology, Neurosurgery and Psychiatry* **55**: 181–184.

Ikeda K, Ikeda S, Yoshimura T, Kato H & Namba M (1978) Idiopathic parkinsonism with Lewy-type inclusions in the cerebral cortex: a case report. *Acta Neuropathologica* **41**: 165–168.

Ikeda K, Hori A & Bode G (1989) Progressive dementia with 'diffuse Lewy-type inclusions' in cerebral cortex. *Archiv für Psychiatrie und Nervenkrankheiten* **228**: 243–248.

Jankovic J, Kirkpatrick JB, Blomquist KA, Langlais PJ & Bird ED (1985) Late-onset Hallervorden–Spatz disease presenting as familial parkinsonism. *Neurology* **35**: 227–234.

Joachim CL, Morris JH & Selkoe DJ (1988) Clinically diagnosed Alzheimer's disease: autopsy results in 150 cases. *Annals of Neurology* **24**: 50–56.

Kamo H, McGeer PL, Harrop R et al (1987) Positron emission tomography and histopathology in Pick's disease. *Neurology* **37**: 439–445.

Kayano T, Funada N, Okeda R et al (1980) An autopsy case of Parkinson's disease with dementia and a wide distribution of Lewy-like bodies in cerebral cortex. *Neuropathology (Tokyo)* **1**: 27–28.

Kono C, Matsubara M & Inagaki T (1976) Idiopathic orthostatic hypotension with numerous Lewy bodies in the sympathetic ganglia. Report of a case. *Neurological Medicine (Japan)* **4**: 568–570.

Kosaka K (1978) Lewy bodies in cerebral cortex. Report of three cases. *Acta Neuropathologica* **42:** 127–134.

Kosaka K (1990) Diffuse Lewy body disease in Japan. *Journal of Neurology* **237:** 197–204.

Kosaka K & Mehraein P (1979) Dementia–parkinsonism syndrome with numerous Lewy bodies and senile plaques in cerebral cortex. *Archiv für Psychiatrie und Nervenkrankheiten* **226:** 241–250.

Kosaka K, Shibayama H, Kobayashi H, Hoshino T & Iwase S (1973) An autopsy case of unclassifiable presenile dementia (in Japanese). *Psychiatria et Neurologia Japonica* **75:** 18–34.

Kosaka K, Oyanagi S, Matsushita M, Hori A & Iwase S (1976) Presenile dementia with Alzheimer-, Pick- and Lewy-body changes. *Acta Neuropathologica* **36:** 221–233.

Kosaka K, Matsushita M, Oyanagi S & Mehraein P (1980) A clinicopathological study of the 'Lewy body disease'. *Psychiatria et Neurologia Japonica* **82:** 292–311.

Kosaka K, Yoshimura M, Ikeda K & Budka H (1984) Diffuse Lewy body disease: progressive dementia with abundant cortical Lewy bodies and senile changes of varying degree—a new disease? *Clinical Neuropathology* **3:** 185–192.

Kuroda S, Hosokawa K, Iguchi K & Tateishi J (1978) An autopsy case of presenile dementia with numerous Lewy bodies in the cerebral cortex. *Clinical Neurology (Tokyo)* **18:** 346–350.

Kuyama K, Kuroda S, Otsuki S et al (1987) An autopsy case of 'diffuse Lewy body disease' presenting dementia. *Clinical Neurology (Tokyo)* **27:** 94–98.

Lantos PL, Luthert PJ, Hanger D, Anderton B, Mullan M & Rossor M (1992) Familial Alzheimer's disease with the amyloid precursor protein position 717 mutation and sporadic Alzheimer's disease have the same cytoskeletal pathology. *Neuroscience Letters* **137:** 221–224.

Leake A, Perry EK, Perry RH et al (1991) Neocortical concentrations of neuropeptides in senile dementia of the Alzheimer and Lewy body type: comparison with Parkinson's disease and severity correlations. *Biological Psychiatry* **29:** 357–364.

Lees AJ (1987) The Steele–Richardson–Olszewski syndrome (progressive supranuclear palsy). In Marsden CD & Fahn S (eds) *Movement Disorders 2*, pp 272–287. London: Butterworth.

Lennox G, Lowe J, Landon M et al (1989a) Diffuse Lewy body disease: correlative neuropathology using anti-ubiquitin immunocytochemistry. *Journal of Neurology, Neurosurgery and Psychiatry* **52:** 1236–1247.

Lennox G, Lowe J, Morrell K, Landon M & Mayer RJ (1989b) Antiubiquitin immunocytochemistry is more sensitive than conventional techniques in the detection of diffuse Lewy body disease. *Journal of Neurology, Neurosurgery and Psychiatry* **52:** 67–71.

Lewis AJ & Gawel MJ (1990) Diffuse Lewy body disease with dementia and oculomotor dysfunction. *Movement Disorders* **2:** 143–147.

Lowe J & Mayer RJ (1991) Ubiquitin and the molecular pathology of chronic degenerative diseases. *Journal of Pathology* **163:** 279–281.

Lowe J, Aldridge F, Lennox G et al (1989) Inclusion bodies in motor cortex and brainstem of patients with motor neurone disease are detected by immunocytochemical localisation of ubiquitin. *Neuroscience Letters* **105:** 7–13.

Lowe J, Landon M, Pike I, Spendlove I, McDermott H & Mayer RJ (1990) Dementia with β-amyloid deposition: involvement of αβcrystallin supports two main diseases. *Lancet* **336:** 515–516.

Lowe J, McDermott H, Pike I et al (1992) αβ crystallin expression in non-lenticular tissues and selective presence in ubiquitinated inclusion bodies in human disease. *Journal of Pathology* **166:** 61–68.

Mann DMA, Jones D, Snowden JS, Neary D & Hardy J (1992) Pathological changes in the brain of a patient with familial Alzheimer's disease having a missense mutation at codon 717 in the amyloid precursor protein gene. *Neuroscience Letters* **137:** 225–228.

Mayeux R, Chen J, Mirabello E et al (1990) An estimate of the incidence of dementia in idiopathic Parkinson's disease. *Neurology* **40:** 1513–1517.

Minagawa M, Maeshiro N, Taguchi K & Shioda A (1980) An autopsy case showing dementia and Shy–Drager syndrome with Lewy bodies and spheroids in the substantia nigra and senile plaques in the cerebral cortex. *Neuropathology* **1:** 28–29.

Mitsuyama Y, Fukanaga H & Yamashita M (1984) Alzheimer's disease with widespread presence of Lewy bodies. *Folia Psychiatrica et Neurologica Japonica* **38:** 81–88.

Monma Y, Takamatsu K, Itoh T et al (1981) An autopsy case of atypical presenile dementia with many Lewy bodies in the cerebral cortex. *Clinical Psychiatry* **23**: 267–275.

Morris JC, Cole M, Banker BQ & Wright D (1984) Hereditary dysphasic dementia and the Pick–Alzheimer spectrum. *Annals of Neurology* **16**: 455–466.

Morris JC, Drazner M, Fulling K, Grant EA & Goldring J (1989) Clinical and pathological aspects of parkinsonism in Alzheimer's disease. *Archives of Neurology* **46**: 651–657.

Muenter MD, Howard FM, Okasaki H et al (1986) A familial parkinson–dementia syndrome. *Neurology* **36** (supplement 1): 115 (abstract).

Munoz-Garcia D & Ludwin SK (1984) Classic and generalised variants of Pick's disease: a clinicopathological, ultrastructural and immunocytochemical comparative study. *Annals of Neurology* **16**: 467–480.

Okazaki H, Lipkin LE & Aronson SM (1961) Diffuse intracytoplasmic ganglionic inclusions (Lewy type) associated with progressive dementia and quadriparesis in flexion. *Journal of Neuropathology and Experimental Neurology* **20**: 237–244.

Perry RH, Irving D & Tomlinson BE (1990a) Lewy body prevalence in the aging brain: relationship to neuropsychiatric disorders, Alzheimer-type pathology and catecholaminergic nuclei. *Journal of the Neurological Sciences* **100**: 223–233.

Perry RH, Irving D, Blessed G, Fairbairn A & Perry EK (1990b) Senile dementia of Lewy body type. A clinically and neuropathologically distinct form of Lewy body dementia in the elderly. *Journal of Neurological Sciences* **95**: 119–139.

Perry EK, Marshall E, Smith CJ et al (1990c) Cholinergic and dopaminergic activities in senile dementia of Lewy body type. *Alzheimer's Disease and Associated Disorders* **4**: 87–95.

Perry EK, Marshall E, Kerwin J et al (1990d) Evidence of a monoaminergic-cholinergic imbalance related to visual hallucinations in Lewy body dementia. *Journal of Neurochemistry* **55**: 1454–1456.

Philpot M, Colgan J, Janota I & Levy R (1986) Dementia without Alzheimer pathology. *Neurology* **36**: 133.

Popovitch ER, Wisniewski HM, Kaufman MA, Grundke-Iqbal I & Wen GY (1987) Young adult-form of dementia with neurofibrillary changes and Lewy bodies. *Acta Neuropathologica* **74**: 97–104.

Quarrell O & Harper P (1991) The clinical neurology of Huntington's disease. In Harper PS (ed.) *Huntington's Disease*, pp 37–80. London: WB Saunders.

Quinn NP (1989) Multiple system atrophy—the nature of the beast. *Journal of Neurology, Neurosurgery and Psychiatry* (special supplement) 78–89.

Quinn NP, Rossor MN & Marsden CD (1986) Dementia and Parkinson's disease: pathological and neurochemical considerations. *British Medical Bulletin* **42**: 86–90.

Schaffert DA, Johnsen SD, Johnson PC & Drayer BP (1989) Magnetic resonance imaging in pathologically proven Hallervorden–Spatz disease. *Neurology* **39**: 440–442.

Sima AAF, Clark AW, Sternberger NA & Sternberger LA (1986) Lewy body dementia without Alzheimer changes. *Canadian Journal of Neurological Sciences* **13**: 490–497.

Spampinato U, Habert MO, Mas JL et al (1991) (^{99m}Tc)-HM-PAO SPECT and cognitive impairment in Parkinson's disease: a comparison with dementia of the Alzheimer type. *Journal of Neurology, Neurosurgery and Psychiatry* **54**: 787–792.

Tiller-Borcich JK & Forno LS (1988) Parkinson's disease and dementia with neuronal inclusions in the cerebral cortex: Lewy bodies or Pick bodies. *Journal of Neuropathology and Experimental Neurology* **47**: 526–535.

Yagishita S, Itoh Y, Amano N & Nakano T (1980) Atypical senile dementia with widespread Lewy-type inclusions in the cerebral cortex. *Acta Neuropathologica* **49**: 187–191.

Yamamoto T & Imai T (1988) A case of diffuse Lewy body and Alzheimer's diseases with periodic synchronous discharges. *Journal of Neuropathology and Experimental Neurology* **47**: 536–548.

Yoshimura M (1983) Cortical changes in parkinsonian brain: a contribution to the delineation of 'diffuse Lewy body disease'. *Journal of Neurology* **229**: 17–32.

Yoshimura M (1988) Pathological basis for dementia in elderly patients with idiopathic Parkinson's disease. *European Neurology* **28** (supplement 1): 29–35.

Yoshimura M, Shimada H, Nagura H & Tomonaga M (1980) Two autopsy cases of Parkinson's disease with Shy–Drager syndrome (in Japanese). *Transactiones Societatis Pathologicae Japonica* **69**: 432.

10

Corticobasal degeneration

P. D. THOMPSON
C. D. MARSDEN

Corticodentatonigral degeneration with neuronal achromasia (Rebeiz et al, 1968), corticonigral degeneration with neuronal achromasia (Case Records of the Massachusetts General Hospital, 1985), cortical degeneration with swollen chromatolytic neurones (Clark et al, 1986) and corticobasal (Gibb et al, 1989) and corticobasal ganglionic (Riley et al, 1990) degeneration are terms used by different authors to refer to the distinctive pathological findings of frontal and parietal lobe atrophy associated with atrophy of the basal ganglia and other subcortical nuclei. The pathological hallmarks of this condition are focal cortical and subcortical degeneration, with pale swollen neurones in cortical and subcortical structures, as first described in three cases by Rebeiz et al (1968). The clinical features of this condition are so striking that it is strange that the illness has been recognized, with increasing frequency, only in recent years. Its cause is unknown, but there is no evidence of inheritance. Up to now some 15 cases have been described with pathological verification.

Symptoms in the majority of cases reported to date with this pathology have been dominated by an asymmetric extrapyramidal and frontal motor disorder with elements of apraxia, rigidity, involuntary movements, dystonia, the alien limb sign, dysarthria and a supranuclear disorder of eye movement. Some authors have preferred to describe this clinical syndrome as progressive apraxic rigidity (Watts et al, 1985; Le Witt et al, 1989). In addition to corticobasal degeneration, it has been suggested that other pathologies, such as Alzheimer's disease (Le Witt et al, 1989), may produce this constellation of neurological signs. Also, there have been other case reports of focal cortical syndromes with pathological change similar to that of corticobasal degeneration in which the major symptoms have been related to a disturbance of language with dysphasia and only subtle motor signs in the limbs (Lippa et al, 1990, 1991), and of cases with combinations of dysphasia and limb apraxia (cases 1, 4 of Sawle et al, 1991).

The severe cortical cell loss with associated gliosis of the subcortical white matter and the large swollen achromatic cells are similar to the findings in Pick's disease. Argyrophilic inclusions (Pick bodies), typical of Pick's disease, are not found in corticobasal degeneration. Similarly, the distribution of atrophy is frontoparietal in corticobasal degeneration, in contrast to the frontotemporal lobar atrophy of Pick's disease. Although extension of

Baillière's Clinical Neurology—
Vol. 1, No. 3, November 1992
ISBN 0–7020–1631–4

the pathological change in Pick's disease to the basal ganglia is common and degeneration of the pyramidal tracts may also occur (Kosaka et al, 1991), descriptions of florid motor disorders in Pick's disease are uncommon (Akelaitis, 1944; Winkelman and Boor, 1949; Cambier et al, 1981). Nevertheless, the extent of overlap between Pick's disease and corticobasal degeneration is at present not known. Amongst the 32 cases of Pick's disease reported from the psychiatric hospital of the University of Geneva by Tissot et al (1985), 14 exhibited lobar atrophy in a distribution that centred on the posterior frontal lobe with prominent involvement of the precentral gyrus. The clinical presentation of these patients was of an extrapyramidal and pyramidal syndrome associated with dysarthria, in contrast to the mood, personality and memory disturbance of classical Pick's disease. The relationship of these pathological findings to other focal cortical degenerations such as posterior cortical atrophy (Benson et al, 1988) will not be considered further. The remainder of this chapter will concentrate on the spectrum of motor and other disorders that may accompany corticobasal degeneration.

PATHOLOGY

The pathological findings consist of severe focal cortical atrophy centred on the peri-Rolandic posterior frontal and parietal cortex with lesser involvement of adjacent cortex, and relative sparing of the temporal and occipital regions. Accordingly, the motor and sensory areas of the cerebral cortex are most severely affected, and there is secondary degeneration of the corticospinal tracts. The cortical atrophy tends to be asymmetric, being most marked opposite to the most affected limbs. In the affected cortical regions, the normal cortical architecture is destroyed, the definition of the layers of the cerebral cortex is lost, and there is intense fibrillary gliosis. The white matter beneath the affected cortical areas is atrophic and gliotic. Neuronal degeneration with nerve cell loss and gliosis are present, particularly in the pyramidal cell layers 3 and 5 of the cortex.

A characteristic feature of the degeneration is the presence of large pale neurones, from which the term neuronal achromasia was derived (Rebeiz et al, 1968). The affected cortical neurones are medium to large pyramidal cells. They are found most frequently in those cortical regions moderately, rather than severely affected. They are also found in subcortical and brainstem nuclei. These cells, which are indistinguishable from Pick cells, have been variously referred to as ballooned, swollen, chromatolytic-like or achromatic cells (Gibb et al, 1989). They are most prominent in the third, fifth and sixth laminae of the cerebral cortex. The swollen achromatic nerve cells are filled with homogenous material which shows faint and variable eosinophilia (Rebeiz et al, 1968) and argyrophilia (Clark et al, 1986). Nissl substance is not detected within the neurones, distinguishing the degeneration from that seen in central chromatolysis (Rebeiz et al, 1968; Case Records of the Massachusetts General Hospital, 1985). Lewy bodies, granulovacuolar degeneration, extensive plaque and neurofibrillary tangle formation have not been features of the cases reported. The cytoplasm of such achromatic cells stain positively for phosphorylated neurofilaments, but not for tau (Gibb et al, 1989). Ultrastructurally, the cytoplasm of the swollen pale neurones is filled with aggregates of 10 nm intermediate filaments (Watts et al, 1989).

Atrophy and cell loss, accompanied by gliosis, is also marked in the lateral two-thirds of the substantia nigra with loss of pigmented cells (Rebeiz et al, 1968; Gibb et al, 1989) and swollen pale cells may be found. Gibb et al (1989) also described basophilic inclusions, referred to as corticobasal inclusions, in the swollen cells of the substantia nigra, but Lewy bodies usually were not seen. The degeneration also affects the medial third of the subthalamic nucleus, the striatum and globus pallidus, the posterolateral thalamus, the red nucleus and other brainstem nuclei. In two of the original cases reported by Rebeiz et al (1968) there was marked atrophy of the denta-torubrothalamic tract; the dentate nucleus was abnormal in these cases but the cerebellar cortex was normal. In subsequent reports, involvement of the cerebellum has been infrequent and the 'dentate' component of the original description has been omitted (Case Records of the Massachusetts General Hospital, 1985). Corticospinal tract degeneration has been present in some cases (Rebeiz et al, 1968; Gibb et al, 1989). The spinal cord has otherwise been normal.

Few neurochemistry studies have been undertaken. A profound reduction in the concentration of dopamine in the substantia nigra, caudate nucleus and putamen was found in one patient (Riley et al, 1990), corresponding to the nigral pallor.

CLINICAL FEATURES

Symptoms are of insidious onset and begin in the sixth to eighth decades. Males and females are equally affected, and there is no family history of a similar disorder. The clinical features are summarized in Tables 1 and 2. One of the most striking findings in the early stages of the illness is the asymmetry of limb involvement. The typical presentation is of a subtle motor disorder of one arm or hand. Less commonly, involvement of one leg is the presenting symptom. At the onset symptoms may be vague and related to an inexplicable loss of hand function with clumsiness, loss of dexterity of fine finger movement or stiffness. Formal testing at this time may reveal slowness in hand and finger movement, difficulty in using objects or mimicking gestures or producing sequences of movement with the affected hand. In attempting to perform manual tasks there may be perseveration of one part of the movement. These findings are consistent with an apraxia. Difficulty in walking is the presenting complaint if the lower limb is affected first. The foot may tend to stick to the floor as walking is initiated, or it may drag and cause the patient to trip, especially on uneven surfaces or if attention is diverted. As with the upper limb, examination of the affected leg may reveal slowness of rapid alternating movements and difficulty in performing sequences of leg movement when lying down. Leg and foot movement when

Table 1. Clinical features of corticobasal degeneration.

Asymmetric onset
Progressive course
Apraxia–rigidity of arm (or leg)
Alien limb phenomenon
Myoclonus (stimulus-sensitive)
Sensory loss
Progression to rigid dystonic (functionally useless) limb
Akinetic–rigid syndrome
Dysequilibrium
Dysarthria and dysphagia
Frontal release signs
Unresponsive to levodopa
Other features (sometimes seen):
  Pain
  Postural and action tremor
  Other involuntary movements
  Supranuclear gaze palsy
  Blepharospasm
  Levator inhibition
  Late dysphasia and memory impairment
  Hyperreflexia and Babinski signs

Table 2. Incidence of clinical features of corticobasal degeneration in 28 cases (includes clinically and pathologically diagnosed cases).

Movement disorders	
Akinetic–rigid syndrome	28 (100)
Dysequilibrium	24 (86)
Postural-action tremor	22 (79)
Limb dystonia	16 (57)
Reflex myoclonus	15 (54)
Cerebral cortical signs	
Sensory loss	20 (71)
Apraxia	20 (71)
Alien limb	14 (50)
Frontal release signs	13 (46)
Dementia	12 (43)
Dysphasia	6 (21)
Other manifestations	
Hyperreflexia	18 (64)
Babinski signs	13 (46)
Supranuclear gaze palsy	13 (46)
Levator inhibition	10 (36)
Dysarthria	6 (21)
Other dyskinesias	5 (18)

Values in parentheses are percentages.
Data from Rebeiz et al (1968), Case Records of the Massachusetts General Hospital (1985), Watts et al (1985), Gibb et al (1989) and Riley et al (1990).

walking is slow and steps are of small amplitude so that walking is accomplished by a series of small shuffling steps. An interesting observation is that some patients experience the greatest difficulty in engaging the leg in motion to start walking and that, once underway, or if climbing stairs, their walking improves somewhat, at least in the very earliest stages. These findings also are those of an apraxia. Alterations in muscle tone with either lead pipe rigidity or *gegenhalten* of the affected limbs is a common finding. The affected arm does not swing in the normal manner during walking. The motor signs may remain unilateral for many years, but as the illness progresses the rigidity and apraxia slowly become more severe and eventually spread to the contralateral side. The hand may progressively adopt a flexed, often fixed, dystonic posture with clenching of the fingers into a fist, often closing around the thumb, which is held adducted in the palm. Eventually the affected limb becomes virtually useless. Truncal movements become slow and laboured, with difficulty standing from a seated position or turning in bed. Truncal equilibrium is also impaired, with falls when standing or turning that cannot be accounted for by clumsy movements of the feet or by tripping.

In addition to limb apraxia, other frontal lobe motor signs become more evident with progression of the disease. *Gegenhalten* is often present from an early stage as are frontal release signs, such as grasp reflexes in the hands and feet, sucking and rooting reflexes. Patients may complain of an inability to release objects from their grasp in addition to the loss of fine motor skills. The alien limb phenomenon may be one of the most striking features of the syndrome. This refers to slow, involuntary, wandering, levitation-like movements of the arm, which often are associated with a prominent grasp reflex, forced groping, magnetic hand movements and intermanual conflict. First described in association with tumours of the corpus callosum (Brion and Jedanyk, 1972), alien limb behaviour has since been reported in association with infarction of the medial frontal cortex (Goldberg et al, 1981; McNabb et al, 1988). The movements are slow and may appear quasi-purposeful; the hand typically rises slowly at the side of the patient, who may be unaware of this movement. The unexpected appearance of the patient's hand beside their face gave rise to the term 'le main étranger' (Brion and Jedanyk, 1972) or alien limb. This description also conveys the apraxic difficulty in using the hand to perform even simple tasks; patients often describe the limb as 'not doing what I want it to', or state that it 'has a mind of its own'. Another striking feature of the alien limb is intermanual conflict, in which the affected limb reaches across to interfere with the voluntary activities of the contralateral normal hand (see case 2, Rebeiz et al, 1968). Alien leg movements also occur with the leg rising while the patient is seated. With increasing rigidity, difficulty walking, bradykinesia and facial immobility, the clinical picture becomes one of an akinetic rigid syndrome. The akinesia and rigidity do not respond to dopamine replacement therapy, despite the profound nigrostriatal pathology and the demonstration of dopamine depletion in these structures.

In addition to the asymmetric akinetic–rigid dystonic syndrome there may be involuntary movements. Alien limb movements have been described above. Superimposed on these there may be chorea, tremor and action and stimulus sensitive myoclonus. In case 2 of Rebeiz et al (1968): 'whenever he moved the hand, it took on a curious athetoid posture with the wrist flexed and the metacarpophalangeal joints stiffly extended, and it underwent a series of alternating athetoid movements'. Gibb et al (1989), in their report of case 3, noticed that her hand tended to 'levitate and the fingers wandered like tentacles'. Tremor and myoclonus interfere with any attempts to use the arm and hand (or leg and foot). The tremor is not the classical rest tremor of Parkinson's disease, but a more jerky irregular tremor most evident in posture or movement. The myoclonus begins firstly in the affected limbs. It may also be exquisitely sensitive to cutaneous stimuli and muscle stretch. The precise origin of this reflex myoclonus is uncertain. Some authors have drawn attention to the similarity of the focal stimulus sensitive myoclonus to that seen in cortical reflex myoclonus (Riley et al, 1990), although there are several differences (Thompson et al, 1990). Myoclonus in corticobasal degeneration is not associated with enlarged cortical somatosensory evoked potentials, and the latency of the reflex myoclonus following effective stimulation, of the order of 40ms, is shorter than the reflex latency of 50–60ms in cortical reflex myoclonus (Obeso et al, 1985). Seizures are not a feature and the electroencephalogram does not show epileptic activity. The site of origin of this myoclonus may well be cortical but appears to be generated by mechanisms different from those operating in cortical reflex myoclonus.

True weakness is not a feature to begin with, but with the passage of time the limb(s) become useless because of rigidity and apraxia. In addition pyramidal signs appear with hyperreflexia and extensor plantar responses.

A supranuclear gaze palsy may be an early and prominent sign leading to confusion with the Steele–Richardson–Olszewski syndrome. The ocular motor disorder is progressive. It may take the form of a gaze apraxia with difficulty initiating saccades, but with preservation of spontaneous reflexive saccades and eye movements elicited by the oculocephalic reflex. Fixation spasm may be evident. Patients may be unable to initiate eye movements to command without using head thrusts or a blink to engage their eyes in motion. There also may be marked saccadic hypometria, in both horizontal and vertical directions of gaze, and slowing of voluntary saccadic eye movements. Gaze impersistence has also been described. Pursuit eye movements are often jerky at an early stage, but with progression of the disease voluntary smooth pursuit deteriorates and finally all voluntary eye movements may be lost. Even at these stages it is usually possible to demonstrate that the ocular movement disorder is supranuclear in origin. Blepharospasm and levator inhibition may produce difficulties in eye opening. Dysarthria is usually present and becomes increasingly severe, as does dysphagia.

Sensory signs and symptoms may appear at an early stage with complaints of pain often suggesting a radicular syndrome. These symptoms are progressive and may lead to loss of both basic (pain and temperature) and discriminatory sensory modalities. The patterns of sensory loss with accompanying pain are suggestive of a thalamic sensory disturbance, rather than a cortical sensory loss. It is of interest that in one of our patients with stimulus induced myoclonus there was dense anaesthesia in the affected arm, yet a peripheral nerve stimulus at intensities below motor (and sensory) thresholds was capable of eliciting a train of reflex myoclonic jerks.

Cognitive changes are unusual early in the disease, the intellect being preserved. With the passage of time, however, memory impairment and dysphasic speech disturbance may emerge slowly, although accurate assessment of this is difficult because of the severe dysarthria and other motor incapacity. In some cases there has been prominent and early disturbance of language (Lippa et al, 1990, 1991).

CLINICAL COURSE

The most common mode of presentation in the cases reported to date is a slowly evolving motor disorder involving the arm or the leg, particularly the arm (Tables 1 and 2). Occasional patients have presented with an akinetic–rigid syndrome, a supranuclear gaze palsy, an alien limb or a focal movement disorder, or a sensory syndrome. However, with the passage of time most patients accumulate a 'full house' of the clinical signs described above. With progression of the motor disorder the patient becomes severely disabled and bed-bound. Severe rigid immobility is likely within 3 to 5 years of the start. The duration of the disease to death is usually about 7 to 10 years.

IMAGING STUDIES

A variety of imaging studies have been undertaken in patients with a clinical diagnosis of corticobasal degeneration. Computed tomography and magnetic resonance imaging of the brain may disclose localized and asymmetric frontoparietal atrophy. Atrophy tends to become more severe as the disease progresses. Positron emission tomography has shown a typical pattern of an asymmetric reduction in the uptake of $[^{18}F]$-6-fluorodopa in the striatum (caudate and putamen) and in the medial frontal cortex (Riley et al, 1990; Sawle et al, 1991). This is consistent with the loss of nigrostriatal projections as predicted by the nigral cell loss demonstrated pathologically (Rebeiz et al, 1968; Gibb et al, 1989) and the striatal dopamine depletion in the case reported by Riley et al (1990). The failure of patients to respond to levodopa therapy further suggests a loss of postsynaptic striatal dopamine receptors, which also is consistent with the presence of striatal degeneration on pathological examination. Characteristic patterns of asymmetric cerebral cortical hypometabolism are seen, with decreased oxygen metabolism in the superior and posterior temporal, inferior parietal and occipital visual association cortices (Sawle et al, 1991). Significant regional asymmetries in cerebral glucose metabolism also have been found in the thalamus, inferior parietal lobule and hippocampus (Eidelberg et al, 1991). The interhemispheric metabolic asymmetry in frontal and parietal regions was found to correlate with the asymmetry in thalamic metabolic rate (Riley et al, 1990). These findings are all consistent with the distribution of neuropathological change. In particular, the asymmetry of thalamic metabolism may be related to both direct pathological involvement, and the loss of corticosubcortical input, due to the cortical disease. In the study of Sawle et al (1991), the thalamic asymmetry was most marked in the two patients who exhibited myoclonus in the contralateral limbs.

OTHER INVESTIGATIONS

Routine laboratory studies of blood, urine and cerebrospinal fluid are normal. Heavy metal toxic screens in urine have been negative. Watts et al (1985) described decreased levels of somatostatin in cerebrospinal fluid in three cases, but this has not been replicated.

Initially the electroencephalogram is usually normal, but may develop asymmetric slowing, maximal over the hemisphere contralateral to the most affected limbs. Nerve conduction studies and electromyography have not revealed consistent evidence of peripheral nerve involvement. Visual and brainstem evoked potentials have been normal.

DIFFERENTIAL DIAGNOSIS

Features that distinguish the akinetic–rigid syndrome of corticobasal degeneration from Parkinson's disease include the early onset of gait and postural abnormality with falls, dysequilibrium and loss of truncal mobility, the alien limb phenomenon, apraxia and other frontal lobe motor signs, a supranuclear gaze palsy, myoclonus and, finally, the lack of response to levodopa therapy. The presentation with a supranuclear gaze palsy associated with an akinetic–rigid syndrome raises the possibility of Steele–Richardson–Olszewski syndrome. Indeed, some of the reports of dystonia in the Steele–Richardson–Olszewski syndrome, in the absence of pathological proof, may well have represented further examples of corticobasal degeneration. Differentiation between these conditions may be difficult since frontal-type motor and subtle cognitive deficits are seen in both (Lees, 1987). Myoclonus, when present, may be one feature in favour of corticobasal degeneration. It is also of interest that the distribution of cerebral hypometabolism on positron emission tomography is different in these conditions (Sawle et al, 1991). The combination of an akinetic–rigid syndrome and myoclonus may be seen in the multiple system atrophies and spongiform encephalopathies. Electrophysiological studies may be of value since the characteristics of the myoclonus differs in these diseases: that in multiple system atrophy tends to be cortical reflex in type (Obeso et al, 1985) and in spongiform encephalopathies it is presumed to be subcortical in origin (Shibasaki, 1981). The presentation of a unilateral frontal lobe motor syndrome with an alien limb or a frontal gait disorder ('gait apraxia') or focal myoclonus should always raise the possibility of a structural lesion of the contralateral cerebral hemisphere. The presence of a supranuclear gaze palsy or dystonia of the affected limbs may be helpful distinguishing features. Dementia and apraxia may be seen in Pick's disease and Alzheimer's disease. As discussed above, the relative prominence of the cognitive deficits in these diseases should allow their distinction from corticobasal degeneration where the motor disorder is the most conspicuous finding. However, this distinction must be made with the reservation that a small number of patients with the pathology of neuronal achromasia have presented with symptoms of cognitive decline and behavioural change. Until the full spectrum of the clinical presentation of corticobasal degeneration is known, any clinical distinction between these conditions should rest on other signs.

TREATMENT

Unfortunately, there is no cure for this condition, which is relentlessly progressive. Levodopa and dopamine agonists have little effect, but are tried. Baclofen and/or an anticholinergic may help the rigidity a little, but they produce unwanted side-effects. Clonazepam may dampen the myoclonus a little. Other drugs such as dopamine antagonists, propranolol, anticonvulsants and serotonin agonists have, in our hands, been of no help. The main thrust of management is thus confined to measures to assist mobility and relieve distress.

CONCLUSION

Corticobasal degeneration is a rare but distinctive entity. The pathology, apart from the absence of Pick bodies and its distribution, is reminiscent of Pick's disease. Whether corticobasal degeneration is a variant of Pick's disease with a different emphasis of anatomical distribution remains to be established. The possibility that corticobasal degeneration is transmissible, or is associated with mutation of prion protein genes, must be tested. The cellular pathology of the neuronal achromasia indicates a disturbance of cytoskeletal metabolism, but whether this is primary or secondary is unknown. The presence of intracytoplasmic phosphorylated neurofilaments is a non-specific finding, being found in many other neurodegenerative conditions.

REFERENCES

Akelaitis A (1944) Atrophy of the basal ganglia in Pick's disease: a clinicopathologic study. *Archives of Neurology and Psychiatry* **51**: 27–34.
Benson DF, Davis RJ, Snyder J et al (1988) Progressive cortical atrophy. *Archives of Neurology* **45**: 789–793.

Brion S & Jedanyk C-P (1972) Trouble du transfert interhemispherique à propos de trois observations de tumeurs du corps calleux: le signe de la main étrangère. *Revue Neurologique* **126**: 257–266.

Cambier J, Masson M, Dairou R & Henin D (1981) Etude anatomo-clinique d'une forme parietale de maladie de Pick. *Revue Neurologique* **137**: 33–38.

Case Records of the Massachusetts General Hospital (1985) Case 38-1985. *New England Journal of Medicine* **313**: 739–748.

Clark AW, Manz HJ, White CL, Lehmann J, Miller D & Coyle JT (1986) Cortical degeneration with swollen chromatolytic neurons: its relationship to Pick's disease. *Journal of Neuropathology and Experimental Neurology* **45**: 268–284.

Eidelberg D, Dhawan V, Moeller JR et al (1991) The metabolic landscape of corticobasal ganglionic degeneration: regional asymmetries studied with positron emission tomography. *Journal of Neurology, Neurosurgery and Psychiatry* **54**: 856–862.

Gibb WRG, Luthert PJ & Marsden CD (1989) Corticobasal degeneration. *Brain* **112**: 1171–1192.

Goldberg G, Meyer NH, Toglia JU (1981) Medial frontal cortex infarction and the alien hand sign. *Archives of Neurology* **38**: 683–686.

Kosaka K, Ikeda K, Kobayashi K & Mehraein P (1991) Striatopallidonigral degeneration in Pick's disease: a clinicopathological study of 41 cases. *Journal of Neurology* **238**: 151–160.

Lees AJ (1987) The Steele–Richardson–Olszewski syndrome (progressive supranuclear palsy). In Marsden CD & Fahn S (eds) *Movement Disorders 2*, pp 272–287. London: Butterworths.

Le Witt P, Friedman J, Nutt J et al (1989) Progressive rigidity with apraxia: the variety of clinical and pathological features. *Neurology* **39** (supplement 1): 140.

Lippa CF, Smith TW & Fontneau N (1990) Corticonigral degeneration with neuronal achromasia: a clinicopathologic study of two cases. *Journal of the Neurological Sciences* **98**: 301–310.

Lippa CF, Cohen R, Smith TW & Drachman DA (1991) Primary progressive aphasia with focal neuronal achromasia. *Neurology* **41**: 882–886.

McNabb AW, Carroll WM & Mastaglia FL (1988) 'Alien hand' and loss of bimanual coordination after dominant anterior cerebral artery territory infarction. *Journal of Neurology, Neurosurgery and Psychiatry* **51**: 218–222.

Obeso JA, Rothwell JC & Marsden CD (1985) The spectrum of cortical myoclonus. *Brain* **108**: 193–224.

Rebeiz JJ, Kolodny EH & Richardson EP (1968) Corticodentatonigral degeneration with neuronal achromasia. *Archives of Neurology* **18**: 20–33.

Riley RE, Lang AE, Lewis A et al (1990) Cortico-basal ganglionic degeneration. *Neurology* **40**: 1203–1212.

Sawle GV, Brooks DJ, Marsden CD & Frackowiak RSJ (1991) Corticobasal degeneration. A unique pattern of regional cortical oxygen hypometabolism and striatal fluorodopa uptake demonstrated by positron emission tomography. *Brain* **114**: 541–556.

Shibasaki H, Motomura S, Yamashita Y, Shii H & Kuroiwa Y (1981) Periodic synchronous discharge and myoclonus in Creutzfeldt–Jakob disease. *Annals of Neurology* **9**: 150–156.

Thompson PD, Day BL, Rothwell JC & Marsden CD (1990) Clinical and physiological findings in corticobasal degeneration. *Movement Disorders* **5** (supplement 1): 43.

Tissot R, Constantinidis J & Richard J (1985) Pick's disease. In Frederiks JAM (ed.) *Handbook of Clinical Neurology*, vol. 2 (46), pp 233–246. Amsterdam: Elsevier.

Watts RL, Williams RS, Growdon JB et al (1985) Corticobasal ganglionic degeneration. *Neurology* **35** (supplement 1): 178.

Watts RL, Mirra SS, Young RR et al (1989) Cortico-basal ganglionic degeneration (CBGD) with neuronal achromasia: clinical-pathological study of two cases. *Neurology* **39** (supplement 1): 140.

Winkleman NW & Boor MH (1949) Asymptomatic extrapyramidal involvement in Pick's disease: a clinicopathologic study of two cases. *Journal of Neuropathology and Experimental Neurology* **8**: 30–42.

Index

Note: Page numbers of article titles are in **bold** type.